ANABOLIC MEN

Master Your Testosterone

4th Edition (TestShock Program)

Published by: Anabolic Men, LLC
Copyright © 2016

by
Christopher Walker and Ali Kuoppala

"A man is not just a thing to be - it's also a way to be, a path to follow, a walk to walk."

-Jack Donovan

Acknowledgements

We would like to acknowledge all of the men and women who have devoted their lives to conducting the countless research studies that we've pulled information from over the last five years of self-education on the topic of natural human testosterone optimization. Your work gave us a base of knowledge to digest, understand, and use to educate the millions of men who have read our work online in recent years, and impacted their lives positively because of it.

Dedication

This program is dedicated specifically to every guy who reads its pages and is forever impacted with a renewed sense of control over their own destiny & health. Remember that you have complete control over your body and mind. You merely need to accept this, and you step into power beyond what you could ever imagine before.

Enjoy this book!

Share it with a friend after reading, or send them to **MasterYourTestosterone.com**.

Get 10% Off On The Anabolic Men Marketplace Online Store Today

Open up your internet browser and go to **store.anabolicmen.com** today and use the coupon code MASTER10 to get 10% off every order.

Our mission with the Anabolic Men Marketplace is to create a 100% trusted source for research-backed nutritional, supplemental products that actually give you the results you're seeking.

We only put items in our Marketplace that are backed by peer-reviewed scientific research in humans showing positive results for the intended purpose.

https://store.anabolicmen.com

Use Code MASTER10 Today for 10% Off

Table Of Contents:

Time To Change Your Life Forever (Starting Now)

There will come a time when enough is enough... when you're fed up with listening to doctors whose only prescription is pharmaceuticals... not helping you use your own body to achieve the natural balance it craves.

It's time to take measures into your own hands, because there is nobody on Earth who cares as much as you do about your own health.

And believe it or not, <u>every single person reading this right now is equally equipped to succeed</u>.

You don't need loads of money, or time, or good genetics to make this happen. You just need to educate yourself, work hard at changing the right things, and be consistent over time and you will succeed.

Our Master Plan

We love setting goals – and achieving them.

If you're anything like us you know the feeling... that adrenaline rush and deep sense of satisfaction that comes with "success" of any kind – big or small.

And like anything else we do – with Anabolic Men we've set some big goals for the coming years, now that this book is changing lives so rapidly.

Our master plan has two major targets:

1.) Help a million men naturally optimize their testosterone. We still remember the feeling of getting this book into the hands of our first 1000 clients. Since then, then numbers have grown to the tens of thousands. So why stop there? We want to help 1 million guys completely, radically change their lives for the better by naturally optimizing their testosterone levels using AnabolicMen.com. One million men with more confidence, more self-worth, no depression, and fully natural alpha authority – and the world is going to be a better place. If you know any friends or family members who would love this book, please share it with them. Let's get to that 1 million mark together.

2.) Lead the fight against charlatans. Unfortunately, the testosterone-boosting industry has become one of the most popular playgrounds for scammers and charlatans, selling you their sugar pills with huge promises that they can never deliver. We want to be your go-to guys in the industry. There are a small handful of awesome educators in this industry, and we will always point you to the best resources. But be wary of most "T-boosting" products out there... they're almost always just flashy marketing with no real substance, created by people with no expertise, just trying to make a quick buck off you.

Dishonesty is rampant in the supplement industry, especially the testosterone supplement niche. Companies make huge promises, but rarely deliver. When we started the Anabolic Men Marketplace my business partner said, "We will only sell supplements that work. If it doesn't work, we're not selling it."

It's like he read my mind... Here's the deal: those "testosterone boosters" you see everywhere… most of them DON'T actually boost your testosterone. They're designed to increase your libido, and nothing more. As you'll learn in this book, libido and T are not the same thing. So what WILL increase your testosterone? Supplements that are designed to do very specific things, like eliminate key vitamin and mineral deficiencies, decrease chronic cortisol levels, and increase hormonal output from training. These are specific examples of things we manufacture. We focus in specific areas of T production that actually make a big impact on your hormone levels. If it doesn't work, we don't sell it.

We hope you love this book. We hope the information in these pages changes your life as much as it has changed both of ours.

This information is gold…

So let's start digging.

PART 1:
THE MASCULINE OPTIMIZATION PYRAMID

It's highly likely that you're reading this book right now because you're searching for answers.

You're searching for *help*.

Over the years, we've come to see some very predictable patterns in hormonal health optimization. We've focused much of our effort to this point on mastering natural testosterone enhancement and fully understanding the collective body of research on the subject.

In doing so, we developed a simple system that thousands of men have since used to optimize their T without drugs – rather, by using nutrition, training, lifestyle, and strategic supplementation.

We realized this system was not limited to *just* testosterone enhancement, but instead signified a protocol that could be used to optimize any number of hormones and biomarkers in the human body.

To illustrate the system itself, we came up with the **Masculine Optimization Pyramid.**

The steps on the Pyramid embody the different levels of focus, in order of importance (from foundation upward), that you must adhere to if you want to fully optimize key hormones, and in doing so optimize your health in general.

It's such a simple system, but we had no way of accurately conveying it graphically…

Until now, that is.

The Pyramid now solves that problem, making it easy to visualize:

MASCULINE OPTIMIZATION PYRAMID

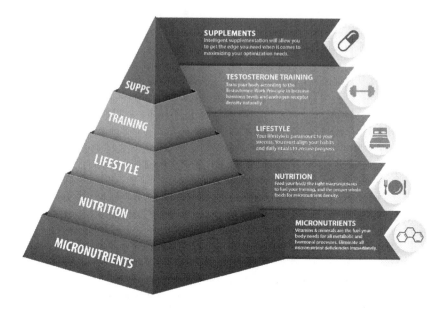

We've also organized the content in this book in a manner so that you can easily navigate through information relevant to educating yourself around specific levels of the Pyramid.

So now you're probably wondering what the Pyramid is... Let's break it down:

Level 1: Micronutrients (The Foundation)

Statistically, you're deficient in a handful of micronutrients which are causing issues for hormone optimization.

Now, you may not be deficient in ALL of them – but there are likely between 5-7 of them that you ARE deficient in that are negatively impacting your hormone production.

These are the top 5 micronutrient deficiencies we've seen in nearly all men. Statistically speaking, you're deficient in these - so this is a great place to start in your self-education and supplementation to eliminate the deficiencies:

- Vitamin D
- Zinc
- Magnesium
- Boron
- Choline

Level 2: Nutrition (Macronutrients And Micronutrients)

There are micronutrients – which we've just covered – but then there are *macronutrients*, which are **proteins, fats and carbs**. And above that is the overall calorie intake (which is based on your body and your goals, fat loss or muscle building/recomposition). Are you eating whole foods in a ratio ideal for hormone optimization?

The following is a list of specific things you need to focus on when it comes to nutrition:

- Overall Caloric Intake
- Macro Intake (fats, carbs, and protein)
- Macro Ratio and Specific Sources
- Increasing Micronutrient Consumption from Whole Foods

Level 3: Lifestyle (Sleep, Sex, Chemicals, Mindset, etc)

Living correctly involves doing a handful of of the right things daily that will facilitate progress (either bringing towards a goal or being counterproductive). These include getting adequate sleep, developing a dominant worldview, controlling your habits, and pursuing healthy relationships.

This level of the Pyramid focuses on these areas:

- Sleep
- Mindset & Meditation
- Habits (Alcohol, Smoking, Marijuana)
- Sex (Real Sex vs. Masturbation)
- Avoid Chemical Exposure

(We'll get into all of these a little later in this book.)

Level 4: Testosterone Training (Train Like A Man Should)

Train in a way that activates as much muscle tissue in as short a time as possible, facilitating adaptive change without over-stressing your body. Bonus points if you focus that training on Androgen Receptor dense muscle tissue, like in the THOR Program.

Training concepts to focus on:

- Resistance Training & Androgen Receptor Density
- Testosterone Work Principle
- Staying Below The Stress Threshold
- Daily Physical Activity

Level 5: Intelligent Supplementation (Get An Edge With Proven Compounds)

If you're doing everything else correctly and want to get the extra edge without pharmaceuticals, then leveraging particular supplements backed by clinical research may amplify your results towards hormonal optimization.

- Supplements/Herbs that actually work for increasing testosterone (and ones that don't)
- Cognitive Enhancers and Nootropics
- General Health
- Specific Issue Problem-Solving Supplements
- Estrogen (blockers, etc)

Total Hormone Optimization (The End Result)

As a result of systematically working your way up the MOP, you'll naturally optimize your overall hormonal health and achieve Hormonal Mastery.

We'll be digging into thoroughly into the Pyramid and all the levels specifically in this book... And after reading these pages, you'll have everything you need to optimize:

- Testosterone
- DHT
- Cortisol
- SHBG, Free Testosterone
- Estrogen

Last Note Before We Begin...

With this broad overview of how the Masculine Optimization Pyramid works, hopefully you can now understand how to use this simple framework to solve your testosterone-related issues.

This book is organized according to providing specific information to you along the lines of this Pyramid, and therefore we encourage you jump around and read in order of specific help you need.

Many of you may need to read from cover to cover, but others may find it helpful to jump ahead to specific sections, like supplements or nutrition, for example. Feel free to explore this book how you see fit.

Now, before we get into the actual levels of the Pyramid, we first need to understand how the body and endocrine system work.

Understanding this is the foundation of everything inside this book.

Without further ado, let's get started...

PART 2:
THE ENDOCRINE SYSTEM

— Chapter 1 —

The Endocrine System Explained

If you're experiencing any of the following in your daily life, your endocrine balance needs some attention:

- Irritable bowel syndrome
- fibromyalgia
- chronic stress
- anxiety disorders
- bipolar disorder
- insomnia
- borderline personality disorder
- excessive fat/muscle gain/loss
- post-traumatic stress disorder
- alcoholism
- attention deficit
- chronic fatigue syndrome
- burnout
- overtraining
- major depressive disorder
- loss of sex drive
- low testosterone

…Yes, the list continues.

If you can relate to any of these, then I'd suggest reading on…

What Is The HPA Axis & Why Should You Care?

Philosophically, I believe we should operate upon solid principles before worrying about details. Most people take the opposite approach, unfortunately.

The outcome is that they do not see results, or their results are transient. Then they wonder why. The only way to understand the why is to take the time to learn the underlying system of principles upon which the details rely.

Everyone reading this book should, at worst, have a basic understanding of what the HPA axis is and why it is so important to your everyday health, and at best, a thorough understanding of the neurobiology that underlies the important reactions and feedback loops within it.

This chapter gives you the scoop.

An understanding of the HPA axis will equip you with the principle-based knowledge that'll serve as the most important tool in your toolbox as you move forward with balancing/optimizing your endocrine system - which, in turn, will lead to lower body fat, increased muscularity, and a heightened sense of well-being.

The HPA Axis is the Hypothalamic-Pituitary-Adrenal axis. It is the line of action between the hypothalamus, the pituitary gland, and the adrenal glands.

The hypothalamus sits at the 'top' of the axis. It is the brain substrate that serves a primary purpose of linking the nervous system to the endocrine system via your pituitary gland. The hypothalamus is roughly the size of an almond and you can find it in all vertebrate nervous systems. It sits just below the thalamus (hence, the hypo-) and above the brainstem.

The direct aim of the hypothalamus when it releases neurohormones is to either stimulate or inhibit the actions of the pituitary gland. A few functions that are more commonly attributed to its control are hunger, sleep functioning, fatigue, thirst, & circadian cycles.

As you can probably assume from the magnitude of regulation that it's responsible for, the hypothalamus is extremely important in terms of creating a homeostasis (balance) within your endocrine system - and therefore entire body.

Symptoms of an unhealthy hypothalamus include inexplicable hunger, insomnia, weight problems, dehydration/hyponatremia, excessive fatigue, etc...

The pituitary gland is next in line. It is shaped like a pea and sits right below the hypothalamus, basically at the center, near the base of your brain.

It is also referred to as the hypophysis but, since I don't even know how to pronounce that correctly, we're just going to use 'pituitary' here.

It is divided into an anterior and posterior lobe and is responsible for secretion of vitally important homeostatic hormones into your body.

The hormones that it releases are:

- Growth Hormone (GH or HGH)
- Thyroid-Stimulating Hormone (TSH)
- Adrenocorticotropic Hormone (ACTH)
- Beta-Endorphin
- Prolactin (PRL)

- Luteinizing Hormone (LH)
- Follicle-Stimulating Hormone (FSH)
- Intermedins (MSHs)
- Oxytocin
- Antidiuretic Hormone (ADH)

The next and final 'stop' in the HPA axis is the adrenal glands, which sit far from your brain, atop your kidneys. They are mainly responsible for releasing hormones - such as cortisol and the catecholamines - into your bloodstream in response to stress.

What are catecholamines *(kat-eh-cola-meens)*?

Epinephrine and norepinephrine: more commonly known as adrenaline and noradrenaline.

Your adrenal glands are also responsible for the secretion of small amounts of androgens (male steroid hormones). The hypothalamus and pituitary gland also communicate directly with the testes (gonads) so this axis is sometimes referred to as the HPG axis as well.

While some testosterone is secreted by the adrenal glands, the bulk of it is secreted from the Leydig cells of the testes in men.

The pituitary gland is known as the 'master' endocrine gland.

The Basic Pathways and Feedback Loops

The HPA axis, as a whole, is incredibly complex.

There are (very very smart) people who devote their entire lives to studying its effects on the human body & behavior (ie endocrinologists, neuroscientists, etc) who still do not understand everything, nor will they ever.

Keep in mind that I am making grossly simplified generalizations when I say that the HPA axis is responsible for not only the above functions, like regulating stress & secreting sex hormones, but also controlling your mood & emotions, your immune system, your energy metabolism, and very importantly - digestion.

In fact, this entire chapter is grossly simplified.

But the point, once again, is not details for the sake of details, but to grasp a general understanding of how this all works.

However simplified the generalizations may be, just believe me that the HPA and HPG axis' are power players in these processes.

Neurons in the paraventricular nucleus of the hypothalamus synthesize and secrete vasopressin & CRH (corticotropin-releasing hormone). The release of these peptides stimulates the secretion of ACTH in the pituitary gland which acts to produce glucocorticoids (ie cortisol - synthesized from cholesterol) in the adrenal glands.

These glucocorticoids now act back on the hypothalamus to suppress any more release of CRH & ACTH. This is what we refer to as a negative feedback loop. It regulates itself when everything is healthy and working properly.

Keep in mind that the hypothalamus is only one of several targets in the brain for glucocorticoids.

Stress hormones such as cortisol act on many different tissues and substrates within both your brain & your body - a big reason why keeping this feedback loop working properly is VITAL to maintaining a healthy body.

One positive feedback loop within the HPA axis that you should be aware of is the excitatory effect of the catecholamines (Epinephrine &

Norepinephrine) on the pituitary gland to increase the production of ACTH and Beta Endorphins.

Remember that the HPA axis is not a self-contained unit - it spans much of the body anatomically but it is also influenced by other substrates in your brain and body, specifically those tied to sensory processing - both on the front end (ie eyes, ears, nose, mouth, skin) and on the back- end (ie amygdala, hippocampus, etc).

Basically what I am trying to say is that it is crucial, *absolutely crucial,* to have a well-functioning HPA axis in order to be healthy, get and stay lean, have good sex, and be happy.

— Chapter 2 —

Testosterone 101

Pharmaceuticals are big business. BIG business.

So I was absolutely not surprised when, a couple years ago, a pharmaceutical company named Abbvie jumped all over the somewhat recent trend of men experiencing low testosterone - packaging their 'solution' and branding the issue as an epidemic, conveniently funneling thousands and thousands of men into doctors' offices, where they were handed prescriptions for hormone replacement therapy solutions & gels (Androgel, to be precise).

Boom, billions of dollars.

So what happened to all of the men, most likely many of you reading this program right now, who are on HRT? Well, your testosterone levels are likely back in the 'normal' range, in many cases on the low side still, depending on where you were starting from. That's good, right?

Not exactly.

What happens if you stop using the gel?

Will your body naturally produce enough testosterone to keep your levels where they are?

Probably not.

So here's the situation: you're chained to rubbing an expensive smelly goo on your chest for the rest of your life - or at least as long as you care about getting a boner.

That's no way to live.

The goo is a band aid. What we need to do is get to the root of the issue, learn and understand the cause of the malaise, then take action based upon what we know. That's the process I used several years ago to take my own T levels from basically nothing to way above normal - out of the medical reference range even.

The first thing the doctor gave me when I was diagnosed with the brain tumor (that was blocking testosterone production) was a prescription for Androgel. I took it for a few weeks, but decided to chuck it, and all of my other medications shortly thereafter, when I made the decision to uproot the problem directly and solve it with a natural solution. Best choice of my life.

That was a few years ago, and since then I've educated myself, then put that knowledge into action in my life. The results speak for themselves.

I'm very confident I will have high testosterone for my entire life because I now understand how to keep it that way. It will naturally decline with age, yes, but it will never reach the point of having to ever think twice about whether it's negatively affecting my life in any way.

Right now my wellbeing is high. So is my morning wood. (Couldn't resist)

I can put on muscle fairly quickly and stay at a low body fat percentage year round without any trouble. I sleep like a bear in hibernation every night and can grow a decent beard if I choose to. I always gain strength and power in training (actually an important cause of the high testosterone, more on that later on) and I'm pretty sure women can smell it.

Oh I also grew 2 inches in the meantime.

The task at hand for me at the moment is distilling this into a replicable process that you can use in your own life.

I'm a believer that things happen for a reason, and it would appear as though all the trouble I went through personally, and the years of self-experimenting, learning what works and what doesn't, then my decision to become a blogger, may have just led us all right to this moment. So yep, I think I was meant to share this knowledge with the world.

Know this: medications and gels are not your only option.

You also don't need to eat a dried tiger penis (apparently a common practice in ancient Chinese herbalism |o_o|).

You can naturally increase your testosterone and growth hormone and then sustain your levels without "assistance".

It is a process, and will take anywhere between 6 months to 2 years most likely. But once you learn it and put it into action, you'll be set.

It's time to begin building the foundation. Let's learn.

What is Testosterone?

Testosterone is the principal male sex hormone. An androgen.

It is found in both males and females, and acts anabolically. While females naturally produce small amounts of testosterone, and have far greater sensitivity to the introduction of additional testosterone into their systems, males, clearly, are where testosterone is most prevalent (7- 10+ times the natural amount of females), and in whom higher testosterone is most often desired.

It is secreted in the testes of males, and ovaries of females, with small amounts also coming from the adrenal glands.

Androgens are steroid hormones, and can be produced naturally and synthetically. The presence of androgens in tissues that have androgen receptors promotes protein synthesis in those tissues, giving it anabolic influence.

Androgenic effects include much of what we consider to be human maturation, especially in sexual tissues/organs. For example, androgens heavily influence maturation of male secondary characteristics such as growth of the penis and scrotum, body hair, vocal sound depth, etc. Anabolic effects are characterized by things like muscle growth and strength, as well as bone maturation, increased density, and increased strength.

Testosterone gets to work, in both males and females, before we're even born and carries out its influence heavily first during the sexual differentiation process, then into infancy, prepubescence, puberty, adolescence, and adulthood.

T plays a role in many processes in the body, one of the more prominently known being spermatogenesis.

Without the presence of testosterone and/or the androgen receptor, spermatogenesis can't proceed past meiosis (ie. you can't produce sperm). In non-sciency terms, you're infertile.

So now that we know where testosterone is produced, let's venture a guess at what may be the cause of low testosterone production.

There are two common culprits, and they're medically recognized as primary and secondary hypogonadism.

The first, primary hypogonadism, is caused by deficient testosterone production in the testes. The boys aren't working properly.

The second, secondary hypogonadism, is caused by hypothalamic-pituitary irregularities. They regulate your endocrine system. So for example, secondary hypogonadism can be caused when a piece of this puzzle isn't functioning properly. I'm of the opinion that these processes (primary + secondary hypogonadism) do not operate independently, as evidenced by the strong influence of the hypothalamus and pituitary gland on the gonads directly.

So in the end, it all comes back to brain health. And therefore... gut health.

Your gut is your second brain. And you can directly influence its health with what you put into your body for nutrition.

NOW we're getting somewhere.

You'll recall that testosterone is produced in the testes by cells called Leydig cells. The average plasma concentration of testosterone in human males typically falls between the range of 200 – 1000 ng/dl. In terms of timeline vs plasma concentrations over a lifetime, T levels rise sharply during adolescence, peak in a man's 20's, then begin a slow decline with age.

While its most potent and widely recognized effect on the human male body is its influence over the growth/development of sexual tissues, your testosterone level is also a good indicator of lean body mass (ie. muscle) potential, with the right stimuli. Elevated testosterone levels will increase red blood cell production, bone density, sugar uptake into muscle tissue, muscle glycogen storage, and protein synthesis associated with muscular growth.

The Feedback Loop

The cascade of events leading to testosterone production begins in the hypothalamus with the release of GnRH (gonadotropin releasing hormone) which acts on the pituitary to produce two hormones: LH (luteinizing hormone) and FSH (follicle stimulating hormone). These are the gonadotropins.

Once in the bloodstream, LH makes its way to the testicles where it exerts its influence on the Leydig cells, triggering a series of events that turns cholesterol into testosterone.

As testosterone levels increase, LH production & transport slows. A negative feedback loop.

The body and brain are communicating constantly in order to regulate important processes. This is one of countless feedback loops (there are many positive feedback loops as well) in the human body.

With this negative feedback loop, the brain can constantly keep hormone levels in check – in this case, testosterone, LH, FSH, and GnRH – under normal, healthy circumstances. When a problem arises anywhere on this pipeline, be it from a tumor, traumatic stressor, or summative build-up of small, unnoticeable toxic stress (super common) – not only is everything downstream affected, everything period is affected.

Because it's a loop.

You'll notice that testosterone doesn't only linearly exert its influence back on the hypothalamus alone, it can also work directly back on the pituitary (essentially "skipping" a step) if your body is looking to quickly regulate gonadotropin release.

When this little system is working properly, everything's good in the 'hood. When something goes wrong down the line is when we run into noticeable issues (more on that later).

FSH, the other gonadotropin, is chiefly responsible for stimulating (or regulating) production of sperm in the Leydig cells in the testes.

At this point we understand that testosterone production is regulated by the brain, namely the hypothalamus and pituitary, via a handful of powerful hormones. And it's synthesized after a number of intermediate steps, from cholesterol in the Leydig cells. And this process is all tied together in a negative feedback loop.

Now it's produced. What happens next?

When testosterone is released into the wild – your bloodstream – it is actually entering a molecular game of 'tag,' to put it metaphorically. A carrier protein named SHBG, or Sex Hormone Binding Globulin, is released from the liver, and SHBG is 'it.'

SHBG's role is to regulate the level of freely circulating testosterone in your bloodstream. So when it binds a testosterone molecule, that testosterone cannot effectively enter and exert its influence on a cell.

So the more SHBG is in the bloodstream, the fewer testosterone molecules actually reach a cellular target. This isn't inherently a bad thing, it's just the way things work. Another negative feedback loop meant to regulate your endocrine function.

However, now I hope you're beginning to realize the sheer amount of self-limiting processes that occur along the line in this cycle... and none of our testosterone has actually had an effect on anything yet!

With SHBG in this role, we now understand that testosterone levels and SHBG levels are inversely correlated: the more SHBG in your system, the lower amounts of free, active T.

Again, if something small is affecting ANYTHING along this pathway, you're likely going to experience an issue, manifesting itself as lower-than-optimal testosterone (and related hormone) levels.

For example, you may have very high levels of free, circulating testosterone, but with an imbalance in SHBG production, much of that free T won't reach a target. That sucks. We'll discuss free testosterone and total testosterone further in a little bit.

— Chapter 3 —

How Is Testosterone Produced?

In case you got lost about exactly how T is produced in the human body, this quick chapter is meant to condense all the important variables in an easy-to-understand manner.

A lion's share of about ~95% of your testosterone is produced inside the testicles, in the testicular leydig cells to be more precise. The remaining ~5% is synthesized from DHEA (precursor androgen) in the adrenal glands.

Obviously the molecule doesn't just magically appear in the testicles, there's a strategic cascade of events that leads to the production of the hormone. And like everything in the body, it starts from the brain.

Here's how the natural "feedback loop" of testosterone production operates:

1. It all starts from the hypothalamus, which is an almond sized brain substrate that links your nervous system to the endocrine system. The first step of the process is simply when the hypothalamus releases a hormone called gonadotropin releasing hormone (GnRH). Keep in mind that this is the master hormone that starts everything.
2. GnRH then stimulates the pituitary gland, which is a small pea sized endocrine gland protruding from the bottom of the hypothalamus. When the gland is stimulated by GnRH, it

releases two hormones: luteinizing hormone (LH) and follicle stimulating hormone (FSH). These are the gonadotropins, and this is exactly why they first hormone is called gonadotropin releasing hormone.

3. After the pituitary gland has released LH and FSH to the bloodstream, both of the hormones make their way from the brain, down to the ballsack. When they have reached their destination they enter the testicular leydig cells.

4. Inside the leydig cells, the following events take place: FSH starts the process of spermatogenesis, whereas LH – through an extremely complex process – converts cholesterol into testosterone.

That's how the big T is produced... But wait, why is it called a *"feedback loop?"*

Answer: After the fresh testosterone molecules are produced, your brain constantly monitors the amount of the hormone in blood, if it gets to be too high, it slows down the release and transportation of LH. And that's how the loop is completed.

How Testosterone Exerts its Effects in The Body

Now the testosterone is freshly produced and your leydig cells release it to the bloodstream. What happens next?

How does the hormone exert the effects? It doesn't just float around the blood for nothing. Right?

Well of course not... Here's what happens next:

1. As the fresh baby testosterone enters the bloodstream, it's called "free testosterone". This is because it's literally free, as it's not bound to anything yet. But then your liver also releases this carrier protein called sex hormone binding globulin (SHBG). And this is where things get complicated.

2. About ~98% of the fresh "free testosterone" is bound to either SHBG or albumin (another carrier protein), and when testosterone is bound to either one of these proteins, it cannot effectively enter cells anymore, and it has really hard time binding to the androgen receptors. Meaning that ~98% of the testosterone is not really that "active". Simply put, the more of the carrier proteins (SHBG and albumin) you have in your bloodstream, the fewer testosterone molecules actually remain bio-available.

3. The remaining testosterone that isn't bound to carrier proteins (free testosterone), freely circulates around your body, just waiting to be bound into a receptor. Then for example, let's say that you're lifting weights at the gym. Your androgen receptors in the muscle tissue activate and free testosterone molecules will be bound to the receptors. This is when the effects start to take place.

4. Once the free testosterone molecule is bound to androgen receptor, the receptor goes through a structural change, making it able to enter your DNA. Once it actually enters the DNA, the effects of testosterone finally take place. When it happens in your muscle tissue, you'll get increased protein synthesis and muscle growth as a result. If this takes place in your face, your beard growth might increase, or facial bone structure might become more dense and angular, etc.

Wherever there are androgen receptors in the body (muscle tissue, penis, bones, etc) free testosterone can bind to it and then enter DNA, and that's where the hormone finally works its magic.

— Chapter 4 —

The Benefits Of High Testosterone

We have all heard the most common benefits of having high T. Such as the increased ability to build lean muscle mass, increased ability to burn fat for fuel, or the improved sexual performance and libido, bone health, etc. But there are also so many other awesome benefits that come along with high testosterone…

… And most people simply don't know about them.

Just take a look at these 5:

Benefit 1: Reduced Facial Fat

It's a quite well known fact that increased testosterone levels make the facial muscles more prominent, and the bone structure more "chiseled" and angular.

But what most people don't know, is that in men, testosterone also controls the fat distribution of the face.

In fact there's quite a large pool of evidence suggesting that the higher the testosterone level, the less subcutaneous fat on the face.

I personally believe that high testosterone is the main ingredient to awesome facial aesthetics. T makes the the bone structure of the face more angular, and it increases the size and thickness of the facial muscles. The reduction of subcutaneous fat in the area amplifies the effect, creating a strong, angular, defined face.

Basing my assumption only on facial aesthetics, I would say that the model on the image above, has quite high serum testosterone levels.

Benefit 2: Improved Mood

I have scanned through thousands of testosterone related studies through Pubmed, and a few trends have caught my eye on multiple testosterone replacement studies...

1. Men who have low – even hypogonadal – testosterone levels are often complaining about depression, feelings of irritability, anger, and poor quality of life (1, 2, 3).

2. When these men increase their testosterone levels (often through TRT) their quality of life, mood, and motivation increase dramatically (4, 5, 6).

I can relate to the studies on a personal level too. I never had clinically "low" testosterone levels, but they weren't exactly high either at the time I started this journey of boosting T naturally...

...As my testosterone levels have gradually gone up throughout these years, my mood, success, and quality of life have all followed the trend.

I actually believe that the success of AnabolicMen.com, could be traced back to the testosterone driven thrive for success and competition.

Benefit 3: Increased Basal Metabolic Rate

Men who have higher testosterone levels, can literally eat a bit more food without gaining weight, than men with low testosterone can.

There are actually two main reasons to this.

1. The first one is more well known, it's the fact that testosterone directly inhibits the formation of new fat cells (7).
2. The second one is not that well known, and it's the fact that testosterone greatly increases the basal metabolic rate (8, 9, 10).

As a guy who has an appetite of an elephant, I appreciate findings like these.

Benefit 4: Women Love Testosterone

This is something that can be easily understood just by using common sense: women – especially when they're ovulating – are more attracted to masculine men.

More in detail, women are attracted to men who have high testosterone charasterics (11), that or just high testosterone, as one study even suggests that women can also be attracted to the "smell" of high testosterone (12).

There's an evolutionary reason for that. As women subconsciously seek the best "genes" to their children, and a man who has high testosterone levels, is exactly what their subconscious mind is looking for.

If you're a feminist, the above statement probably got you really mad. But hold on to your horses, it goes the other way around too. Men are subconsciously attracted to feminine women who have high estrogen levels (13).

Benefit 5: Improved Circulation

Improved blood flow all-around the body is one of the not so well known – but awesome – benefits of high T.

Testosterone directly stimulates the enzyme nitric oxide synthase (eNOS)(14). This is a fancy way of saying that it increases the production of nitric oxide, a molecule that both widens and relaxes blood vessels and arteries.

This is one of the reasons why high testosterone is a good thing for your cardiovascular health, and one of the reasons why it's borderline unhealthy and even dangerous to have clinically low T.(15)

Nitric oxide improves your workouts, improves your erectile quality, shortens your recovery time after workouts, and simply just makes your body to operate much more efficiently as blood is flowing more freely.

— Chapter 5 —

What Is The Optimal T Level?

Testosterone is without a doubt the most important hormone in a man's body. It make's a man happy, motivated, strong, virile, and basically much more of a man.

And it comes not as a surprise that one of the most commonly asked questions I've received so far is this:

What is the optimal testosterone level for my age?

And in all honesty, it's extremely hard to tell.

Labs give different reference range, experts give all sorts of numbers, studies have come to different conclusions, and I have my own opinions based on personal experiences and the emails that I've been getting for the past 6 months.

However the most common reference ranges for average testosterone level seems to fall between the numbers of 250-1200 ng/dl.

And on top of that the common mantra seems to be that testosterone levels will start to decline at around the age of 30 due to "normal aging process".

However that's bullshit in my opinion. Older men are simply having lower testosterone levels because they become sedentary, they stop having sex, and they "settle down".

I base this claim on the following facts:

a) In rural populations, older men have just as much testosterone as the younger guys do. (16)
b) In several studies, research have found out that there's a lot of guys who are 70+ years old but still have testosterone levels of a 17 year old.
c) Several respected doctors and scientists won't buy the claim either. (17)

That's why I believe that the real reason why testosterone levels usually start to decline at the age of 30 is the fact that men around that age are often sedentary, don't have sex, settle down, can't sleep as well as younger guys, and start taking prescription medications for various "illnesses"...

...Thus, in this chapter you're not going to see any charts about what would be the optimal level for certain age, as I simply believe that whether you're an old man or a young gun, you should aim for the same levels.

And based on the emails that I've gotten, my 5-year research, and personal experience, I've put up my own ideas for optimal testosterone levels:

0-400 ng/dl – This is the area that I personally see as the zone of "low testosterone". It's because most of the men who have all the classic signs and symptoms of low testosterone, often fall into this range (some younger guys have had the symptoms even at close to 500 ng/dl).

500-700 ng/dl – This is the area that I see as "normal testosterone". It's a range where there's normally no symptoms or signs of low testosterone present, and everything should function effortlessly.

700-1,000 ng/dl – This is what I'd like to call high testosterone in the modern standards (our ancestors probably had double or even triple this amount). It's a point where missing a morning erection is a rare event, and building muscle is a breeze.

1,000+ ng/dl – This is the line of optimal for me. Everything above this point is pretty awesome, and if you're past the 1,000 ng/dl point naturally, I can only congratulate you for a job well done. However, it's a sad fact that most men in the modern world of processed foods, chemical estrogen mimics, and high obesity rates will never see these numbers.

So that's how I feel. The above is only my personal view of the optimal levels, and doctors or health care professional may disagree, I don't care. This is simply what I've found to be the most accurate view of the situation so far.

NOTE: That's only the optimal for total testosterone. Other factors that play their parts are the amount of free testosterone, total estrogen, free estrogen, DHT, prolactin, cortisol, etc.

— Chapter 6 —

Optimizing Free Testosterone & Lowering SHBG Levels

This section is vitally important for you to read if you want to fully understand how to maximize the effectiveness of the testosterone in your system.

Free testosterone is different from *total testosterone*.

So what's difference?

Well, if you can recall the discussion earlier on SHBG (Sex Hormone Binding Globulin) you'll remember that SHBG binds specifically to androgens.

When testosterone is SHBG-bound (or bound to any other molecule or protein) it can no longer be utilized by other tissues.

Free testosterone is unbound, and active in the bloodstream. It can travel to the necessary tissues and exert its effects on them.

You should strive to have a balance between free and total testosterone levels. Some individuals have normal testosterone levels, but super low free testosterone. This may leave them perplexed if they do not know how little free testosterone they have, and they will very likely still experience the common symptoms of low testosterone such as low libido, trouble losing body fat, low muscularity, trouble sleeping, depression, and low well-being.

The conventional wisdom would say to simply take measures to lower your SHBG levels in order to increase your free testosterone.

If you search on the "male vitality" or "anti-aging" forums online for SHBG issues you'll almost immediately come upon countless threads where guys talk about all of the drugs they're taking to lower their SHBG levels.

This is overly simplistic in its approach, and for many guys even ends up lowering their overall T levels even further.

How can that happen?

Well, the part of the equation that they're neglecting to remember is that SHBG doesn't only bind testosterone. It is an androgen binding protein, therefore it will also bind estrogen.

If you take a drug that specifically inhibits binding (or production) of SHBG, then you will also increase the amount of free estrogen in your bloodstream, which will negatively impact your testosterone levels.

Bad news... So what should you do instead?

Well, SHBG is produced in the liver. An abnormal amount of SHBG in the bloodstream, binding androgen molecules to the point of negatively affecting your testosterone levels indicates that your liver is out of balance.

The most important thing to do at this point is address your liver health.

Specifically, stop drinking alcohol for a while, and use intermittent fasting with pure water as way to allow your body a specific amount of time every day to heal itself. Depending on how messed-up your liver is, this may take months, and it may take years before things are fully restored to homeostatic levels. However, just make small steps forward, progressing slowly while you take the other necessary steps in terms of nutrition, training, and lifestyle.

You'll see an upward trend over time.

If you have a specific known liver disease then now you know that it is likely the cause of your low free testosterone levels as well. Cirrhosis can be caused several ways, including very serious conditions like hepatitis and chronic alcohol abuse. Your liver will also be ravaged from tumors, liver cancer, cysts, fatty liver disease (caused by obesity in general), parasitic infection, portal vein thrombosis, and bile duct obstruction. These conditions require professional medical attention beyond the scope of this program.

Some warning signs that you may be experiencing liver problems are:

Jaundice, discolored skin and eyes (yellowish), abdominal swelling and pain, dark urine, pale stools, itchy skin, bloody stools, chronic fatigue, loss of appetite, and chronic nausea.

See a doctor to run some lab tests to check on your liver health if you think this may be the issue.

Also, and potentially a very likely cause of liver imbalance, is excessive acetaminophen (i.e. Tylenol) intake. Acetaminophen is in many over the counter medications (so check the label before ingesting). The fact that it is seemingly benign makes it even more dangerous because you are more likely to consume excessive amounts - enough to damage your liver.

Acetaminophen causes free radical damage by creating a hydrogen peroxide foaming, depleting the liver of glutathione, its primary defense against free radicals.

So just be careful. If you regularly consume acetaminophen, reduce your intake or find an alternative.

The good news...

If you take the necessary steps in this program and apply the knowledge you learn to your everyday life, you'll naturally bring your endocrine system back into balance, which will in turn encourage liver balance (if you're not in an extreme medical case as noted above).

You will, over time, optimize the ratio of free T to total T, bringing it all back into balance so your body can operate the way it should, and your "low T" symptoms will gradually disappear in the process.

10 Ways To Lower SHBG Levels Naturally

We have testosterone which is bound to two different proteins, albumin and sex hormone binding globulin (SHBG). This bound up testosterone is unavailable to be used by our androgen receptors and it's basically like a "reserve" of our male hormones.

Then we have "free testosterone", which isn't bound to proteins. It floats around the bloodstream and is constantly ready to bind into the androgen receptors, creating masculinizing effects (free testosterone only accounts 1-2% of our total testosterone but experts agree that it's the most important kind as it's the one that creates the effects of testosterone).

Now if you're smart, you're probably thinking, *"How could I get more of this free testosterone then?"*

That's what this article talks about. You see, science has shown that we can naturally reduce these binding proteins from our bloodstream, resulting in more free testosterone.

That's why this section is about how to lower SHBG, which is the protein that binds most of your total testosterone making it unavailable for the receptors.

By simply learning how to lower SHBG count in your body, you will free up testosterone and make it more powerful.

> NOTE: Albumin, which is the other binding protein, is much weaker and less abundant than SHBG, thus I don't feel the need to focus on it as much as we should on sex hormone binding globulin.

1. Boron for Free Testosterone

Boron is a trace mineral that most people have never even heard of...

It's present in our natural soil due to the fact that it comes to earth from cosmic ray spallation.

Given that we don't eat foods grown in nutrient rich soils anymore (because of the processed shit), we're depleted in multiple important minerals...

...And one of them is boron, which has a valuable role in our endocrine system:

a) This human study found out that 10 mg's of boron taken daily for a week was enough to increase free testosterone levels by 28%. SHBG count in serum also decreased significantly which probably explains the increase in free T. (18)

b) In this human study the researchers gave their subjects 6 mg's of boron daily for 60 days. The results showed a similar 29,5% increase in free testosterone, which was again caused by a significant drop in SHBG count. (19)

I'm personally supplementing with the boron in Testro-X everyday.

2. Eat Plenty of Carbs

Many guys like to think that low-carb dieting would be the best way to go when boosting testosterone.

It makes some sense as insulin (a hormone that increases when we eat carbs) and sugar (which is a carb) are both known for their testosterone lowering effects…

…And actually there was a point in my life when I also believed that a low-carb diet would be the way to go.

However that's not true, studies constantly show that low-carb diets decrease testosterone levels, whereas high-carb diets significantly increase the big T while they simultaneously decrease estrogen, cortisol, and SHBG (20, 21, 22).

Therefore eating a diet moderately high in carbohydrates would be a good way to lower SHBG count (and increase testosterone).

3. Take Vitamin D

Vitamin D is one hell of an awesome vitamin. Most commonly it's associated with cardiovascular health, bone health, and immune function.

And while vitamin D is called a "vitamin", it's not It's really a steroid hormone that regulates more than 1,000 bodily functions, mistakenly named a vitamin.

Best part about the bone vitamin however is the fact that it increases testosterone levels (23, 24, 25)...

...And this study (26) found out that 3332 IU's of vitamin D3 was enough to significantly reduce sex hormone binding globulin (SHBG) count.

Therefore if you want to increase testosterone (both total and free), and reduce SHBG count, start supplementing with high quality vitamin D3 supplement, be out in the sun, and eat plenty of fish.

4. Fiber is Not Really that Important

It's a common mantra from the governmental health panel that we need to eat huge amounts of dietary fiber in order to be "healthy". However there's no reason for that. There's absolutely no scientific evidence that we would need so much fiber daily.

Kellogg's and other cereal giants are just paying millions of dollars to various influential organizations (such as the AND) in order to get their message of "healthy breakfast with plenty of fiber" out there, which will then only increase their revenue, not our health.

I'm personally avoiding fiber, and the reason is simple: high fiber diets are known for their testosterone lowering effects. They also increase SHBG which binds up testosterone making it unable to bind to the receptors (27, 28).

5. Certain Prescription Drugs can Skyrocket SHBG

Few months ago I wrote a big list of prescription drugs that were scientifically proven to decrease testosterone levels…

…Then I followed up with a post about Finasteride and other hair loss drugs which were shown to be even more harmful for your testosterone levels. Quite many of those meds in the list also increased SHBG levels, resulting in lowered free T.

These drugs for example: statins (29), beta blockers (30), antifungals (31), antidepressants (32), and hair loss drugs (33).

6. Natural Hormone Optimization in General

Testosterone in itself will reduce SHBG count. It's not exactly clear why, but men with higher testosterone levels usually have lower SHBG levels.

Estrogen also impacts SHBG, as lower levels of the female hormone will lower SHBG, which is an awesome thing…

...This means that simply following the teachings of this blog (which in all of its simplicity is to boost testosterone and reduce estrogen), could significantly lower your SHBG levels as your hormonal health improves.

So just boost that T and get rid of that overblown E.

7. Fish Oil Favorably Impacts SHBG count

Fish oil in general is pretty awesome. I supplement with it daily and also eat plenty of fatty fish, for a good reason though...

Firstly, it's been shown to increase luteinizing hormone (LH) production. (34) LH is the hormone that stimulates the gonads to produce testosterone.

Secondly, this in-vitro study (35) found out that omega-3's are anti-estrogenic.

Thirdly, this Japanese study (36) found out that fish oil reduces SHBG count.

I'm personally using and recommending Pure Fish Oil from Norway (pharmaceutical grade) (now available in the Anabolic Men Marketplace **store.anabolicmen.com**).

8. Magnesium Increases Free Testosterone

Magnesium is one of the most important elements for the human body.

It's essential for our survival and regulates hundreds of enzymes in the body.

We're also somewhat deficient in the mineral due to the fact that most of us eat shitty diets. However we shouldn't be as magnesium has shown to be pretty awesome in regards of free testosterone and SHBG:

a) This study (37) found out that magnesium makes testosterone more bio-available via decreasing SHBG.
b) This study (38) found out that a gram of magnesium a day in combination with exercise is enough to raise free testosterone levels by 24%.
c) This study (39) examined several health parameters of 400 men. The researchers found out that the men who had highest serum magnesium levels, also had lowest SHBG and highest testosterone and IGF-1 (growth hormone) levels.

I highly recommend pure magnesium oil which is applied transmedially to the skin. It has much higher bio-availability than oral supplements.

9. Zinc for Everything

Zinc is literally the master mineral of the endocrine system...
...Several studies show that it increases testosterone, reduces estrogen, increases dihydrotestosterone (DHT), and improves sperm parameters (40).

But these studies made zinc even better of a mineral, now it's also seen to reduce SHBG count (41, 42).

My recommendation for zinc is Thorne Research's Double Strength Zinc or the Zinc from Testro-X by Truth Nutraceuticals.

10. Don't Go Overboard With Alcohol

Binge drinking has its downsides, such as the fact that it significantly reduces testosterone levels, testicular weight, and sperm parameters (43).

It also skyrockets the female hormone estrogen and the stress hormone cortisol (44).

And that's not even all, as binge drinking impairs the P45 enzyme system of the liver which skyrockets SHBG (45).

In other words, binge drinking is pretty damaging for your endocrine system.

Chapter 7

Cortisol

Cortisol gets a lot of play in the blogosphere, especially in the fitness realm.

"Keep your cortisol low," is the mantra.

But how many of us actually know what it is, much less understand the way it works? How can we expect to keep it at a healthy level if we don't even understand what we're trying to manipulate?

Well, let's address that issue together right now.

After reading this chapter, you will no longer be one of the blind lemmings following what you hear proclaimed by gurus and mass periodicals. Instead you'll be capable of making decisions based on your innate knowledge of your own body and lifestyle coupled with a general understanding of how the system you're looking to manipulate actually works.

Let's begin.

What Is Cortisol?

Cortisol is a glucocorticoid, a class of steroid hormone, released from the adrenal cortex.

Its release is regulated by the hypothalamus (in a similar series of steps as we saw with testosterone) and the influence of CRH (corticotropin-releasing hormone).

The hypothalamus uses CRH to signal the anterior pituitary to release another hormone called ACTH (adrenocorticotropic hormone), which enters the bloodstream and acts on the adrenal glands downstream to begin production, and subsequent release, of cortisol (which is also known as hydrocortisone).

What Does It Do?

Baseline levels of cortisol are required for healthy functioning of the body. Chronically elevated levels are what we need to look out for. You'll understand why when you understand what it does.

Cortisol plays a key role in a process called glycogenolysis, the breaking down of muscle glycogen in the liver and muscle tissue, by triggering the activation of an enzyme called glycogen phosphorylase. This entire process is triggered by the presence of epinephrine and/or norepinephrine (E/NE), also known as adrenaline and noradrenaline.

E/NE are released in response to stress (commonly associated with the 'fight or flight' response). This little process is why cortisol is also associated with stress.

Under times of stress, the body needs to have a mechanism of action for allocating resources away from less important things, such as the immune system, and toward more immediately important processes such as breaking down muscle glycogen.

Evolutionarily this is important because it allows the human under pressure or external threat to quickly evade danger.

Cortisol is responsible for this.

However, now we can see why elevated levels of cortisol can be a bad thing. In terms of muscle wasting, chronically elevated cortisol will lead to a catabolic process known as proteolysis.

It's also known to suppress lipolysis (breakdown of fat tissue) and decrease bone formation (by reducing calcium absorption in the intestines and facilitating an exchange of potassium for sodium in the cells).

Hopefully you can see the trend: it appears to act antithetically to testosterone.

An elevated cortisol level also facilitates insulin resistance by decreasing the amount of glucose transporters that get shuttled to the surface of the cell membrane, and inhibits collagen formation, which subsequently inhibits protein synthesis due to a decreased ability of muscle tissue to uptake amino acids.

Cortisol also suppresses the immune system via a negative feedback effect on a group of cytokines (interleukin-1) which disables production of T-cell growth factor. T-cells are known to actually secrete a "modifying factor" (GRMF) that regulates cortisol release, so by disabling T-cell production, cortisol has less of a checks & balances system to answer to (to anthropomorphize it all).

In terms of brain damage, chronically elevated cortisol levels can damage cells in the hippocampus, creating a memory-deficit effect. While it works hand-in-hand with E/NE to create "flash bulb" memories (short, highly emotionally salient memories under stress), at chronically high levels, it will also severely hamper your ability to recall basic information.

This is why you feel "brain fog" during prolonged periods of stress at work or in family life and you may feel absent- minded and forgetful. Cortisol is damaging your hippocampal neurons, inhibiting your ability to recall information you've already "stored".

Okay, now that the doomsday picture has been painted, let's take a look back at the process briefly and identify where we may want to exert some influence in order to control cortisol production, keeping production at a healthy level.

My vote is for the pituitary gland.

Remember, the pituitary secretes ACTH into the bloodstream to signal to the adrenal cortex to secrete cortisol.

So now that we understand quite a bit about cortisol itself, and possess a basic understanding of the system, let's take a look at the interplay between cortisol and testosterone.

Recall that when cortisol is released in response to stress, it triggers the reallocation of resources away from other body processes. One effect of this is actually a decrease in testosterone. They work inversely.

Under normal conditions this is completely fine; processes such as spermatogenesis are low on the totem pole compared to jumping out of the way to avoid getting smacked by a speeding taxi, for example.

Once the external stressor is gone, the body restores its homeostasis, lowering cortisol levels and increasing the testosterone levels back to normal.

However, under the influence of chronically elevated cortisol levels, that homeostasis is not restored.

Testosterone is chronically suppressed.

This manifests in all manner of the symptoms that we commonly associate with today's "low T" epidemic.

— Chapter 8 —

Growth Hormone

Now let's talk about growth hormone. First, what is it?

GH (or HGH) is a peptide hormone secreted from the anterior pituitary and regulated by GHRH (Growth Hormone Releasing Hormone) and GHIH (Growth Hormone Inhibiting Hormone) – both secreted from the hypothalamus.

These two 'neurosecretory' hormones actually get released into the blood surrounding the pituitary and, in combination with physiological balance (heavily influenced by things like sleep, nutrition, exercise) they act upon the pituitary gland to initiate secretion of GH in a pulsatile manner.

Hopefully by now you're noticing a trend in how this works in terms of the HPG (Hypothalamus-Pituitary- Gonadal) axis. They also use pretty self-explanatory names for these hormones, which is nice.

Growth hormone is responsible for facilitating cellular growth, regeneration, and reproduction in humans and its effects are anabolic in nature. The bulk of your GH release occurs while you're asleep, with around half of it occurring between stages 3 and 4 NREM sleep. During the day it's been found to secrete in surges every 3 to 5 hours.

Here's a nice little sketch of the general path of action GH can take.

There are multiple ways to manipulate your GH secretion. Even just from what we've just learned we can easily see that by influencing the balance of GHRH to GHIH we'd be able to stimulate more GH secretion. Those neurosecretory hormones are also heavily influenced by the physiological downstream effects your body experiences from sleep, nutrition, and exercise – so those are some other things we'll explore.

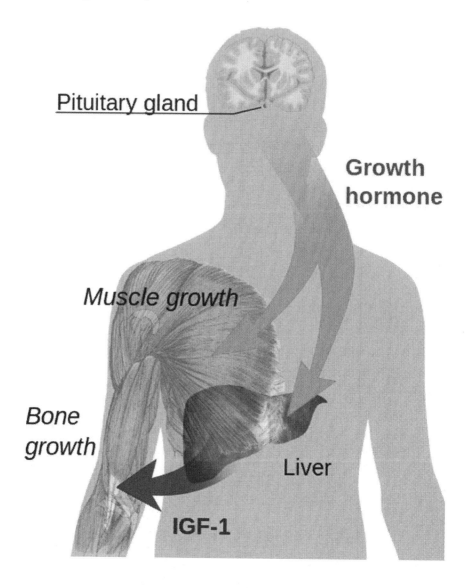

Why? Mostly because they're the easiest to control and measure.

Ghrelin is another lead. It was found to be a ligand for the growth hormone secretagogue receptor back in 2000, I believe... which in layman's terms means its presence can stimulate GH release.

A couple other natural GH release-stimulators are deep sleep, L-DOPA, fasting, and nicotinic acid (vitamin B3).

On the flip side, common GH inhibitors are 1) high circulating levels of GH itself or IGF-1 (due to the negative feedback loop), 2) glucocorticoids (ie. cortisol), and 3) DHT.

Elevated (or even just normalized) levels of GH will make it much easier for you to build muscle (via increased ability to synthesize proteins), drop fat (via promotion of lipolysis), and spare glycogen (via reduced uptake of glucose in the liver).

Chapter 9

Insulin

Insulin is a hormone secreted by the pancreas that is mainly responsible for shuttling glucose in the blood to muscles, fat, and the liver.

This glucose provides energy for these cells (or is stored as glycogen & fat).(46)

Here are more things Insulin does for us:

- Prevents hyperglycemic toxicity in neurons (which can lead to brain cognition issues) (47)
- Promotes muscle protein synthesis
- Metabolic processes (including the breakdown of fat and protein)

Knowing how important insulin is for our bodies, it's not difficult to figure out how poor insulin sensitivity can be a problem. Insulin resistance (IR) is a condition in which the body's cells become resistant to the effects of insulin.

Knowing how important insulin is for our bodies, it's not difficult to figure out how poor insulin sensitivity can be a problem.

Insulin resistance (IR) is a condition in which the body's cells become resistant to the effects of insulin. Because of this, More insulin is needed for it to have its proper effects.(48)

Some of the most notable symptoms of insulin resistance include:

- Weight gain, particularly around the middle
- Lethargy
- Fatigue and tiredness (*especially after eating a carb heavy meal*)
- Excessive Hunger
- Difficulty concentrating (*brain fog*)
- High blood pressure (due to elevated levels of circulating insulin in the blood)
- Low Testosterone Levels

If you have experienced any one or combination of the above symptoms, poor insulin sensitivity is likely the culprit.

Because of the importance of insulin in our bodies – and the adverse side effects of being insulin resistant – It is imperative that you do everything you can to make your body as insulin sensitive as possible.

When you are more insulin sensitive, you can utilize carbs better for energy, building muscle, and will help you store less fat.(49) What's more is that greater insulin sensitivity has been shown to promote higher testosterone levels in men.(50)

Luckily, there are natural ingredients that have been shown to have powerful effects for improving insulin resistance and increasing insulin sensitivity! Even better, there is a plethora of peer-reviewed scientific research backing these ingredients and their effectiveness.

Berberine and Insulin Sensitivity

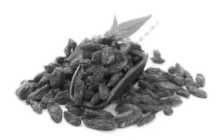

Berberine is an alkaloid extracted from various plants and has been used in Traditional Chinese Medicine for its anti-inflammatory and anti-diabetic effects.

Some other notable benefits include its ability to improve intestinal health, lower cholesterol and decrease glucose production in the liver.(51)

The science behind berberine is incredibly promising as well. **Human and animal research have shown that supplementing with berberine is equally as powerful as taking pharmaceuticals prescribed for treating type II diabetes!**

(Specifically Metformin and Glibenclamide).(51,52,53,54) In fact, berberine is one of the few supplements with human evidence that show it to be as efficient as pharmaceuticals.

Cinnamon and Insulin Sensitivity

Cinnamon is commonly used as a spice, but also for its numerous biological effects on the body. Supplementing with cinnamon has been shown to reduces the rate at which glucose enters the body, improves glucose use in the cell, reduce fasting blood glucose and potentially improve cholesterol levels.(55)

The best type of cinnamon is Ceylon, which is its original source. The reason for this is that Ceylon cinnamon has the lowest Coumarin content (Coumarin is carcinogenic in high quantities, so Ceylon is the safest form of cinnamon.(55)

Chromium and Insulin Sensitivity

Chromium is a mineral that the body uses to regulate glucose metabolism and insulin sensitivity.(56) Chromium deficiency impairs the body's ability to use glucose to meet its energy needs and raises insulin requirements. Supplemental chromium may also help to treat impaired glucose tolerance and type 2 diabetes. (57) Because of its interaction with glucose, it is recommended to use Chromium alongside a carbohydrate rich meal.

When taken in the correct dosages, these three ingredients have the potential to drastically improve your ability to utilize insulin and receive all of the amazing benefits that being more insulin sensitive provides.

Unfortunately, the majority of natural supplements for treating insulin resistance either include ingredients that are not scientifically proven to be effective or include one of these three ingredients in an inadequate dose. Neglecting these two things ultimately results in a supplement that provides little to no benefit for improving insulin sensitivity.

I've helped thousands of men naturally increase their testosterone and health over the years and have seen just how many people suffer from poor insulin sensitivity.

The number of individuals who have insulin issues is much larger than you'd think and, unfortunately, most of these people are unaware that poor insulin sensitivity is the cause of their problems.

Rather than jumping on the pharmaceutical bandwagon or taking ineffectively formulated supplements, I wanted to create something that allowed people to increase their insulin sensitivity naturally.

The Natural Solution To Insulin Resistance

Sensolin is a great supplement for naturally improving insulin resistance and boosting insulin sensitivity.

Unlike most insulin sensitivity supplements that include a laundry list of ineffective ingredients, Sensolin only includes three core ingredients.

However, these three core ingredients have been shown in multiple peer-reviewed scientific studies to be effective at improving insulin sensitivity.

What's more is that Sensolin provides all three of these core ingredients in clinically effective dosages – *so you can be rest assured you are getting the most benefit possible.*

Sensolin Ingredients:

The ingredients in Sensolin have been demonstrated in multiple peer-reviewed scientific studies to be effective at decreasing insulin resistance and improving insulin sensitivity.

Berberine HCl

Berberine is an alkaloid extracted from various plants and has been used in Traditional Chinese Medicine for centuries.

The benefits of berberine Include:

- Anti-inflammatory and anti-diabetic effects.
- Improved intestinal health
- Improved cholesterol levels
- Decreased glucose production in the liver
- Increased exercise performance
- Decreased blood pressure

The recommended dosage for berberine is 900-2,000mg with 500-1,500mg showing effectiveness in multiple human-based studies (It's also recommended you split this dosage over 2-3 servings throughout the day).

Sensolin provides 500mg per serving to be taken 2-3 times daily.

Cinnamon Ceylon Oil

Cinnamon is commonly used as a spice, but also for its numerous biological effects on the body. The best type of cinnamon is Ceylon because of its lower coumarin content.

The benefits of cinnamon include:

- Reduce the rate at which glucose enters the body
- Improved glucose usage in cells
- Lower fasting blood glucose
- Improve cholesterol levels

The recommended dose of cinnamon that provides its anti-diabetic and insulin sensitivity improving effects is 1-6g of cinnamon daily, taken with carbohydrate containing meals.

Sensolin includes 1g of Ceylon cinnamon per servings (taken 2-3 times daily).

Chromium

Chromium is an essential mineral consumed through the diet. It is found in plant products and grains.

The benefits of Chromium include:

- Regulation of glucose metabolism
- Improved insulin sensitivity
- Treat impaired glucose tolerance and type 2 diabetes.
- Reduction of appetite
- Improved symptoms of depression
- Increased Libido

The recommended dosage for chromium is 800 mcg-1,000 mcg taken in two doses daily.

Sensolin includes 300mcg of chromium per servings (taken 2-3 times daily).

When we set out to create Sensolin, we knew we wanted to create the greatest medical-alternative, natural supplement for people with poor insulin sensitivity. To achieve this goal, we knew that Sensolin had to meet the following standards:

- Include 100% natural herbs and ingredients.
- Only include natural ingredients that were backed by multiple scientific peer-reviewed studies.
- Provide these ingredients in their proven clinical effective dosages.

Sensolin meets all three of these standards and then some.

Sensolin is designed to help folks who are experiencing the unfavorable symptoms of poor insulin sensitivity. Things like low energy, lethargy, low testosterone, high blood pressure, brain fog, insatiable hunger and excess fat storage.

Using Sensolin, along with living a healthier lifestyle through proper nutrition and exercise, can help to improve insulin sensitivity and drastically increase your ability to lose fat, build muscle, stay focused, and feel full of energy.

If you are tired of dealing with the undesirable symptoms of poor insulin sensitivity, then Sensolin may be the answer you're looking for.

— Chapter 10 —

DHT (Dihydrotestosterone)

Dihydrotestosterone (DHT) optimization is a controversial topic among men. Some say that it's a "bad hormone" that causes hair loss and prostate enlargement, while others praise it for being the ultimate male hormone, since it's significantly more potent than its little brother, testosterone.

In fact, DHT has 2-3 times higher affinity to the androgen receptors and it's known to be bound and active in the receptor sites for five times longer than testosterone. (58) Dihydrotestosterone also has much higher androgenic activity than testosterone, whereas testosterone on the other hand has significantly higher anabolic (muscle building) activity than that of DHT.

While it's known that overly high DHT levels – in combination with chronically high estrogen and the male-pattern baldness gene – are associated with scalp hair loss, (59) it's also known that in men with no MPB-gene, DHT levels at the top of the reference ranges are not associated with any rate of increased hair-loss (this study of 316 men actually showed that high DHT was associated with 35% LOWER risk of developing baldness). (60)

Another claimed side-effect of high DHT hormone levels is prostate enlargement (BPH), and while some studies have linked high dihydrotestosterone levels to that condition, it must also be noted that many have not found any correlation between DHT and prostate enlargement markers (even 10-fold increases in DHT were noted to have no significant effect on prostate size in this study). (61)

Bottom line on side-effects: If you are having prostate issues and are going bald, its likely that you possess the genotype for those conditions, and that overly high DHT levels can in some (but not all) cases aggravate them. The gene explanation also makes sense, if you look at the studies which often show extreme variances between the effects of androgens on hair loss and prostate enlargement.

Take this study for example (62) where DHT was identified as a compound that had an important role in the development and progression of prostate enlargement, and compare it to this one where men rubbing 70mg/day of DHT-gel to their scrotum for 3 months showed no signs of prostate enlargement (no increases in prostate volume or PSA levels). (63)

One factor that has always confused me about these claimed side-effects is that hair-loss and prostate problems become increasingly more common as men get older, whereas androgens are known to go down as men age. If DHT is the only culprit, why don't all men in their 20's have prostate problems?

If those side-effects above are possible, why would anyone purposefully want to increase the DHT hormone?:

- *Dihydrotestosterone is necessary for the growth of body hair (64) and linear beard growth (65)*
- *Unlike testosterone, DHT cannot be converted into estrogen by the aromatase enzyme (66)*
- *Exogenous DHT administration is known for its mood, energy, and confidence boosting effects in men (67)*
- *By increasing cAMP levels in tissue, (68) dihydrotestosterone stimulates lipolysis (fat burn) and thyroid function*

- *Although DHT is not highly anabolic it still promotes muscle gains by increasing nervous system and muscle strength (69)*
- *Dihydrotestosterone and testosterone are responsible of ALL masculine body and facial characteristics (70) (wide jaw, broad shoulders...)*
- *Increased DHT levels are strongly linked to higher brain GABA-levels, (71) promoting that calm "alpha male" relaxation in any situation*
- *DHT (being the main androgen in male sexual organs) is even more potent than testosterone at promoting libido and erection quality (72)*

Condensed version? DHT makes you look, act, and feel like a damn man, even more so than testosterone.

Before we get in to ways to boost dihydrotestosterone levels, here's how the hormone is made:

1. Your body produces three different types of an enzyme called 5-alpha reductase (type I, II, and III).
2. Those enzymes then convert – varying on the type – testosterone into DHT inside the penis, testicles, skin, nervous system, and many organs such as liver, kidneys, and brain (this conversion normally occurs to 5% of the testosterone produced). (73)
3. One weaker adrenal androgen – androstenedione – can also be directly converted to DHT by 5-a enzymes, this conversion however is more notable in women than men (74) (yes women have some low amounts of DHT too).

Now that the rambles have been done, here's finally your 20 ways to boost DHT levels naturally:

1. Drop the Fat Pounds

It has already been established in this book that being fat just doesn't cut it for testosterone production (and a bunch for other good things in life).

You need to be at a reasonable point of lean to have your body pump out a good amount of testosterone on a daily basis, and also to make sure that the extra adipose tissue won't convert most of that T into estrogen by increased aromatase activity.

It has been well-documented that fat men have significantly lower testosterone levels than lean men (75, 76, 77, 78) accompanied with higher aromatase enzyme activity. (79)

Since ~5% of the testosterone you produce converts to DHT by the actions of 5-a enzyme, it would make sense to get to around 8-14% fat percentage in order to maximize that T production, which would also lead to higher turnover to DHT, since you would simply have more to convert from.

But it doesn't end there. Increased body fatness will also break DHT down to a weaker metabolite; 3α-diol, (80) which is again, why you don't want to be fat. Fatness suppresses T and DHT, and promotes estrogen production, and that's a no-no for men.

<u>Bottom line:</u> *Get to the "sweet spot" of 8-14% body fat, which maximizes testosterone production, reduces testosterone turnover to estrogen, and reduces DHT turnover to 3α-diol. Mind you I didn't even have to mention the plethora of other benefits that come when you're lean, such as: better looking body, improved insulin sensitivity, better cardiovascular health…*

2. Boost that Testosterone

Like said few times above already, ~5% of your testosterone will turn over to DHT thanks to the 5-alpha enzyme.

Therefore logically, as your testosterone production gets higher, so does your DHT production.
Good example of this are studies of men undergoing testosterone replacement therapy (TRT), these guys are administered exogenous testosterone and as a result their serum T levels as well as DHT levels increase (81, 82, 83).

Simply provide your body more of the "raw material" – which in this case is testosterone – and the 5-a enzymes will do the rest to convert a chunk of that to dihydrotestosterone. Simple. Effective.

This works with natural testosterone optimization, as well as synthetic alternatives (TRT). For the latter, a novel way to increase the turnover rate would be using the testosterone gel to the area of the scrotum (a method that's proven to increase the turn over %). (84)

NOTE: *This book you're reading is absolutely chock-full of ways to naturally increase your testosterone levels, it's a great way to start learning how from to boost testosterone naturally.*

3. Start Lifting

Weight lifting is one of the best ways to naturally stimulate hormone production.

I have written about the effects that resistance training has on testosterone levels before in detail in the THOR Program (**thorprogram.com**). This boost in testosterone alone is enough to improve DHT levels by increased turnover rate…

…But resistance exercise works also on skeletal muscle tissue to increase the basal DHT levels in rodents, (85) and tissue levels of 5-alpha reductase and DHT in humans. (86) So a mix of good things happen inside of your muscles when you lift.

All this while you're getting stronger, more ripped, and healthier. Therefore resistance training is a no-brainer and every man interested in their hormonal health should practice some regularly.

4. Sprint Fast

HIIT exercise or basically any type of exercise where you do quick explosive spurts is really good for testosterone, DHT, and growth hormone.

I have previously talked about HIIT training and its effect on testosterone levels here, (87) and as you might guess the effect is as positive as it gets. Now again as ~5% of testosterone converts to DHT, this boost in testosterone alone should positively impact dihydrotestosterone levels.

Looking specifically at studies where the researchers have examined the effect of quick bouts of exercise on DHT levels, we can see that in young men DHT goes through the roof acutely after sprinting. (88) And in another study it was noted that all anabolic/androgenic hormones skyrocket with sprints, but it has to be an all-out spurt to actually stimulate DHT production. (89)

NOTE: In THOR (**thorprogram.com**) the bulk of "cardio" is sprinting or walking, simply because they're both so good for hormonal output.

5. Intermittent Hypoxia

A few months ago when I was searching through Pubmed for nothing special, I accidentally stumbled upon some studies about training in a low-oxygen state, aka hypoxia.

Hypoxia happens when there's a deficiency of oxygen reaching the tissues of the body...

...One example of this would be training in high altitudes, where there is naturally lower amounts of oxygen in the air. Another example would be simply holding the breath for a while or breathing into a bag, both of these are good ways to enter short-term hypoxia. Then there's also those goofy "altitude masks", they probably work, but seriously who the hell wants to walk around looking like Bane in a gym?

Why hypoxia? What has this low-oxygen stuff have to do with DHT hormone?

It has been studied in animals that intermittent hypoxia (short-term low-oxygen exposure) stimulates testosterone production by upregulating cyclic adenosine monophosphate (cAMP) and testicular enzymes. (90)

It has been also shown that hypoxia activates androgen receptors in human tissue (91, 92). Lastly, low-oxygen states have been shown to increase the turnover rate from testosterone to DHT in skin and hair follicles (93) and promote growth hormone release by increasing CO_2 levels of the blood. (94)

How would one get to short-term hypoxia? *That's a good question, and honestly it's kind of hard to answer. You could do bag breathing, or go train in a mountain like many professional athletes do. Or you could do "breath-stop" sets in the gym, where you would very slowly inhale through your nose and exhale through your mouth during movements, making your body deprived of oxygen for a short duration.*

6. More Calories, More Dihydrotestosterone

Everyone knows that your body needs energy (calories) to maintain many of its functions. And over long-term if you suppress the intake of calories, your body will begin to slow down and shut some of the mechanisms not vital for survival.

One of these mechanisms that first takes a hit is the reproductive system, and with that, testosterone production and DHT production. An extreme example of this can be seen from this case study following a contest preparation for natural bodybuilding competition, (95) the ruthless low-calorie diet accompanied by huge amounts of working out resulted in near castrate level hormones.

Another study (96) – likely closer to normal conditions – had a group of men eating a calorie deficit (1350–2415 kcal/day) for 7-years and compared their hormones to men who ate at caloric maintenance/surplus (2145-3537 kcal/day).

As to be expected, the long-term restriction of calories had caused the calorie restriction groups testosterone level to be 31% lower than the normal caloric intake guys had (the researchers didn't test for DHT, but if T drops by that much its likely that DHT also took a hit). The only study I found directly examining DHT levels and caloric intake was conducted on rodents, in it the researchers found out that caloric restriction was associated with significant drops in dihydrotestosterone levels. (97)

Bottom line: *If you need to lose weight, follow this guide and go on a caloric deficit until you reach 8-14% bodyfat, (98) then return to normal maintenance calories to keep that T and DHT high. If you're already lean, then my good man, make sure that you eat enough to support your hormones.*

7. Up the Carbs

Here's some not so good news for the low-carb folk; carbohydrates are important for both healthy testosterone and healthy DHT production.

It has been shown in many studies that diets higher in carbohydrates, result in more favorable free-testosterone to cortisol (fTC) ratio, more total testosterone, and higher 5-alpha reductase activity.

For example, this study from Anderson et al. (99) found that when caloric intake and fat intake are kept identical, a diet where the carbohydrate to protein ratio was kept at 2:1 showed 36% higher free-testosterone levels along with significantly reduced cortisol, when compared to a diet where the ratio was switched to 1:2.

A study by Volek et al. saw similar results, (100) eat twice as many calories from carbs as you do from protein and you will be at a "sweet spot" to increase free testosterone and lower cortisol secretion.

This effect is even more pronounced in athletes, who will see major drops in their T-levels after lowering carb intake (101, 102).

One previously done study from Anderson et al. (103) examined the effects of carbohydrate on DHT, and found out that on a high-carb diet 5-alpha activity and dihydrotestosterone levels will be significantly higher than those seen on diets with lower amounts of carbs.

Bottom line: *A scientifically sound amount of carbs for optimal T, C, and DHT production would be to eat 2 times as many carbs as you eat protein. So 2:1 ratio, which is why you can always see me recommending ~40% calories from carbs, ~20% from protein, and ~40% from dietary fat.*

8. Protein in Moderation

I know this statement always freaks out the neurotic bodybuilders who believe that protein is the be-all end-all macronutrient, but protein really is the LEAST important of the three main macronutrients when it comes to testosterone and DHT optimization.

Sure you want to get some amounts of protein because it's vitally important for maintaining and increasing the rate of protein synthesis and muscular health, while its also known that chronic protein malnutrition leads to lowered testosterone levels and thus also lower DHT. (104) So yes do get moderate amounts of protein…

…But again, not too much. If you paid any attention to the studies in the above subheading, you can see how it's obvious from the studies of Anderson et al. (99) and Volek et al. (100) that high protein intake is able to suppress testosterone, 5-alpha enzymes, and DHT levels.

So like said above, try to aim for carb to protein ratio of 2:1 for optimal DHT production.

NOTE: *It's worth noting that soy isolate has been found to lower dihydrotestosterone production (105, 106), so if you're not a vegan/ vegetarian, consider getting the bulk of your protein from animal sources, preferably red meat.*

9. Fat is Your DHT Raising Friend

Study after study has shown that increased amount of dietary fat in the diet, results in increased testosterone – and as to be expected – higher DHT levels too (107, 108, 109, 110, 111).

This is not a surprise, since the "backbone" of every steroid hormone is a 17-carbon fat molecule called *"gonane"*.

So I should just pound all kinds of fats to naturally boost DHT then, right?

Not exactly. The types of fats that are most commonly associated with higher testosterone and dihydrotestosterone levels are the saturated fatty-acids (SFA) and monounsaturated fatty-acids (MUFA). When it comes to polyunsaturated fatty-acids (PUFA) the effect is often the complete opposite, a reduction of androgens. (112)

When it comes to DHT, there are some in-vitro studies available on the effect of different types of fats, allow me to quote my older article: (113)

It's a well known fact that PUFAs, aka. polyunsaturated fatty-acids (especially the rancid ones from processed vegetable oils) lower testosterone levels, and therefore also DHT levels. (114) PUFAs also directly inhibit the formation of 5-alpha reductase enzyme in the following inhibitory potency: Gamma-linolenic acid -> Alpha-Linolenic acid -> Linoleic-acid -> Palmitoleic-acid -> Oleic-acid -> Myristoleic-acid. (115)

Bottom line: *Since ~20% of your calories should come from protein and ~40% from carbs, the remaining ~40% shall be reserved for fats. The bulk of your fats should come from eggs, butter, animal organs, and red meat, with moderate amounts of coconut oil, olive oil, and avocados. Also for higher DHT consider minimizing the usage of all PUFAs (mostly vegetable oils), these harm your testosterone, DHT, and also thyroid. (116)*

10. The Caffeine Fix

There have been few human studies where caffeine taken before a workout has resulted in 12-21% higher testosterone levels, which is great since coffee is freaking awesome. (117)

This small increase in testosterone should alone slightly increase the turnover amount to dihydrotestosterone, but that's not all caffeine is capable of...

...In a rodent study, (118) it was noted that a single caffeine administration (undisclosed amount) was able to increase 5-alpha reductase activity by ~30% via an unknown mechanism.

Another rodent study (119) used human equivalents of 2-4mg/kg caffeine and noted up to 57% higher DHT levels.

NOTE: *One possible mechanism behind caffeine's ability to boost T, DHT and 5-alpha enzyme activity is its stimulatory effect on cyclic adenosine monophosphate (cAMP), (120) which theoretically should result in improved messaging between cells and hormones, but it could also be something else, all I know is that I'll be sure to drink my coffee.*

11. Organic Foods May Boost DHT

Organic foods might not look different, and frankly their nutrition profile isn't that much better than that of many conventional foods, but when eating organic it shouldn't be about what more you will be getting, but instead what you aren't getting.

To clarify, I'm talking about pesticides, insecticides, herbicides, and fungicides. The chemicals generously sprayed on conventional – and in some cases organic – foods.

The problem with these chemicals is that many of them have been identified as anti-androgens, aka. compounds that block androgen production and receptor activity.

Several pesticides have been found to disrupt testosterone synthesis, DHT conversion, and 5-alpha reductase enzyme activity in the body (121, 122, 123).

Bottom line: *I'm not going to be the woo'ster who fear-mongers everyone into neurotic avoidance of everything conventional, but it's a fact that many man-made chemicals used to preserve and protect foods are also endocrine disruptors.*

12. Use Sorghum Flour, Syrup, Etc

Sorghum (S.Bicolor) is a gluten-free grain native to Africa.

It's not very common in Europe and United States, but you can still find products like whole sorghum poppies, sorghum flour, and sorghum syrup from various online retailers. What I've personally tried are sorghum pancakes, popping popsorghum, and making a tincture from the grain with vodka. The ways to use this grain are endless.
Why sorghum?

This might be a long shot, since there's only one study available about the subject, but a study examining the effect of alcohol extracts of multiple grains on 5-α reductase activity, (124) found that the ethanol infused brans of rice and safflower had very high potency to inhibit 5-α reductase activity, whereas sorghum increased the activity of the 5-a enzyme by 54%.

Bottom line: *The high amounts of Gamma Linoleic Acid (GLA) in rice and safflower bran were likely the main cause behind reduced 5-alpha activity (remember that GLA is the most potent PUFA for 5-alpha inhibition). Sorghum on the other hand lacks GLA and apparently has something in it which is able to promote 5-alpha activity. Still remember that these studies were done on crude alcohol extracts of the* brans of these grains, so eating white (branless) rice probably doesn't have a similar DHT blocking effect, but safflower oil likely has.

13. Be Cautious with 5-alpha Inhibitors

This section of the chapter might be the most important for some readers. Depending on your diet and lifestyle, you could be absolutely hammering your DHT levels with natural stuff like foods, herbs, and mushrooms, as well as things like prescription drugs.

Heck, some "T-booster" supplements are actually loaded with compounds that inhibit the 5-a enzymes, so no wonder why they can raise testosterone levels if less will be converted to DHT, duh.

Below I will list you some foods, herbs, and prescription drugs that are known for their DHT blocking effect. Now I don't want you to become neurotic with avoiding all that stuff because so many natural compounds can slightly inhibit 5-α, but if your goal is to boost DHT naturally, then it may be wise not to swim in the stuff below.

Foods
- Nearly all polyunsaturated fatty-acids (PUFAs)
- Foods high in beta-sitosterol
- Foods high in lycopene
- Soy isoflavones
- Pumpkin Seeds
- Green tea
- Curcumin

Supplements
- Fenugreek
- Astaxanthin

- Reishi mushroom
- Saw Palmetto
- DIM

Drugs
- Finasteride
- Dutasteride
- Turosteride
- 4-MA
- Statins
- SSRIs

Other
- Phthlates in plastics
- Bisphenol A
- Many pesticides
- Aryl-acid dyes such as blue-25, red-11, orange-1, yellow-1, and violet-13

14. Opiates, Really?

This isn't something I necessarily recommend, but just a mere interesting fact.

As you might already know, long- and short-term use of opiate painkillers like morphine, codeine, and oxycodone have been linked to lowered testosterone levels in human males. (125)

Previously I thought that this was due to direct suppression of T production, but then *Mika from Anax* shared some studies about opiates actually increasing 5-alpha reductase and the conversion from T to DHT (126, 127).

At first this might sound like a cool idea to try, but at the same time, opiates can also increase aromatase activity, cause addiction, and mess with the gut flora.

Bottom line: *Opiates are a no-no for me but if I ever am in such excruciating pain that I need them, at least – amidst all the side-effects – I know that my DHT might go up, haha*

15. Nicotine for Extra DHT

Dihydrotestosterone is eventually metabolized down into less effective form called 3a-diol, which is then eventually followed by glucuronidation and clearance via the kidneys and urination.

As explained in the beginning of this list, this DHT breakdown is significantly increased in fat people, since the adipose tissue (fat mass) increases the rate of dihydrotestosterone reduction to 3a-diol. (128)
Aside from being lean, there's one surprising compound that can inhibit this breakdown and leave more active DHT to the body; nicotine.

It was seen in an in-vitro study that nicotine and a breakdown product of nicotine called cotine were able to suppress the enzymes that metabolize DHT into 3a-diol, (129) thus causing DHT accumulation in tissues. This might also explain why smokers are often found to have higher levels of DHT than non-smokers. (130)

Bottom line: *No, I'm not recommending anyone to start smoking cigarettes, but something like nicotine gum could be a way to increase dihydrotestosterone levels.*

94

16. Creatine

If you've been actively hitting the gym, changes are that you already use creatine.

It's somewhat of a "staple" supplement in the bodybuilding, powerlifting, etc circles due to its massive amount of scientific literature promoting creatine as a supplement that ACTUALLY works to increase strength and lean mass. (131)

More impressively, creatine has been shown to increase testosterone levels in many studies, and it does so even at rest, (131) without even needing the exercise induced T stimulation to actually be effective.

When it comes to dihydrotestosterone levels, a study of 20 college-aged rugby players (132) showed that a 7-day loading phase – followed by a 14-day maintenance supplementation – led to 56% higher DHT levels during the first seven days, and 40% elevation for the following fourteen days. NOTE: *When buying creatine, do remember that the plain and cheap basic monohydrate has been found to be just as effective as the more expensive forms of the compound.*

17. Butea Superba

Butea Superba (Red Kwao Krua) comes from Thailand and is widely used as a pro-erectile herb. It's also known for its androgenic effects in research animals and possibly also in humans.

The animal studies on Butea have shown that the herb comes with a dose-dependent reduction of testosterone, however these effects are accompanied with increased androgenic effects (higher hepatic liver enzymes, increased spleen weight), suggesting that the decrease of T might be caused by increased turnover to DHT (133, 134).

One case study (135) of a Thai male who reportedly took Red Kwao for a "few weeks" and after that complained of a side-effect; too high sex drive, was noted of having unnaturally high DHT levels of 1512 pg/mL (reference ranges being 250-990 pg/mL).

The medical professionals eventually tracked this down to the Butea Superba supplement and recommended him to stop supplementation immediately. The study reports that 1-week after the cessation of B. Superba the subjects DHT levels – as well as his libido – had returned to normal.

The effects of the above study might be caused by illegal "spiking" of the supplement with some steroids (after all this was in Thailand), but then again there was this comment on the blog some time ago:

M · 10 months ago

Don't know if anyone will see this but hey why not.

Me: 28, male, military, cannot implement many natural testosterone methods due to my job. On TRT, pellet therapy, puts my total T about 1100. Been on for a year feel great. Through your blog started reading about DHT, ran across this article and got interested. Got tested. DHT was low despite zinc and other mineral supplementation. Test scale was 16-79, mine was at 16. Changed nothing, started taking 2gm of Butea Superba a day, 1gm morning 1gm night for one month. Got tested, DHT was at 65. All in all id say thats scientific enough finding that this is a supplement that actually does something.

2 ^ ⌄ · Reply · Share ›

18. Phosphatidylserine

Phosphatidylserine (PS) is a phospholipid, a naturally occurring serine present in almost all of the cells of our bodies. Its main function is to deliver bodily signals between cells and hormones, but it can also reduce oxidative stress,improve the testosterone to cortisol ratio, promote DHT turnover, and even improve cognitive functions.

Due to many studies linking PS with improved brain processing abilities (136, 137, 138), the compound has received a qualified health claim from the FDA stating: *"consumption of phosphatidylserine may reduce the risk of dementia and cognitive dysfunction in the elderly"*

When it comes to hormones and performance, a few studies have shown that PS supplementation can reduce exercise induced oxidative stress in the body (139, 140, 141) and even increase testosterone levels while simultaneously suppressing cortisol during exercise, therefore increasing the T:C ratio by up to 180% (142, 143).

What about DHT you ask? Well, there's some evidence that in test-tubes, PS can increase 5-alpha activity by up to 2.5 fold (144, 145).

19. Forskolin

Forskolin (Coleus Forskohlii extract) is often hyped up as a fat burner in the Dr. Oz show. Unfortunately this only makes the herb seem like a steaming pile of bullshit, since you know, Oz is one hell of a woo-peddler.

Anyway, don't throw your axe to the well just yet. Scientists actually use forskolin as a positive control for testosterone inside test-tubes, due to its well-known stimulatory effect on cyclic adenosine monophosphate (cAMP). In fact, up to 200% increases in testosterone have been seen in test-tubes with forskolin, (146) and increases of 33% in a human study. (147)

As you might remember from the coffee-subheading above increased cAMP has been theorized to be the reason why caffeine increases 5-

alpha levels, and since forskolin is much more potent at boosting cAMP, (148) one could easily think that its also potent at increasing DHT.

Bottom line: *Some in-vitro research suggests that when cells are incubated with forskolin, 5-a activity increases, (149) but so far there's no in-vivo human studies showing what happens to DHT when human subjects consume oral forskolin supplements. At this point I would say that it's plausible that forskolin could be a potent DHT booster.*

20. Boron

When talking about vitamins and minerals most people are sure to mention magnesium, zinc, vitamin D, calcium… But what about boron? A trace mineral with not that big of a popularity, but perhaps the most impressive results in terms of testosterone and DHT in scientific studies.

Yes that's right, a dirt-poor trace mineral has been shown to induce some significant improvements in your androgens. A study from Naghii et al. (150) showed that 10mg/day of boron for a week, was able to increase free testosterone levels by 28%, reduce estrogen levels by 39% and boost DHT by 10%.

Another study from Mjilkovich et al. (151) showed similar results with 12mg/day boron for 2-months, free-T increased by 29% and the adrenal androgen DHEA shot up by 56%, unfortunately DHT or 5-alpha levels weren't examined in this study.

Bottom line: *Boron is relatively cheap and if it works as well as in the studies above, then why not.*

— Chapter 11 —

How To Lower Estrogen Naturally

The female hormone estrogen is a nasty one, as it's also present in men. That's right, us men are filled with female hormones!

Tiny amounts of estrogen are actually needed in the male body. However in this modern society we are exposed to thousands of chemicals and other estrogenic compounds that act as endocrine disruptors in the male body, effectively boosting female hormone levels way above the levels that are "normal" in males.

I'd say that 99.5% of the male population has too much estrogen in their system, and I'm not even joking here. That's how bad the situation is nowadays as everything is filled with estrogenic compounds from our foods to our personal care items all the way up to the receipts we get from the grocery stores.

That's the truth, and it's a scientifically proven fact. Estrogen is everywhere.

So why is estrogen so harmful to men? And why would you need to lower estrogen levels in the first place?

That's a good question and every man should be aware of the answer: Estrogen and estrogen mimics are notorious for their ability to completely crush male testosterone levels.

You see, estrogen and testosterone are constantly battling for the same androgen receptors.

If you're having overblown estrogen levels, which is also called with a fancy name: "male estrogen imbalance", you're missing those receptor spots to the female hormone.

And when that happens, you're hormonally screwed.

And that's not even all there is to overblown male estrogen imbalance because there's this enzyme called *aromatase* which will convert your testosterone straight into estrogen.

So essentially when we're boosting testosterone we need to make sure to lower estrogen levels as low as possible, and also make sure that our aromatase enzyme will be as low as possible. Because high testosterone combine with high aromatase enzyme means that your beloved male hormones will be effectively converted into estrogen, and that's really really bad for us guys.

The good news are that it's pretty easy to lower estrogen levels naturally, and if you're doing it successfully, then your testosterone levels are bound to increase significantly, so obviously you as a man do need to decrease your male estrogen levels.

So how on earth can a man lower estrogen naturally?

And how can we keep aromatase enzyme at bay?

You'll find that out soon as here comes the list of 20 ways to naturally decrease estrogen levels in the male body:

1. Get Rid Of That Spare Tire

Estrogen molecules practically live inside your *fat cells* and it's a scientific fact that the more fat a man has, the more estrogen he's bound to carry.

Another scientific fact is that the more fat a man carries, the lower his testosterone levels are. See a link here or what?

First, to lower estrogen naturally and begin the removal process, you should start with weight loss. Or not necessarily even weight loss, but more specifically fat loss.

It doesn't matter if you're not that heavy, as it's the fat that you need to get rid of, not the weight. So you could be *"skinny fat"* and still have the estrogen profile of a woman.

So start melting that fat away. The more you do it, the more your estrogen will decrease.

2. Eat Some Cruciferous Vegetables

Cruciferous Vegetables like broccoli, kale, brussel sprouts, cauliflower, maca, and so on are filled with some very favorable compounds to decrease your estrogen levels.

1. They're rich in zinc which is a mineral known to boost testosterone. Zinc also stops the aromatase enzyme from doing its damage on your testosterone levels, so that your T doesn't convert so easily to estrogen anymore.
2. They're rich in a compound called Indole-3-Carbinol (I3C) which converts into 3,3-Diindolylmethane (DIM) in your

stomach. DIM is known best for its ability to regulate estrogen, which means that it effectively flushes out estrogenic compounds and xeno-estrogens from your body.

Many people like to eat their cruciferous vegetables steamed. However, I believe that when you expose those veggies to too much heat, they'll lose some of the beneficial nutrients.

That's why I usually eat them plain or frozen with a garlic dip. After all, you should do what suits you the best, just make sure that you eat these!

3. Avoid Exposure to Unnecessary Chemicals

In the modern world, we're constantly bombarded with chemicals. They're in our faces 24/7 and it's a cold hard fact that we can't completely avoid them no matter how hard we try to.

Fortunately, this doesn't mean that we can't do anything, as we still can avoid them as much as possible, and we also can avoid the worst kinds of them, and I'll be going into more detail with the worst ones as we move further with this list.

As a rule of thumb, you should avoid all the possible chemicals you can because almost all of them are known to disrupt our extremely sensitive endocrine system. Bunches of those chemicals are also straight on estrogen mimics in the body.

Interesting fact: The US database has over 50,000,000 chemicals listed in it, which makes it completely impossible to make sure that they're safe to consume in any way, shape, or form.

4. Don't use Plastic Products

It's believed that the increased plastic usage is the leading cause of the feminine outlook of young men in this modern era.

This is caused by the incredibly strong estrogenic effect that plastics have on the male body, as they're filled with Phthalates, compounds that make all plastics flexible.

Phthalates are known to mimic estrogen inside the male body, and that's why it's only a sign of weakness if you're still after reading this post using plastic water bottles or eating those plastic micro-ready disasters.

The easiest way to get your body <u>filled with phthalates and xenoestrogens</u> is to drink a lot of soda.

Here's why:

When a plastic bottle is made it would take a full year for it to "cool down" so it wouldn't leak those estrogen mimics into its contents any more.

However when those big soda companies manufacture thousands upon thousands of those bottles a day, do they really wait for a full year before filling them?

Hell no! What a waste of money would that be right?
Instead, those bottles are instantly filled with acidic soda that furthermore dissolves those fresh phthalates into your "refreshing" beverage.

Remember that when you're gulping down on that Coca-cola next time.

5. Avoid Parabens

Parabens are the chemicals used in almost all of our personal care items. They're also strong estrogen mimics in the male body and if you're serious about decreasing estrogen levels naturally, then you have to eliminate these endocrine disrupting chemicals.

The easiest way to eliminate parabens is to switch to natural personal care items.

If you want to see those parabens for yourself then take a look at the ingredient labels on your personal care items and look for the following chemicals:

- Butylparaben
- Ethylparaben
- Heptylparaben
- Methylparaben
- Propylparaben

6. Start Eating Organic foods

Commercial foods found in your favorite grocery store are mostly shit. That's the reality. As they're over processed microwaveable wonders with no nutrients and a huge list of unnecessary chemicals, endocrine disruptors, estrogen mimics, and low-quality ingredients.

There's no real reason to eat these foods as there are organic options available, which are free from those harmful estrogenic chemicals.

Organics may cost a bit more, but they'll pay themselves back in increased lifespan and a much healthier life, along with a much better hormonal profile, and I'd dare to say that they'll also improve your sex life.

More testosterone with lower estrogen = Much better sexual performance, stamina, erections, and pleasure.

So start eating organic and watch your body heal itself as food really is medicine, and by this, I mean <u>real organic foods and herbs</u>.

7. Avoid Bisphenol-A

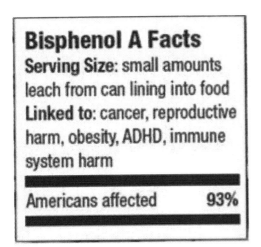

Bisphenol A Facts
Serving Size: small amounts leach from can lining into food
Linked to: cancer, reproductive harm, obesity, ADHD, immune system harm

Americans affected   **93%**

Bisphenol-A or BPA is a chemical compound found in the linings of our canned goods, it's also in the ink in our newspaper, the ink that's in your grocery store receipt, and in a bunch of other places like multiple varieties of plastics for example...

The reason why this chemical is so bad is the fact that in animal studies it's capable of transforming males into females. Yes, this is no bullshit. BPA is so highly estrogenic that it can change the sex in some animals, think it was frogs that they studied if I recall correctly.

Feminizing effects of BPA have also been noted in human males, and that has drawn researchers to believe that BPA is also one of the leading causes behind the increased feminine features of modern day males.

The last research study reported that 93% of the Americans have way too much BPA in their system, so don't think that you're safe from it mate.

You can read more about chemicals and BPA on my post called chemicals and testosterone levels.

8. Consume some Calcium-D-Glucarate

Calcium-D-Glucarate is a fiber present in the skin of many berries. Juniper and blueberry, for example, are very rich sources of Calcium-D-Glucarate.

This fiber effectively binds into the "bad estrogen molecules" in your gut, and this will help your body to remove those xeno-estrogens via your intestines.

To get adequate amounts of this male estrogen lowering fiber you can either supplement with it or eat a bunch of berries.

I'd suggest the latter but both of them are valid options.

9. Consume a Methylator

This is a bit tricky to explain but what the heck I'll try:

Your estrogen molecules are all missing one methyl group, once you consume something that acts as a methylator, you'll "complete" the molecule and it can then be "chelated" by your body.

The chelation process basically means that it's being flushed out from your body, so in a way you're flushing out estrogen by eating something that acts as a methylator. Therefore you're also lowering male estrogen levels naturally.

So what's the best methylator?

Choline and Betaine and the best ones, and beets are ridiculously high in betaine. Beets also boost nitric oxide. So eat tons of beets. Both choline and betaine are available on the Anabolic Men Marketplace at store.anabolicmen.com

10. Skip those Processed Meats

I have 2 rules regarding meats:

1. Meats are great for your testosterone.
2. Meats are bad for your testosterone.

Don't lynch me just yet, I'll tell you what I mean by that:

Meats are great for your testosterone if they're grass-fed, organic, and filled with natural cholesterol and saturated fat with some nice amino acids.

Meats can also be bad if they're un-organic, processed, and factory farmed.

Those meats are filled with trace estrogen and synthetic hormones, along with some trace antibiotics and other medications.

You can thank the greedy "power farmers" and big ass companies for that. As those pigs for example, are fed with antibiotics for their whole life so that they don't get infections.

They're also injecting synthetic estrogen to those pigs to make them gain fat mass super fast. Those animals are also injected with growth hormone so they can pack on some muscle.

The downside is that all of those trace hormones and antibiotics are present in the final product: processed meat.

When you're eating that meat guess where the trace hormones and antibiotics end up to? Inside of you, that's right.

11. Eat some Citrus Fruits

Citrus fruits like lemons, grapes, limes, and oranges are known to be anti-estrogenic. They're also scientifically proven to lower estrogen in males.

So one super simple and easy way to lower estrogen levels naturally is to just consume those damn citrus fruits. That's it. Almost too easy.

12. Improve your Gastrointestinal Health

Your gut flora has to be in peak condition so it can move those estrogen molecules away from your body faster. If your gut health is not in check (which is very uncommon these days), your estrogen molecules that would normally be exiting your body, will get reabsorbed in the intestines because they're moving too slowly.

So make sure that you're eating those healthy live bacteria and stuff like that, but don't fall victim on those "lactic acid pills", as the bacteria in those is already been dead for too long and it doesn't do shit in your body anymore.

Instead try this trick to improve your gastrointestinal health, (152) which significantly helps you to decrease those male estrogen levels.

13. Supplement with Wild Nettle Roots

Wild nettle roots are great because they're known for their ability to decrease your male estrogen levels quite well.

However, that's not all there's to nettle roots as they're also able to significantly decrease SHBG (Sex Hormone Binding Globulin) count in the male body.

SHBG is a protein that binds to your free testosterone molecules and makes it "unavailable" to be used by your body. So basically it's not able to enter androgen receptors after it's bound to SHBG.
So to lower estrogen naturally and lower SHBG, supplement with wild nettle roots.

Nettle roots are also able to stop the conversion of testosterone to estrogen, by stopping aromatase enzyme from working.

This furthermore improves the condition called male estrogen imbalance.

You can read more about free testosterone and SHBG in other chapters of this book.

14. Consume Some Maca Root

Maca is a great herb that is commonly used for boosting male libido… (not necessarily T levels).

However it's also very good at removing estrogen levels from the body, as it's a cruciferous vegetable and extremely high in DIM.

Maca is also known for its ability to significantly improve sperm count and testicular health, also it's incredibly high in nutrient density.

I highly suggest that you start supplementing with Maca as soon as possible.

15. Avoid the use of Soy Products

Soy is extremely powerful phyto-estrogen or plant-estrogen.

Which means that it's filled with estrogenic activity and it increases estrogen levels in the male body, and that's not a good thing at all…

I remember when I was having a vacation in Thailand couple years ago, that I always felt super amazing in the morning when I woke up, and me and my girlfriend were really eager to take those long tuk-tuk rides into some bigger cities and do bunch of cool stuff.

However always after I had a meal there, I suddenly started to feel like crap, and I just was like *"Fuck it, let's not do anything"*.

I first though that it was the carbohydrates that were always present in the form of rice (which came in every meal), but then it hit me.

Everything was laden with soybean oil and soy sauces and shit like that. So I was cramming some serious loads of estrogen into my body.

Boy I'm glad that I figured it out, because after that I started to avoid most of that soy, and my energy levels and overall being improved 110%.

So no matter what the vegetarians are trying to prove, soy is, and will always be estrogenic. And it just downright isn't good for males.

16. Don't Binge Drink

Excessive alcohol consumption has been shown to significantly decrease your testosterone levels, while simultaneously it will be skyrocketing your estrogen.

This happens for a bunch of reasons, but the main reasons are these two:

1. Your liver is too busy filtering that excess alcohol, so it has no time to regulate your estrogen.
2. Alcohol is notorious for boosting the activity of aromatase enzyme, which converts testosterone into estrogen.

That's why alcoholism is a sure way to get yourself a nice condition called: male hormone imbalance.

17. If you Drink Make sure it's not Beer

Beer might be the ultimate man drink and I do have to admit that I'm constantly breaking this rule myself.

However the fact is that beer is extremely estrogenic. The hops in it can contain up to 300,000 IU's of phytoestrogens per 100 grams and that's a lot.

I can't remember the source but I recall reading an article about the history of beer, and in it the author stated that beers masculinity link dates back hundreds of years. As it was originally a blend of herbs that made men aggressive and virile lovers.

However in the dark ages the church didn't like the idea of virility and aggressiveness, so they ordered a law that forced breweries to add certain amount of estrogenic hops into this masculine beverage, so that men would finally calm down and behave.

I can't say for sure that this story is true, because I can't recall the source, so can't check it out. However it makes a lot of sense.

18. Get yourself a Faucet Filter

Tap water is often said to be extremely clean.

However that's not the case at all, as they have found traces of numerous chemicals in the US tap water recently.

Some of these include: estrogen from the birth control pills, rocket fuel traces (what the fuck), bromide, fluoride, chlorine, BPA, pthalates, and a whole bunch of other nasty chemicals.

So obviously those chemicals will interfere with your sensitive endocrine system, and that will cause: hormonal imbalance, male estrogen imbalance, low testosterone, and several other conditions.

So a super easy and a pretty cheap way to avoid those nasty conditions, is to get yourself a solid faucet filter.

19. Strength Training

Strength training with big ass weights is awesome and in my opinion it's one of the manliest forms of exercise you can do.

The best part is that resistance training has been scientifically proven to: decrease male estrogen levels, increase male testosterone levels, and increase human growth hormone levels.

That's awesome. So stop making excuses and get yourself a gym card. If you're seriously afraid of going into a gym, then build yourself a cheap home gym with these tips.

Then when you're got that done: Lift big weights with incredible intensity and your body will thank you in numerous ways.

20. Maximize Your Sleep Quality

Sleeping is the best thing that you can do for your hormones because it's the time when your endocrine system really kicks in and recharges itself.

That's also when your body regulates estrogen and flushes it out of your body. This activity will be extremely high in the REM-stages of your sleep, and that's why it's crucial to maximize the quality of your sleep.

Good sleep also boosts your testosterone and growth hormone levels, and it's also pretty enjoyable thing to do. So sleep much and focus on improving the quality of it.

Conclusion

There you have it. A nice 20 trick list of ways to lower estrogen levels naturally. So you don't have to suffer those nasty conditions like male hormone imbalance, male estrogen imbalance, overblown female hormone levels in the male body, or low T.

I seriously hope that this list helps you to take action and really do this stuff. You don't have to complete all of these 20 tasks today, but make sure that you're doing something, as for men it's hugely beneficial to decrease estrogen levels.

And if anyone you know is suffering from high estrogen and asking you some questions like: "How to lower male estrogen levels naturally?" or "What the fuck is going on with my body? I'm growing tits!" Then send them this book, and we'll help those poor guys with some knowledge.

How To Avoid Excess Estrogen Production

Although the term aromatization sounds like it has something to do with the way you smell different stimuli, it actually is much more important to your body than that... especially if you're dealing with excess estrogen.

What is Aromatization?

Aromatization is the process that converts testosterone into estrogen. (153) This is a natural process your body goes through to maintain homeostasis.

The reason that this process is called aromatization is because aromatization is named after the chief enzyme involved in the conversion – aromatase.

While aromatization mostly occurs in the male body, it also occurs naturally in the female body as well (153) if testosterone levels become out of balance.

Why Does Aromatization Occur?

Aromatization occurs when the body is attempting to maintain homeostasis. Homeostasis is a function that keeps the body at normal levels required to stay healthy.

Homeostasis keeps the body in the average ranges for temperature, hormones, mass, and many other factors. (153) This of course includes the all-important testosterone to estrogen ratio you hear so much about on AnabolicMen.com.

The male body only produces about 7mg of testosterone a day naturally. This small amount of testosterone will naturally come along with a small amount of estrogen production to maintain the optimal testosterone to estrogen ratio.

Aromatization mostly occurs when a large fluctuation of testosterone production occurs, such as when anabolic steroids are injected.

The large amount of testosterone will be seen as an excess by the human body and aromatization will occur in an attempt to balance the new testosterone with a higher amount of estrogen. (153)

When Does Aromatization Occur?

Aromatization can occur for two reasons, both caused by a bodily reaction to maintain homeostasis.

1 – For Natural Causes

If you naturally increase your testosterone production, aromatization will still occur, but at a rate that your body can handle. Natural testosterone production increases occur in a growth, not an all-at-once spike. Because of this, aromatization due to natural testosterone optimization can actually come along with some healthy side effects.

When combined with testosterone, estrogen can actually increase muscle mass and regulate libido.

2 – Anabolic Steroids

Anabolic steroids, in contrast with natural production, will increase your testosterone all at one time. In many cases, testosterone injections can be 100mg at one time which, compared to the 7mg of average natural production is a sharp jump. The aromatization caused by testosterone injections will increase estrogen levels at a higher and less comfortable rate, which could result in some of the negative effects of estrogen spikes. These negative effects include gynecomastia (man boobs) and increased fat around the waist.

The amount of estrogen produced during aromatization will differ between men. Some men will actually have more estrogen produced than is natural due to a testosterone injection and some men will have a more desired increase in the testosterone to estrogen gap.

It all comes down to how much aromatase is present in your body.

What is Aromatase?

Aromatase is a naturally occurring enzyme located in multiple tissues in the body like the brain, muscles, and testicles. In women it is also located in the ovaries, placenta, and lining of the uterus.

Aromatase is the enzyme responsible for converting testosterone into estrogen.

It has also been found to control active amounts of cortisol the body uses to regulate the immune system.

Basically the higher amount of aromatase circulating in the body, the more testosterone will be converted into estrogen during a testosterone spike.

What Causes an Increase in Aromatase?

You will see that an increase in aromatase activity occurs for the same reasons that testosterone levels decrease. For example, aromatase activity increases with age, in line with the testosterone decrease along with age. (154)

Aromatase has also been found to increase with the amount of fatty tissue present. Poor nutrition and weight gain are a common cause of increased aromatase activity.

High stress and lack of exercise also cause increases in aromatase. If you suffer from Metabolic Hypothyroidism, it is probable that you also have a high amount of active aromatase.

A scary finding is that aromatase has been connected to the development of chronic diseases like cancer (154) and autoimmunity.

Many scientists believe that the increase in weight gain and therefore increase in aromatase across the globe has caused the increase in cancer being experienced.

How to Inhibit Aromatase & Naturally Decrease Excess Estrogen

Other than making you a generally healthier person, inhibiting aromatase production will also clearly increase your testosterone levels because less testosterone will be converted into estrogen.

If you look up inhibiting aromatase you will be flooded with results of synthetic aromatase inhibitors, but there are actually several foods that decrease aromatase production naturally.

This study (155) shows that natural aromatase inhibitors are so effective that they can actually prevent breast cancer.

Here are seven foods that can help inhibit aromatase production (156) that every man (and woman) should add to their diets:

Celery - This study (157) shows that the high Luteolin content found in celery is effective in decreasing active aromatase in the body. Not only that, but simply the smell of celery has been found to increase testosterone production in the testes.

Red Wine - This study (158) found that the phytochemicals found in red wine are able to inhibit aromatase production in a dose dependent manner. Watch out though, because too much alcohol can reduce testosterone production, so stick to one or two glasses.

Olive Oil - Olive oil contains a compound called Oleuropen, which gives olive oil very powerful aromatase-inhibiting functionalities.

White Button Mushrooms - This study (159) showed that white button mushroom extract decreases aromatase activity in a dose dependent manner.

Oysters - Oysters are beneficial and healthy for many reasons, but one of those reasons is that oysters are very high in zinc. Zinc is one of the most powerful naturally-occurring aromatase enzyme inhibitors. Load up on those oysters.

Cruciferous Vegetables - By cruciferous vegetables, I am talking about broccoli, cauliflower, maca, kale and Brussel sprouts.

Cruciferous vegetables are high in the compound 3,3'-Diindolylmethane (DIM), which has been found to lower aromatase activity.

Parsley - Parsley is high in apigening. Apigening has been found to be a powerful aromatase inhibitor. Another plus, parsley also increases testosterone production in the leydig cells.

Conclusion

Aromatization can seem like a confusing process at first, but I will try to wrap it up into one small paragraph of conclusion.

Aromatization is the process that turns testosterone into estrogen in an attempt to maintain testosterone to estrogen balance in the body. When testosterone is increased naturally, the estrogen created is not detrimental to the male body.

When testosterone is injected, estrogenic problems may arise. Whether or not estrogen will increase drastically with testosterone is based on how much aromatase is in the body.

Aromatase is a nasty enzyme that anyone would benefit from lowering.

Aromatase can be inhibited synthetically or naturally (recommended) by eating several foods like celery, red wine, olive oil, white button mushrooms, oysters, cruciferous vegetables, and parsley.

Decrease aromatase to make yourself and all-around healthier person and decrease cancer risk.

5 Powerful Supplements That Lower Estrogen Fast

In this final section of this chapter on estrogen, I break down the 5 estrogen supplements that are proven to help lower high estrogen levels.

Now, there are many reasons why high estrogen levels are no good for men. Sure you need some for bone & joint health, and brain function, but most men these days have their levels completely overblown due to high exposure to xenoestrogenic chemicals, storing too much fat in their bodies, and consuming a diet that is not hormonally beneficial in any way shape or form.

In men, 95% of the time elevated estrogen levels are due to having too high level of aromatase enzyme activity. That is, an enzyme directly converting testosterone molecules into estrogen.

High estrogen on the other hand has been found to suppress testosterone production by inhibiting the luteinizing hormone release from the pituitary gland. (160)

This vicious cycle eventually causes very low levels of testosterone, with overblown estrogen – and thus – the testosterone to estrogen ratio shifts far too much to the right, resulting in:

- Feminization of the physique and face.
- Retaining of subcutaneous water under the skin.
- Weakened libido and dramatically increased emotionality.

- In the worst case scenario; development of man-boobs, prostate issues, and hot flashes.

This list consists of five scientifically proven supplements that work by either inhibiting the aromatase enzyme or by down regulating the activity of estrogen towards its receptors.

NOTE: Do remember, that outside of using estrogen supplements, the hands-down the best way to lower high estrogen levels is to get lean, eat real food, and avoid exposure to man-made estrogen-mimic chemicals.

The 5 Natural Estrogen Supplements to Lower High Estrogen Levels

1. Zinc

Zinc is one of the 24 essential micronutrients necessary for human survival.

It's known to regulate hundreds of bodily enzymes, as well as being absolutely necessary for the proper functioning of the immune system.

Some of the scientifically proven benefits of zinc supplementation include (seen up to the point where bodily zinc levels are saturated):

- reduced activity of estrogen receptors and inhibition of aromatase enzyme. (161)
- *Increased thyroid hormone production (162) and lower levels of SHBG. (163)*

- *Increased levels of DHT, (164) total, and -free testosterone. (165)*

For best results consume 15-30mg's of high-quality zinc supplement or have large amounts of some good meat in your diet, best if you do both.

2. Boron

Boron is a mineral and estrogen supplement that can pack an estrogen-lowering punch.

Although it's a trace mineral, and not considered absolutely essential to human survival, it still has some interesting benefits for us.

Study from *Naghii et al.* (166) for example showed the following results after men consumed 10mg's of boron for a week:

- Free-testosterone levels increased by 28%.
- Free-estrogen levels had decreased by -39%.
- Dihydrotestosterone (DHT) levels rose by 10%.
- Inflammation biomarkers (hsCRP, TNF-α) dropped significantly.

Another study saw that 6mg's/day of boron for 2 months can increase testosterone levels by 29% as well as improve serum vitamin D by increased absorption of the vitamin.

NOTE: For best results consume 6-10mg's of high-absorption boron glycinate or eat plenty of raisins.

3. Grape Seed Extract

Grape seeds are high in a valuable compound called procyanidin, this phenol is mostly hailed due to its ability to naturally increase nitric oxide levels (and therefore improve circulation).

One of the lesser-known benefits of grape seed extract is its ability as a natural estrogen supplement to reduce estrogen levels by inhibiting the activity of aromatase enzyme.

Researchers studying ways to prevent and cure breast cancer have identified grape seed extract as a natural compound that blocks estrogen biosynthesis by inactivating the aromatase enzyme (167, 168, 169).

Due to grape seed extract having low bio-availability in the human body, high doses (up to 2000mg/day) of the extract are needed to see these positive effects in studies. This would translate to about a gallon of grape juice or five pills of high-potency grape seed extract supplement.

To counteract the low absorption rate of GSE, take it in fasted-state; one study saw that this improved the bio-availability by up to 5x! (170)

4. Resveratrol

Resveratrol is the antioxidant polyphenol found in red grapes. It's one of the main reasons why red wine is considered healthy. It is also a great estrogen blocker supplement.

Many studies have shown that resveratrol can increase testosterone levels and suppress estrogen by inhibiting the aromatase enzyme in test-tubes (171, 172, 173).

The problem with resveratrol however is that it doesn't seem to work as well in living organisms, ie. when people take it orally. This is due to low bio-availability.

The only two types of resveratrol I've seen to actually work and be properly absorbed in studies are the conjugated form of resveratrol, (174) and this patented resveratrol delivery system called VESIsorb® (absorption rate 100x that of pure resveratrol powder). (175)

5. Tongkat Ali

Tongkat Ali (Eurycoma Longifolia, Pasak Bumi) comes from Malaysia, it has huge popularity as a pro-erectile testosterone booster due to multiple studies supporting its effect at increasing testosterone levels and suppressing the stress hormone cortisol. (176)

There seem to be many claimed mechanisms of action in which Tongkat Ali works, but three of the scientifically proven ones include; stimulation of testicular CYP17-enzymes, suppression of SHBG, and inhibition of aromatase enzyme.

The inhibition of aromatase enzyme has actually been shown in only one rodent study so far, (177) but the results were staggering…

…Injected Tongkat Ali blocked estrogen with comparable potency to Tamoxifen, which is a synthetic – and extremely powerful – prescription aromatase inhibitor.

Conclusion on Estrogen Supplements

If your estradiol is high, and you're looking for ways to suppress it back to a more natural level, consider losing weight, cutting out man-made xenoestrogens from your life, and stacking together the following anti estrogen supplements:

1. Zinc Picolinate
2. Boron Glycinate
3. High Potency GSE
4. VESIsorb® Resveratrol
5. Tongkat Ali Extract

All of these supplements are now available on the Anabolic Men Marketplace at **store.anabolicmen.com.**

— Chapter 12 —

How To Lower Prolactin Naturally

Prolactin is a hormone that triggers the milk production in pregnant women, but believe it or not, most guys have high prolactin levels too. In this chapter I'm going to teach you how to lower prolactin levels naturally.

By now you might already guess what a hormone that induces breast milk production in women does to men?

Answer: High prolactin levels will lower libido and testosterone levels. (178) Prolactin is also highly linked to gynecomastia (man breasts). (179)

I'm personally not even sure what my prolactin levels are currently, but one thing is for certain: I'm actively making sure that I do things to reduce prolactin levels naturally, no matter what the levels might be.

Why should you learn how to lower prolactin levels?

Because I believe that no man should have high levels of a hormone that's notorious for triggering breast milk production and causing low T along with diminished libido in their body.

So that's why today, we're talking about how to lower prolactin levels and get rid of it:

Supplement with Ashwagandha

Ashwagandha is a herb that's mostly used as an "adaptogen" meaning that it lowers stress levels.

But that's not all there is to Ashwagandha for sure…

…This human study (180) found out that 5 grams of Ashwagandha for 3 months increased testosterone levels by 40% in healthy male participants.

Furthermore the same human study (180) also found out that Ashwagandha lowered prolactin levels by a nice 15%.

I personally like experiment with different Ashwagandha tinctures and dry roots from time to time, but if you wan't to leave the guessing work out of your supplementation try KSM-66 ashwagandha, it's a scientifically proven water extract with high potency.

NOTE: a decrease of 15% is a modest reduction, but when accompanied with the 40% increase in T along with the fact that Ashwagandha is extremely nutritious "superfood". It becomes quite obvious that this herb is totally worth supplementing with.

Consume More Vitamin E

Vitamin E is greatly linked to increased sperm production, and there's also some inconclusive evidence that it may boost testosterone levels…

Vitamin E has also many other benefits, such as the fact that it's a powerful antioxidant in the body... And in this study, (181) 300 mg's of vitamin E for 8 weeks, decreased prolactin levels by a staggering 69% when compared to placebo in healthy human subjects.

That's a massive decrease. One that is hard to obtain with strong medications for such purposes.

The best way to get natural vitamin E trough supplementation is without a doubt a combination of natural tocopherols.

NOTE: Never ever get synthetic vitamin E, it's derived from petrochemicals. Also never get "natural" vitamin E that's derived from soy products.

Get Your Dopamine Levels Up

High dopamine levels are extremely beneficial for men. Firstly, it stimulates testosterone production...(182)

Secondly it stimulates growth hormone secretion... (183)

And thirdly if you have high dopamine levels you're most likely having low prolactin levels. (184)

So without a doubt, dopamine is something that you might want to increase if you're a male. Here's few ways to do that. (185)

NOTE: Recent studies have shown that after a guy has an orgasm, prolactin levels will skyrocket and dopamine levels will plummet. This greatly increases the refractory period between ejaculations, and makes you want to go to sleep.

However, if a guy has high dopamine along with low prolactin, then the reduction in dopamine is far less significant, and the time between "mating sessions" is decreased. (this is a fancy way to say that low prolactin levels increase your sexual powers).

Supplement with Vitamin B6

Vitamin B6 is essential part of the B vitamin complex.

It has multiple functions in the human body, the best one probably being the fact that it's essential for testosterone production.

However B6 is not only beneficial for testosterone...

...This study (186) found out that a single dose of 300 mg's vitamin B6 increased serum growth hormone levels significantly while also causing a sharp decline in prolactin levels in human subjects.

Supplement with Mucuna Pruriens

Macuna is one of my all time favorite testosterone boosters, mainly because it has human studies (187) that prove its effects...

...However that's not the only benefit. Mucuna Pruriens also decreased prolactin levels by a very nice 33% in this study. (188)

It's not for certain what causes this decrease in the first place, but most likely it's caused the fact that Mucuna Pruriens is filled with L-Dopa.

And L-Dopa is a precursor of dopamine (as explained above, high dopamine inhibits prolactin).

Mucuna Pruriens would probably be my number #1 choice for lowering prolactin, mainly because it's so beneficial in other areas too.

Sleep Like a Pro

Sleeping well will without a doubt decrease your prolactin levels naturally.

There's multiple reasons for that, as sleeping more and with better quality is beneficial in many areas that correlate with lowered prolactin.

Such as: it increases testosterone levels, increases dopamine levels, decreases estrogen levels, increases growth hormone levels, and so on… So it's quite obvious that quality sleep has a prolactin reducing effect.

> NOTE: The above is not only a theory, as this study (189) proves that better sleep quality truly does decrease prolactin levels in men.

Get Adequate Amounts of Zinc

Zinc is one of the main nutrients behind healthy testosterone production, and it's also not a super big secret that zinc deficiency completely destroys testosterone levels.

What most people don't know is that zinc also reduces prolactin levels.

In this study 50 mg's (190) of daily zinc supplementation, more than halved prolactin levels of the male participants.

If you decide to get zinc as a supplement, I highly recommend this zinc combo. (191)

Conclusion on How to Lower Prolactin

Prolactin is a nasty hormone for you if you're a man, as it decreases testosterone levels and is highly linked to gynecomastia (man boobs). It's not uncommon for men to have high prolactin levels these days, as the "normal" diet is what it is, along with multiple other factors…

Fortunately it's quite easy to learn how to lower prolactin levels naturally. Certain supplements, vitamins, herbs and minerals along with adequate sleep will do the trick, as explained above.

> NOTE: Unnaturally high prolactin levels can also be a sign of pituitary gland tumor. So if your levels are extremely high and you have other hormonal problems, make sure that you get your brain scanned as quickly as possible.

PART 3:
MICRONUTRIENTS
(MASCULINE OPTIMIZATION PYRAMID LEVEL 1)

— Chapter 13 —

Micronutrient Deficiencies

Probably one of the simplest ways to increase natural testosterone production, is just to correct all of your underlying vitamin and mineral deficiencies. That is, since you can often do it effortlessly with a proper diet and a multivitamin supplement, or a cocktail of appropriate minerals and/or vitamins, which can typically be obtained affordably.

Depending on the state of your current micronutrient balance, it's not uncommon to double or even triple your testosterone levels by just correcting micronutrient deficiencies and adding in a good multivitamin for testosterone.

No joke, I have seen it happen with dozens of AM readers who have emailed me their natural T optimization progress along this past year or so.

You'd think that with the current obesity epidemic, any average Joe's vitamin and mineral reserves should be easily topped-up, since we're cramming foods to our mouths more than ever before...

Still, large portions of the US population are deficient in multiple key micronutrients: (192)

- vitamin A (35%)
- vitamin C (31%)

- vitamin E (67%)
- vitamin D (74%)
- vitamin K (67%)
- choline (92%)
- potassium (100%!?)
- calcium (39%)
- magnesium (46%)

Since the state of our Average Joe's micronutrient balance is downright scary, today's article will be devoted to one simple thing.

Correcting your vitamin and mineral deficiencies, since it's likely that you do have some…

How to Fix your Micronutrient Deficiencies

Fixing your vitamin and mineral imbalances for optimal testosterone production starts from optimizing the diet and then using a solid multivitamin for testosterone production.

For starters, you don't want to omit from any macronutrient group (protein, fats, carbs), and you definitely need to eat more real 'whole foods' instead of processed crap.

I'm talking about foods like: *eggs, grass-fed meats, pomegranates, berries, avocados…* A proper 'whole food-based diet' alone covers the intake of many key micronutrients…

…However, speaking from experience, even that is not always enough. To support your diet, I would advise that you also supplement with a multivitamin for testosterone (the one I am using is Vitamin Code Raw One For Men).

Not convinced about the the importance of vitamins to increase testosterone production? Take a look here:

- Vitamin A is stored in testicles (and few other glands of the body). Studies have shown that when there's no active vitamin A in the testes, T levels start dropping rapidly, and estrogen synthesis shoots up. (193) Also in a study of 155 male twins, (194) a clear correlation was found between vitamin A levels and serum testosterone. In prepubertal teens, vitamin A + iron supplementation is as effective in starting puberty as hormone replacement therapy. (195)
- Vitamin B complex (which consists of 8 different water-soluble vitamins), plays an important role in testosterone production and overall bodily energy levels, deficiency in many B vitamins results in increased estrogen levels, increased prolactin levels, and lowered testosterone levels (196, 197, 198, 199).
- Vitamin C has a protective effect on testosterone molecules, and this is because it's a potent antioxidant and able to block some cortisol secretion and oxidative damage (200, 201, 202, 203, 204)
- Vitamin D supplementation with a dose of 3332 IU's for one full year leads to 25% higher testosterone levels in healthy male subjects. (205) The positive correlation with vitamin D levels and serum testosterone have been noted in various other human studies too (206, 207, 208).
- Vitamin E deficient human and rodent subjects both experience a significant drop in LH, FSH, and testosterone levels, conversely, vitamin E supplemented humans and rodents notice significant increases in pituiary LH and FSH, and also in serum testosterone. (209)

- Magnesium intake has had a direct effect on serum testosterone levels in various studies. In this one, (210) 10 mg/kg of magnesium was able to increase free testosterone levels by 24%. Here (211) magnesium intake was positively correlated with high serum T levels, and in this large review study (212) the researchers conclude: *"there is evidence that magnesium exerts a positive influence on anabolic hormonal status, including testosterone, in men."*

- Calcium has its role in controlling neurotransmitter release and the signaling between cells and hormones. Not much is known about its effects on testosterone, but in 1976 a group of researchers found out that calcium stimulates testosterone synthesis in isolated leydig cells. (213) 33 years later another study saw that calcium supplementation didn't alter T levels at rest, but did significantly increase (18%) T levels post-exercise. (214)

- Selenium, mostly due to its glutathione stimulating effects, has been linked to increased testosterone production and improved sperm parameters in few studies (215, 216)

- Zinc has a significant positive effect on testosterone production and a deficiency will hammer the endocrine system. In fact, zinc might be one of the most important micronutrients for healthy testosterone production. It has increased testosterone levels in athletes and exercising 'normal men' (217, 218), in men with zinc deficiency, (219) in infertile men, (220) in animals... (221) It's also noted in one rodent study that zinc deficiency can upregulate the estrogen receptors by 57%, (222) probably due to the fact that zinc has its role in controlling the aromatase enzyme.

- Boron, although not very common mineral to supplement with, has few interesting studies backing up its testosterone boosting effects. In this human study (223) 6 mg's of boron for 60 days increased free testosterone levels by 29%. In another human study, (224) 10 mg's of boron for 7 days increased free testosterone by 28%.

- Manganese appears to have a direct GnRH stimulating effect in the brain, (225) and logic says that it should therefore also increase testosterone levels. However, mega-dosing with manganese should not be an option, since it accumulates in the body and can become neurotoxic at high levels. When taken at too high doses, manganese can actually reduce T levels. (226)

Conclusion on a Multivitamin for Testosterone

The above is just a short list of scientific examples of vitamins for testosterone and why you don't want to be deficient in any of these key vitamins and minerals.

Eat a diet rich in whole foods and always consume foods from all the macronutrient groups (fats, carbs, protein), this alone provides you with many of the essential micronutrients for T production, and also makes sure that your body can absorb them efficiently (for example, fat-soluble vitamins can't properly absorb if you're eating a low-fat diet, etc).

To support your diet, add in a multivitamin for testosterone and perhaps some other vitamin and mineral supplements (though multi is the way to go and definitely enough if you're low on cash).

We now stock the Garden of Life's RawOne for Men on the Anabolic Men Marketplace at **store.anabolicmen.com**

— Chapter 14 —

Vitamin A

Vitamin A, unlike the name indicates, is not a single compound. Instead its a blanket term for a group of active unsaturated molecules including: retinal, retinol, and retinoic acids, along with multiple provitamin A carotenoids such as: α-carotene, β-carotene, lutein, and lycopene, which the human body can convert into active Vitamin A.

The recommended daily intake for vitamin A for a normal sized male is about 900-3000 µg/day of retinal, retinol, or retinoic acid, or about 12-24 times that of carotenoids, since they have a significantly lower bio-availability in the human body and are also poorer sources of the active vitamin A.

Vitamin A is also noted as one of the "24 essential vitamins & minerals for human survival", and this is definitely for a good reason…

…Because without adequate amounts of vitamin A, you would slowly go blind, (227) your immune system wouldn't function normally, (228) not to mention that you would also become infertile, (229) and your body would have a really hard time absorbing dietary fat (230) (which in turn would cause colossal damage all-around the body).

Anyhow, here's what vitamin A does to testosterone levels:

Vitamin A and Testosterone Production

There's not much research behind vitamin A's effect on male testosterone levels, but a handful of studies has shown some positive associations between the vitamin and androgen production.

Vitamin A is found inside the testicular sertoli cells in retinal form and when needed it can be converted to more biologically active form; retinoic acid. It's also seen in rodent studies that if there's no active vitamin A present inside the testicles, testosterone levels drop rapidly and estrogen levels inside the testes shoot up.

If you're deficient in vitamin A, your body cannot properly utilize dietary fat for its many processes. As a good intake of the right fats is one of the utmost important building blocks of testosterone, (231) vitamin A deficiency will more than likely impact T production in a negative manner.

Also, your body uses a compound called *transferrin* to transport cholesterol molecules into the testicular leydig cells in order to convert them into testosterone. Without vitamin A, the body can't synthesize *transferrin*, and the transportation of the principal testosterone precursor gets impaired.

a) There's a lot of evidence suggesting that vitamin A is an essential part of male reproduction, since the synthesis of sperm cannot fully occur without retinoic acid (232, 233, 234).

b) In a human study (235) consisting of 155 twin males, vitamin A was found to have a significant positive correlation with testosterone production.

c) In this animal study (236) (which had guinea pigs as subjects), vitamin A deficiency significantly lowered testosterone production.

d) In this human study, (237) 102 young boys with delayed puberty and short stature were divided into 4 groups: first one was a control group, second group was given synthetic testosterone, third got vitamin A and iron supplements, and the fourth group got a combination of TRT, vitamin A, and iron. As you can imagine the control group didn't gain any significant height or begin puberty at an accelerated rate.

However, both the vitamin A group and testosterone treated group noted similar improvements in height growth, puberty rate, and testicular volume (yes, that's right. Vitamin A + iron was as effective as hormone replacement therapy in jump-starting puberty).

e) In this rodent study, (238) it was noted that the testicular system of rats contains several receptor sites for vitamin A, and that it can be stored in testicular sertoli cells. What's more interesting is that when the rodents diets were cut off from all vitamin A, testosterone production rapidly decreased (up to the point of where sexual organs literally atrophied), and estrogen exposure inside the testes rose rapidly (as humans share nearly identical testicular systems with wistar rats, this becomes very interesting).

There's definitely some evidence that being deficient in vitamin A is not a good thing for your testosterone production or testicular health.

And it's more than likely that men with low vitamin A levels can see significant improvements in their testosterone levels after supplementing with vitamin A or consuming a lot of it in their diets.

However, there's no evidence to support the claim that superloading with vitamin A, or even supplementing with it in the presence of already optimal intake would increase testosterone levels.

It's likely that the same thing happens with vitamin A, as does with vitamin D, (239) where dose-dependent increases in testosterone are seen up until the point where optimal levels of the vitamin in blood are achieved and the rising testosterone stops going higher after that.

"What is the best form to supplement with?"

Answer: The provitamin A carotenoids are the most common form, since they're the easiest ones to extract and/or synthesize in a lab. However they're not as bioavailable as the active forms, and your body has to convert them to actual vitamin A. On a bright side, you can't really overdose on carotenoids since the body converts only what it needs. The active forms however, accumulate in the body since they're fat-soluble and basically "ready-to-use". But, the body can use and absorb them much better than carotenoids. Just don't start superloading with them.

What works fine for me is that I take a multi-vitamin which contains carotenoids, and also liver tablets which have the more active forms of vitamin A. If I would have to choose either one of the two, I'd go with liver tablets though.

What are the best food sources for vitamin A?

Answer: You can fill up your daily intake with provitamin A carotenoids easily by eating a sweet potato (100g is 380% of RDA), or couple carrots (100g is 340% RDA), or a few handfuls of dark leafy greens (100g is 270% RDA).

To get the active forms of vitamin A (retinal, retinol, and retionic acids) your best option would be beef liver (100g is 1411% RDA), or a teaspoon of cod liver oil (which is about 100% of the RDA), or just some salmon (100g is 50% RDA).

Conclusion

Vitamin A has an essential role in testosterone production, and deficiency in the vitamin will most definitely hammer your testosterone levels.

However, deficiency in vitamin A is not that common, unless you live in a developing country or if you're eating a low-fat diet (the body has hard time absorbing vitamin A when there's no fat with it). Anyhow, if you want to make sure that you get enough vitamin A, the simplest way would be to just to buy some liver tablets, or to make your own.

Foods That Contain Vitamin A

NOTE: *It's also worth noting that you need saturated fat with the vitamin A for proper absorption.*

Here's five foods high in vitamin A (both retinoids and carotenoids) that fit a testosterone boosting diet:

1. Animal Liver (Beef, Pork, Turkey, Chicken)

By far the best source of the most bioavailable vitamin A in retinoid form can be most easily attained by eating animal liver.

Not only is it rich in vitamin A, it's also a nutritional powerhouse containing iron, copper, zinc, phosphorus, potassium, vitamins D, E, and C…

Here's the amounts of vitamin A in 100 grams of the following types of liver:

- *Turkey liver (8058 µg 895% RDA).*
- *Beef and pork liver (6500 µg 722% RDA).*
- *Chicken liver (3296 µg 366% RDA).*

Don't like the taste of liver? Try duck liver paste on top of a bread (tastes much better than most other types of liver foods), or consider supplementing with dessicated liver. Either way, if you're not including liver in your life, you're missing out big time.

2. Sweet Potatoes

Sweet potaoes are among the best carbohydrate sources for someone looking to optimize their testosterone levels.

They also happen to be very high in the carotenoid form of vitamin A…

…When the beta-carotene of 100 grams of sweet potatoes is converted into the active retinoid form (using the retinol activity equivalences), we are left with 961 µg of active vitamin A per 100 grams of sweet potatoes, which accounts to 107% RDA.

So sweet potatoes are not only testosterone friendly, but also a viable source of vitamin A in the carotenoid form.

3. Cod Liver Oil

Cod liver oil is often used as a supplement, but really, it's food. It's simply the oil extracted from the liver of the fresh-water cod.

And as to be expected, it's ridiculously high in fat-soluble vitamins A, E, and D.

100 grams of cod liver oil contains a staggering 30000 μg (3333% RDA) of the active retinoid form of vitamin A...

...Obviously nobody eats 100 grams of the stuff. Still, only a tablespoon of cod liver oil is enough to cover the daily need for vitamin A, as it has 340 μg's (136% RDA) of the micronutrient.

NOTE: *Never buy cheap fish oil or cod liver oil in capsules, it's in many cases rancid and oxidized and can have very high levels of mercury. The best and cleanest cod liver oil comes from Norway.*

4. Cheese

Cheese is a source of high quality casein protein, as well as testosterone boosting saturated fat.

It also has a good amount of fat-soluble vitamins, including vitamin A in its retinoid form.

On average, cheddar cheese at 100 grams provides you with 265 μg vitamin A (29% RDA).

So nothing close to liver, but its still good to include some cheddar and blue cheese in your diet for the sake of promoting testosterone production and getting in some much needed micronutrients.

5. Butter

Butter is one of the preferred fat source on a testosterone optimized diet.

It simply has the right type of fatty-acids, with plenty of great micronutrients to fuel the endocrine system.

When it comes to vitamin A, butter is a decent source, as 100 grams give you 684 µg (76% RDA) of active vitamin A...

...Obviously 100 grams of butter is a lot and we're not recommending an intake so high, but including plenty of butter as your main fat source is still a good idea if one aims to increase natural testosterone production. You'll get some much needed vitamin A on the side.

— Chapter 15 —

B Vitamins

When you think of B vitamins and testosterone, you're probably thinking of a B12 shot or supplement that amps you up without jitters.

The truth is, there are eight B vitamins in total, and they all serve similar functions of releasing energy from foods into our body. B vitamins are water soluble, meaning they can be excreted through your urinary system quite easily, so there's no real concern of overdose.

These essential vitamins provide all-around maintenance for your body, including your mental health.

B vitamins aren't produced in your body, so you must ingest them through diet or supplementation. Leafy greens and whole, unprocessed foods are usually great sources for a range of B-complex vitamins, which is why they're usually stressed when it comes to healthy eating.

The eight B vitamins are thiamine (B1), riboflavin (B2), niacin (B3), pantothenic acid (B5), vitamin B6, biotin (B7), vitamin B12, and folic acid.

Low levels of any of these vitamins can lead to anemia-like symptoms and general malnutrition.

What Does The Vitamin B-Complex Have To Do With Your T Levels?

Vitamin B1 – Thiamine:

Thiamine, like all B vitamins, is required daily in a steady dose by the human body to carry out proper function without sacrificing nutrition.

Thiamine serves especially important purposes in the neurological system.

The lack of thiamine can cause permanent cognitive damage in the long term, and affect focus, mental capacity, and neural health in the short term.

Testosterone, a steroid hormone, must bind to androgen receptors through the endocrine and adrenal systems, which are very closely linked to the neurological systems in the body. If neural function is impaired, the production and uptake of testosterone can be severely limited.

In addition to regulation neuron pathways, thiamine is necessary for the indirect upkeep of muscle mass. Thiamine deficiency can lead to a number of issues with muscular atrophy, which can also be attributed to low testosterone levels (240).

Low thiamine levels can also contribute to feelings of muscle fatigue and lack of motivation and focus.

Vitamin B2 – Riboflavin:

Riboflavin presents itself in foods also containing other testosterone-boosting factors like bromelain (241). Riboflavin is one of the essential nutrients needed in testosterone production but also serves an interesting purpose in the inhibition of testosterone 5 alpha-reductase (242).

This enzyme converts testosterone into a more potent form of the androgen, known as dihydrotestosterone (DHT). Riboflavin deficiency can lead to lethargy and fatigue as well, decreasing sex drive and general health.

Bananas are a great source of libido-boosting vitamin B2. This is easy to remember thanks to phallic symbolism.

Vitamin B3 – Niacin:

Niacin is a known booster of human growth hormone. It also produces the right kind of cholesterol that our body needs (high-density lipid or HDL).

Testosterone is actually formed from cholesterol, so it's pretty straightforward to assume that niacin can definitely affect T production. Alongside increased testosterone levels, growth hormone production which is "turbocharged" by niacin, can lead to plenty anabolic muscle growth and a huge increase in muscle mass (244).

Niacin also acts as an antioxidant by binding free radicals and slowing aging processes.

Vitamin B5 – Pantothenic Acid:

Pantothenic acid is well known as a cure for acne.

This is due to its role as a fat metabolizer when bound to a sulfur-based molecule to create coenzyme A. Interestingly enough, B5 also serves as a cholesterol producer, which as mentioned above, is a necessary component of building testosterone.

Pantothenic acid plays a vital role in the adrenal system by helping the basis of sex- and stress-hormone production. It is also a key factor in the manufacture of red blood cells, which are the sites of oxygen uptake in our body (245).

Increased oxygen uptake contributes to better performance in training, which also spikes testosterone levels.

Vitamin B6:

B6 is one of the B vitamins that play a more direct role when it comes to testosterone production. Vitamin B6 works to suppress the synthesis of estrogen in the body, which helps testosterone levels rise.

Vitamin B6 also works directly with the regulation of androgen production, which leads to increased T levels as well. B6 is also important for the production and transport of red blood cells.

A deficiency in vitamin B6 can lead to fatigue, loss of appetite, and decreased immunity (246).

Vitamin B7 – Biotin:

Studies have shown that biotin deficiency can lead to reduced testicular function in rats and that administered biotin treatments can reverse the issues that arise from low testosterone levels (247).

Biotin also improves the utilization of glucose in the body, which can reduce risks for obesity, a big detractor from high testosterone levels.

Vitamin B12:

Also known as cobalamin, B12 is the 'energy vitamin' which is also known to raise testosterone levels dramatically as well as produce a spike in energy levels when injected. For this reason, it is a great nootropic and can be used for pre-workout benefits as well.

This vitamin derives energy in the body through the breakdown of dietary fats, so during a bulking period, it can lead to increased muscle anabolism and less fat production. A study has indicated that B12 can also have a positive effect on sperm motility and concentration, which is tied to testicular testosterone levels (247).

Folic Acid:

While generally regarded as a prenatal supplement, folic acid, or folate, can have a lot of beneficial effects for anabolic muscle processes.

Folic acid is essential for the synthesis and upkeep of new cells in the human body. It also acts to repair damaged musculature and promotes DNA and RNA synthesis. Folate is known to produce nitric oxide in the body, which a key physiological component in bulk training that helps increase muscle mass (249).

Increased muscle mass causes increased testosterone levels, so it's not a big surprise that folic acid can really help to raise your testosterone, like the other B-complex vitamins.

How To Get Higher Levels of B Vitamins

Vitamins in the B-complex can work both individually and synergistically in order to maintain basic bodily function. As mentioned before, these vitamins must be taken dietarily, as they are not naturally produced by the human body.

If your diet leaves something to be desired in terms of B-complex content, a B-complex multivitamin, or specified B vitamin supplements can help.

Good food sources of thiamin include pork, lentils and nuts. Riboflavin can be found in dairy products and lean meats. Niacin-rich foods include pasta and legumes. Folic acid (as well as thiamin, vitamin B6, and riboflavin) is known for its presence in dark green leafy veggies like spinach, chard, and kale, as well as fortified grains and cereals.

Vitamin B6 can be found in poultry, seafood, and root vegetables. B12 is naturally found in shellfish but is also used to fortify grain and soy products. Biotin and pantothenic acid can be found in liver, egg yolk, salmon, and dairy, as well as some legumes and mushrooms (249).

— Chapter 16 —

Vitamin C

Vitamin C (ascorbic acid) is likely the most researched, well known, and most-used nutritional supplement in the whole World. Not only that, but it's also safe, cheap, and available pretty much all-around the globe.

But what about the effects of vitamin C on male testosterone levels? That's a topic not so often talked about.

At least until now...

Ascorbic Acid and Testosterone Levels

Vitamin C is an essential vitamin for human survival, and like I said above, one of the cheapest, safest, and most widely used nutritional supplements in the World.

It's water-soluble, and its main function in the body is to serve as an antioxidant...

...However, what most people don't know, is that vitamin C can also be a pro-oxidant. How it acts depends on what the body needs at any given time.

Ascorbic acid is also needed in the biosynthesis of multiple bodily enzymes...

...And when used in combination with garlic, vitamin C is ridiculously effective at increasing nitric oxide levels, (250) and therefore also blood flow.

But how does the world's most-used vitamin affect male testosterone levels? That's what we're about to find out:

a) First of, there's an in-vitro (test tube) study (251) where it was found that vitamin C as an electron donor, can regenerate damaged testosterone molecules by up to 58%. In a similar in-vitro study, (252) vitamin C was able to increase testosterone levels in testicular leydig cells due to enzyme upregulation.

b) Several animal studies have shown that vitamin C protects the testicular leydig cells from oxidative stressors, and thus, preserves testosterone levels from; alcohol, (253) noise-stress, (254) lead, (255) burns, (256) cadmium, (257) antibiotics, (258) arsenic, (259) PCBs, (260) aluminum, (261) alfatoxin, (262) and endosulfan. (263) Similar protective effects have been seen in humans too. (264)

c) So, ascorbic acid clearly preserves testosterone molecules from oxidative damage, but could it increase testosterone levels in healthy gonads? This rodent study (265) suggests so, and in this human study, (266) vitamin C significantly increased sperm quality, motility, and volume. However the only two human studies that I'm aware of which examined vitamin C's direct effects on testosterone levels, showed no significant increases in T after ascorbic acid supplementation (267, 268).

d) The last thing worth mentioning here, is the fact that vitamin C supplementation is known for its cortisol (stress hormone) lowering effects. This in turn should improve the testosterone:cortisol ratio more in favor of testosterone, creating a more anabolic environment in the body (269, 270, 271, 272).

Who could benefit from Vitamin C supplementation?

Answer: Well, for starters pretty much anyone who wants to protect their balls from oxidative damage. If you're exposed to any of the things in point "b)" above, then increased ascorbic acid intake (and for that matter other antioxidants too) would be advisable, just to preserve testosterone molecules from cellular damage.

Another group that could benefit from extra vitamin C intake would be people who train hard, as ascorbic acid helps in suppressing the exercise induced rise in cortisol, and therefore would improve the testosterone to cortisol ratio in favor of anabolism.

However, if you don't train hard, and if you suspect that your diet and overall health is in such a good order that there's no oxidative damage going on in the ballsack, then vitamin C supplementation is probably not going to do much for your hormones.

How much ascorbic acid should you take?

Answer: In a healthy scenario, the human body has a pool of vitamin C of about 2 grams. (273) This can be maintained with ~100 mg's of daily ascorbic acid supplementation, hence why the RDA of vitamin C is 100-200 mg's.

This low amount can be easily attained through the diet (citrus fruits, kiwi, etc), or from a high quality multi-vitamin.

However, if you're under stress, and/or exposed to compounds that cause oxidative stress in the body, a higher dose (1-5 grams) of vitamin C could be taken to protect the leydig cells from damage. To lower the exercise induced rise in cortisol, 1-3 grams of ascorbic acid should be enough.

What's the best form of vitamin C to supplement with?

Answer: I'm personally a big fan of raw whole-food vitamins and minerals. Thus, why I recommend this 100% food based ascorbic acid supplement (274) which is made from acerola cherries. For a more cost-effective alternative, pure bulk vitamin C powder would be fine too. For people who can't handle acidic compounds (GERD, etc) Ester-C would be the best option.

Also, if your goal is only to maintain the body's natural pool of vitamin C, you should be covered just by eating some citrus fruits on a daily basis, or by taking a multi-vitamin that includes at least 100 mg's of ascorbic acid.

Does vitamin C increase testosterone levels? Not directly if you believe the latest human studies, and this is likely due to the fact that in a healthy scenario, the human body maintains a pool of available vitamin C in various tissues (testicles, pituitary gland, thyroid, liver, etc).

However, supplemental ascorbic acid does protect testosterone molecules exceptionally well from oxidative damage during the times of stress. Probably because the bodily pool is drained faster when exposed to various stressors.

And that's also why I believe most men could benefit from extra vitamin C supplementation. Because of the modern day diet of processed foods, environmental toxins, obesity, and sedentary lifestyles, most men do have some oxidative stress going on inside their gonads.

The best ways to get yourself enough vitamin C would be from a diet consisting of citrus fruits, through a high-quality multi-vitamin, from natural berry powders, or from a bulk ascorbic acid supplement.

Foods Rich In Vitamin C

Vitamin C (ascorbic acid) is pretty awesome. Not only is it a vital micronutrient for human survival, it also maintains testosterone levels and protects hormones from the harmful effects of oxidative damage.

There are many foods high in vitamin C, but for this section I have chosen 5 of them that perfectly fit a testosterone boosting diet, majority of them being fruits.

From time to time we get readers emailing us all confused about why we recommend fruits that are high in fructose, since everyone and their dogs think that fructose would be evil...

...So let us tell you that in reality:

- *Fructose protects the liver cells (275) and increases the rate of carbohydrate metabolism. (276)*
- *Fructose is the main sugar involved in reproductive system function and sperm production. (277)*
- *Fructose lowers SHBG and thus leaves more bioavailable free-testosterone to the blood stream. (278)*
- *Fructose stimulates the conversion from thyroid hormone T4 to T3 in the liver, upregulating metabolism. (279)*

Anyhow, now that your possible fructose paranoia has been hopefully cured, here's five food sources of vitamin C that are also great for testosterone production:

1. Squeezed Orange Juice

Squeezed orange juice is one of the staples in my diet.
I religiously drink 1-2 liters of it per day to supply my body with fructose to blunt SHBG and promote thyroid hormone conversion.
On the side, orange juice is a good natural source of vitamin C.

To be exact, a glass of squeezed OJ contains up to 108mg's of vitamin C, accounting for 120% of the RDA.

2. Pineapple

Who doesn't love pineapples?

Not only are they tasty, but there's also research showing that a proteolytic enzyme by the name of "bromelain" found in pineapples can maintain testosterone levels during strenuous endurance training. (280)

Bromelain also breaks down the peptide chains that bind amino acids, making protein digest better in the body. And then there's the fact that pineapples are rich in fructose, which has numerous hormonal benefits as explained above.

100 grams of fresh pineapple chunks contain 47mg's of vitamin C, accounting for 52% of the RDA. So not quite as dense in ascorbic acid as OJ is, but still a good natural food source of vitamin C that you should be consuming.

3. Sweet Potato

Sweet potatoes are one of the better carb sources on a testosterone optimized diet.

They're incredibly dense in vitamin A, but also contain nice amounts of vitamin C too.

To be exact, 100 grams of sweet potatoes gives you a good 19mg's of vitamin C (21% RDA)...

...So these definitely shouldn't be your sole source of vitamin C, but sweet potatoes are great for replenishing glycogen stores after exercise so why not get some of that vit C on the side too?

4. Mango

Mangoes are one of the most widely consumed fruits in the world.

They're fairly carb dense with majority of those carbs coming in from fructose. Once again this freaks most people out, but as a man looking to improve your testosterone levels as well as to boost metabolic rate, getting that fructose is actually incredibly beneficial. When it comes to vitamin C rich foods, mangoes have some.

They contain 27mg (30% RDA) of vitamin C per 100g.

5. Kiwi

Kiwi fruit is widely known, but not much of its health benefits are discussed.

Maybe people are scared of the high fructose content, but as explained many times now, that is nothing to be scared of.

One interesting study actually looked how kiwi fruit affected sleep quality in healthy adults, (281) and the researchers found out that 2 kiwi's 1-hour before bed time for a month were able to dramatically improve both subjective and objective parameters of sleep quality.

This is great news, since sleeping more and better has been firmly linked to higher testosterone levels.

Now, back to vitamin C. Kiwi is an excellent source, with 92mg's per 100g (155% RDA).

So maybe next time before you hit the sack, eat few kiwi fruits for better sleep, more T, and a good amount of vitamin C.

Conclusion

Vitamin C is great, and getting the currently set RDA% from foods is not hard at all.

However if you're looking for benefits like increased nitric oxide production and a boost in testosterone levels, the dosages go upwards of 1 gram per day.

This is pretty hard to get from foods, and much better achieved through supplementation with something like *Redwood* from Truth Nutraceuticals or ascorbic acid capsules plus garlic extract.

— Chapter 17 —

Vitamin D

Vitamin D is one of the 24 essential vitamins needed for human survival. It regulates more than 1,000 bodily functions. Not to mention the vitamin D testosterone benefits are quite profound. It occurs naturally in fish and eggs, although the best way to get it is through regular sun exposure.

Vitamin D is truly a "wonder vitamin", and most people use it because it's proven to be heart healthy and good for the bones.

But vitamin D is much much more than just a bone vitamin...

Vitamin D increases testosterone levels and maintains optimal endocrine system health in both, men and women:

Vitamin D Testosterone Benefits

Vitamin D is actually not even a vitamin...

...It's a steroid hormone, mistakenly named as a vitamin.
This hormone D like I said above, regulates more than 1,000 bodily functions, including fertility, growth, hormone secretion, and sexual function...

...Needless to say that if your serum vitamin D levels are too low, more than 1,000 bodily functions are also somewhat impaired. Several of these functions that vitamin D regulates are linked to the endocrine system, thus not getting adequate amounts of "the bone vitamin", should in theory reduce testosterone levels.

Recent Studies on Vitamin D and Testosterone Levels:

a) This study (282) found out that vitamin D and testosterone levels were correlated. Men with sufficient vitamin D levels had significantly higher testosterone levels and lower SHBG count, than men who had insufficient amounts of the vitamin (or hormone) in their blood serum.

b) This study (283) found out that when healthy male participants take 3332 IU's of vitamin D daily for a year, they end up having 25.2% more testosterone on average when compared to placebo.

c) This study (284) found out that older men who supplement with vitamin D, are less likely to have low testosterone levels than men who are not supplementing with the "bone vitamin".

d) In this Australian study, (285) the researchers found out that in older men, low vitamin D status is associated with low free testosterone and increased fracture risk.

e) This study (286) examined the already proven positive association between vitamin D and testosterone levels. They had 1362 male subjects, and the results show that vitamin D has a linear positive association with serum total and free testosterone levels. However when the amount of vitamin D in serum goes above ~80 nmol/L (pretty much optimal), the increase in testosterone plateaus. Meaning that vitamin D more than likely does increase testosterone levels, but it won't help if you are already in the optimal range of vitamin D (which is definitely not where most men are).

f) It's actually better to get your vitamin D from sunlight exposure, at least if you believe the results of this 1939 study from Dr. Abraham Myerson, (287) which showed that five days of UV light exposure to men's chest area, increased total testosterone levels by ~120%. When the genitals were exposed to UV radiation for the same amount of time, the increase in testosterone skyrocketed to ~200%.

g) There is also some evidence (288) that bright light exposure signals the brain to release luteinizing hormone (LH), which triggers testicular leydig cells to produce testosterone. So being out in the sun for that vitamin D is definitely not a bad idea.

e) In few studies, it has been noted that in both; humans and animals, blood vitamin D levels are positively associated with sperm quality and motility (289, 290, 291).

What the results of vitamin D and testosterone studies tell us:

1. Men with low vitamin D levels are much more likely to have low testosterone levels when compared to men with adequate amounts of the vitamin.
2. Healthy men who decide to supplement with low dose vitamin D, can expect to have around 25% more testosterone in their bloodstream after a year of supplementation.
3. If your serum vitamin D levels are already in the optimal range, you might not get a testosterone boosting benefit from extra supplementation.

4. UV light exposure seems to skyrocket testosterone production, especially if you expose your genitals to the sun rays.

So we can conclude that vitamin D is really a testosterone booster, at least the science seems to support this idea from multiple view points.

What is the vitamin D testosterone dosage?

Answer: The optimal amount of vitamin D in the blood serum seems to be around 50-70 ng/dl. This can be quite easily achieved when supplementing daily with a low to normal dose of high quality vitamin D3 supplement (this is my recommendation), through a multivitamin, or by spending few hours in the sun each day. Best if you do both.

NOTE: You should avoid the D2 form of the vitamin, it's cheaply made and the chemical process of manufacturing it is questionable. It's also not nearly as good in terms of bio-availability as the D3 form is.

Conclusion on Vitamin D Testosterone Benefits

Vitamin D is a testosterone booster, but if your vitamin D levels are already optimal (most men don't fall into this category by the way), then extra supplementation won't help.

It's also known for its ability to increase lifespan, it improves cardiovascular health, and it even maintains bone health when taken along with calcium and vitamin K2.

So if you're not already living in an overly sunny place, then supplementation with this high quality vitamin D3 supplement might just be a wise decision .

5 Foods To Incorporate Into Your Diet To Get More Vitamin D

Here are five foods rich in vitamin D:

1. Mushrooms

Many types of mushrooms are absolutely loaded with naturally occurring vitamin D.

This vitamin D is in the form of D2 (ergocalciferol), which is significantly less bioavailable for the body than the vitamin D3 found in animal products, (292) but according to research it can still be used to replenish serum vitamin D levels. (293)

But just how much vitamin D2 do mushrooms have? Here's a list:

- Portobello mushrooms, exposed to sun, grilled – 493 IU/ 100g (82% RDA).
- Maitake Mushrooms, raw – 943 IU/100g (157% RDA).
- Chantarelle mushrooms, raw – 178 IU/100g (29% RDA).
- Morel mushrooms, raw – 173 IU/100g (28% RDA).
- Shiitake mushrooms, dried – 129 IU/100g (21% RDA).

The problem with these reference amounts is that according to the research done by Dr. Michael Holick, vitamin D2 is about 30% as effective as vitamin D3 in replenishing serum vitamin D levels, this would mean that you would need to 3x all the amounts above for real "useful" vitamin D amounts.

2. Wild Fish

The flesh of oily fishes is known of being one of the richest natural sources of vitamin D3.

What you should make sure though, is that the fish you eat is wild, and not farmed with soy pellets. This ensures that you get mainly omega-3's from the fatty part of the fish, instead of the inflammatory omega-6 fatty acids that build up in factory farmed fish due to their feed.

Another reason to choose wild over farmed is the ridiculously high amount of toxic heavy-metals and pesticides found in farmed fish.

Anyways, fish and fish liver products have plenty of vitamin D3:

- Cod liver oil – 10 000 IU/100g (1666% RDA).
- Wild salmon – 859 IU/100g (143% RDA).
- Wild mackerel – 250 IU/100g (41% RDA).
- Wild sardines – 193 IU/100g (32% RDA).
- Wild tuna – 230 IU/100g (38% RDA).

As you can see, cod liver oil is loaded with naturally occurring vitamin D3, which makes it a really good food/supplement for replenishing serum vitamin D levels, if you get it, do get the authentic Norwegian kind from clean fish.

Another good supplement option is liquid vitamin D3 drops.

3. Milk

Milk is naturally rich in calcium, as well as good source of high-quality casein protein, and saturated fat (if you buy whole milk).

Naturally milk only contains trace amounts of vitamin D, but ever since it became apparent in 1933 that there's wide-spread deficiency in vitamin D levels, many countries began adding vitamin D3 to foods...

...One of the first ones to be fortified was milk, and ever since then, nearly all brands of milk have contained varying amounts of added vitamin D.

On average, a cup of fortified milk contains 120 IU of vitamin D3 (20% RDA).

4. Egg Yolk

One of the best sources of naturally occurring micronutrients (vitamins and minerals) is the yolk of an egg.

It holds nearly all of the essential vitamins and minerals needed for life, as well as cholesterol and fatty-acids to enhance their absorption.

As we've said many times in this website, only a fool would throw away the yolk!

100 grams of egg yolks contains 225 IU's of vitamin D, which accounts for 37% of the RDA... So eggs solely aren't the best source of vitamin D, but one should still get a chunk of their daily D3 from egg yolks.

5. Oysters

Many mollusks are filled with vitamin D, but easily the best one for testosterone optimization is the oyster.

The legend says that *Casanova* ate 50 oysters every morning to maintain his libido, and some recent evidence suggests that he might of have been onto something. (294)

When it comes to vitamin D content, oysters rank in relatively high. *100 grams of raw oysters contain 320 IU's of vitamin D3, accounting for 53% of the RDA.*

Conclusion

Although certain foods are high in vitamin D, **we still recommend extra supplementation in the form of cod liver oil or liquid vitamin D3 drops** to make sure that you get sufficient amounts of this crucial micronutrient.

Although the RDA is set to 600 IU for now, some researchers believe that the daily requirements for vitamin D have been grossly underestimated, and the real number could be up to 10x higher than the RDA originally calculated many years ago. (295)

Also the importance of sunlight vitamin D synthesis doesn't get the press it deserves, as less than 30 minutes of sun exposure during the summer months is enough to get your daily dose of vitamin D.

Chapter 18

Vitamin E

Vitamin E is one of the 24 essential micronutrients for human survival.

It's a fat-soluble vitamin that comes naturally in the forms of tocopherols and tocotrienols, and is most well-known of having powerful antioxidant properties, but also benefits the body by being an enzyme coactivator and by playing a protective role in neurological function.

One of the lesser known benefits of vitamin E, is its ability to prevent and slowdown the oxidation of polyunsaturated fatty-acids (PUFAs), (296) which is great since the oxidation of polyunsaturated fatty-acids is likely one of the main reasons why high intake of PUFAs lower testosterone levels. (297)

There are many foods high in vitamin E, and in this chapter you'll learn the five that best suit a testosterone boosting diet:

1. Spinach

Spinach is one of the best dark leafy vegetables to consume as a man.

There are myriad of benefits in doing so, mainly the large amount of vitamins and minerals present in spinach, its low calorie content, and the high amount of natural nitrates which have been shown to naturally raise nitric oxide production and erection quality. (298)

When it comes to vitamin E, spinach is considered to be a decent source. We would say it's not high enough in vitamin E to solely get all you need from it, but still with the other benefits and its impressive micronutrient density, you should consume it on a daily basis.

At 100 grams, spinach contains 2mg's of vitamin E in the form of alpha-tocopherol, accounting for 13% of the RDA.

2. Egg Yolk

If you've followed these foods high in [insert micronutrient] articles, you've probably noticed that in nearly all of the articles I recommend eating eggs.

That is also the case for vitamin E, as the yolk has plenty of it, along with some fat and cholesterol to improve its absorption.

Like in the case of spinach above, we don't recommend that you solely get your vitamin E from eggs (as that would mean a lot of eggs), but it's still good to get some of it from this nutritional powerhouse.

100 grams of raw egg yolks contain 3mg's of vitamin E (20% RDA) in alpha-tocopherol form.

3. Brazil Nuts

Many types of nuts are high in vitamin E.

But we're somewhat hesitant to recommend nuts in general due to their high polyunsaturated fatty-acid (PUFA) content which is known of lowering testosterone levels and also increasing the need for vitamin E (due to PUFA causing more oxidative damage in the body). (299)

However, Brazil nuts are off the hook. They're lower in PUFA than most nuts, excellent sources of selenium, boron, and magnesium...
...And also rich in vitamin E, 100 grams providing 7,8mg's (52% RDA).

4. Avocado

Avocado is a nutrient-bomb filled with fat-soluble vitamins.

It also has ample amounts of monounsaturated fatty-acids, which have been found to increase testosterone levels in several studies...

...And avocados also contain a bitter glycoside by the name of oleuropein, which was found to significantly increase testosterone levels in rodents.

When it comes to vitamin E, 100 grams of avocados contain 3,1mg's (20% RDA).

5. Shrimp

Shrimp is great, especially if you're on a cut, since they're so low in calories, filling, and almost purely high-quality protein.

I eat shrimp almost daily, since they're one of the richest natural sources of the amino-acid glycine (which our modern diets are far too low in).

When buying shrimp, make sure to get wild shrimps, not farmed. The latter are loaded with heavy-metals.

When it comes to vitamin E, wild caught shrimp is a decent source at 2,5mg's per 100g (16% RDA).

Conclusion

There are many vitamin E rich foods, some which have even higher amounts than the ones in this post (like almonds, sun flower seeds and oil, etc)…

…But the reason we didn't include them is that they're also high in PUFAs, which increases the bodily need for vitamin E, and also lowers testosterone levels. (300)

If you feel like you can't get enough vitamin E from the diet, consider using a high-quality vitamin E supplement (especially if you eat a lot of polyunsaturated fatty-acids).

— Chapter 19 —

Magnesium

Magnesium is the 11th most-abundant mineral in the human body, and it controls more than 300 bodily functions, along with hundreds of enzyme functions. Most people associate the mineral only with bone and heart health, but it's so much more than just for the heart and bones…

…You see magnesium is also the primary electrolyte used by virtually all of the bodily enzymes. It maintains fluid balance, gives energy to the cells (ATP), activates creatine, improves sleep quality, and increases the amount of bio-active (free) testosterone.

All that's great, but the thing that I'm most interested is the last one. Magnesium increasing free testosterone levels:

Magnesium and Testosterone Levels

Magnesium is very similar to zinc when it comes to increasing testosterone levels…

…Deficiency in both will seriously lower testosterone levels, but if you're already having adequate amounts of the minerals in your system, then megadosing with them will not do much for your hormones.

And this is where it all boils down. Do you actually need more magnesium?

Research suggests that you probably do, as this study (301) shows that nearly 70% of the adults in the United States eat below the recommended RDA of magnesium, 19% eating less than half of the recommended daily value.

On top of that, magnesium evaporates from the body through sweat, so if you're hitting the gym, or living in a hot place, then it's very likely that you're not consuming enough of this essentially important mineral (especially if your eating habits are based around the Western diet)...

...But back to the actual subject, here are some studies:

1. This in-vitro study (302) found out that magnesium frees bound testosterone and makes it more bio-active. This happens because the mineral inhibits SHBG (sex hormone binding globulin), which is a molecule that binds to free testosterone, making it unavailable for the receptors.
2. In this human study, (303) roughly one gram of magnesium was enough to increase free testosterone levels by 24% in combination with intense exercise.
3. In this study (304) which had 400 participants, the researchers found out that in older men, higher serum magnesium levels correlate with higher testosterone levels.
4. The researchers in this review study (305) found out something very similar about magnesium as the studies cited above. This is what they write: *"there is evidence that magnesium exerts a positive influence on anabolic hormonal status, including testosterone, in men."*

5. In this study, (306) the researchers found out that Gitelman's syndrome (which causes imbalances in magnesium and calcium levels) often leads to delayed puberty in young boys, most likely this delay in puberty is caused by low testosterone levels, and the low T is caused by low magnesium and calcium levels.

So all-in-all, it seems that there's a point in supplementing with magnesium, especially if you're exercising...

...However, if you sit at the couch all day, and already consume plenty of magnesium, then it's likely that extra supplementation isn't going to do much.

What is the best form of magnesium to supplement with?

Answer: Magnesium glycinate is the best form of oral magnesium in terms of absorption, whereas oxide is the worst (and most used).

What are the best dietary sources for magnesium?

Answer: Contrary to popular belief, grains are not a reliable source of magnesium due to the high amount of pythic acid. You're far better of by consuming the following foods: <u>Raw</u> cacao products, unprocessed salts, meat, leafy greens, and some nuts.

I've heard that calcium blocks the absorption of magnesium?

Answer: Calcium, zinc, magnesium, and iron all bind to the same receptors inside the body, however the receptors can uptake around

800 mg's of minerals, so unless you're megadosing on all of them simultaneously, you should be fine in terms of absorption

Conclusion

Magnesium is very much like zinc in terms of increasing testosterone. If you're deficient in it, your testosterone levels will decrease quite significantly, but if you have plenty of it in your system already, then consuming even more isn't going to do much...

...But as explained above, majority of us in this planet can't get enough of magnesium to begin with, so supplementation in most cases is going to increase baseline testosterone. If you're looking for high quality magnesium supplement, take a look at Testro-X, which contains a clinical dose per serving.

Magnesium Rich Foods To Eat

However, many magnesium rich foods are actually not that great for testosterone levels.

Things like soybeans, flaxseeds, sunflower seeds, peppermint, and many other dense magnesium sources, can actually end up reducing your T-levels due to other – not so testosterone friendly – compounds found in them.

These five foods however, are high in magnesium, and awesome for testosterone production as well:

NOTE: If you can't use these to meet your daily Mg2+ needs, consider supplementation.

1. Dark Chocolate and Cacao Products

The cacao bean in its unprocessed state is one of the richest known dietary sources of magnesium.

This makes raw cacao powder (and many other products made using cacao bean) great foods to replenish bodily magnesium levels.
100 grams of cacao powder for example contains 520mg's of magnesium which is 130% of the RDA.

> NOTE: *If you opt for dark chocolate or raw cacao nibs which also have the cacao fat intact, you'll deliver your body with an awesome testosterone boosting saturated fat rich in stearic acid (one of the best possible fatty-acids in terms of T-production).*

2. Beef

Animal meat, especially beef, is great source of magnesium.

It's not as dense in the mineral as cacao beans are, as 100 grams of beef patties will give you a decent 50mg's (12% RDA) of magnesium.

However, since beef is one of the best foods to increase natural testosterone levels and should be your main protein source anyway, having it as one of your magnesium sources is a great idea.

Just remember that beef shouldn't be your ONLY magnesium source, as it would take almost a kilo (2.2lb) of beef patties to actually meet the daily magnesium needs.

3. Spinach

Not only is spinach loaded with testosterone boosting apigening and erection quality enhancing natural nitrates...(307)

...It's also a very good natural source of magnesium.

100 grams of cooked spinach will give you 87mg's of magnesium which is 22% of the RDA.

> NOTE: *Aside from eating some dark chocolate and beef, consider adding a cup of cooked spinach to your diet. Not only to supply magnesium, but also because it's an incredibly healthy leafy green that works wonders for your hormones and circulation.*

4. Brazil Nuts

I believe that every man should be consuming a handful of Brazil nuts daily to promote healthy testosterone levels.

This is because they're ridiculously high in the minerals boron and selenium (both of which are crucial for T-production)...

...And also loaded with magnesium, as 100 grams will give you 376mg's of magnesium, which is 94% of the RDA, aka. almost solely enough to meet the daily needs.

Note that you should be getting your Brazil nuts with as much skin as possible, since that's where the majority of the minerals are in.

5. Swiss Chard

Similarly to spinach, Swiss chard is a naturally dense source of nitrates (compounds that have been scientifically proven to increase nitric oxide and erection quality).

On top of that, there's plenty of magnesium in this leafy green.

To be specific, 100 grams of cooked Swiss chard gives you 86mg's of magnesium, covering 21% of the RDA.

So obviously, the testosterone boosting greens of choice for replenishing magnesium levels are spinach and Swiss chard.

Conclusion

Magnesium is essential for humans, and when it comes to testosterone production, doses close to 1 gram (1000mg) have been found to significantly increase free testosterone levels by reducing SHBG. (308)

This amount is relatively easy to get from daily foods, as long as you eat plenty of dark chocolate, spinach and Swiss chard, along with some beef and few handfuls of Brazil nuts.

If however you can't meet your daily magnesium needs, consider using a high-quality magnesium supplement to replenish the serum levels (note that magnesium evaporates through sweat, so athletes require bit more than sedentary guys).

── Chapter 20 ──

Zinc

Zinc is one of the 24 essential minerals needed for human survival. The human body can't synthesize its own – nor does it have a storage system for it – so you must get adequate amounts of zinc through foods or dietary supplementation daily.

It's involved in numerous actions of the cellular metabolism, up-regulates more than 100 enzymes, supports healthy growth, helps with DNA synthesis, and is deeply tied to reproductive system health.

Zinc is also – up to a certain point – a testosterone booster, which inhibits the aromatase enzyme, thus reduces the conversion from testosterone to estrogen.

Here's what I'm talking about:

Zinc Can Increase Testosterone Levels and Block Estrogen

Zinc as I said above, is a testosterone booster up to a certain point...

...As it increases testosterone levels in healthy men, if they're depleted in the mineral. If your serum zinc levels are already in balance, it's likely that extra supplementation will not yield any extra benefits, in fact, too much zinc is not a good thing either.

What's considered depletion then?

Well, you need at least 15 mg's of daily zinc to even maintain the most crucial endocrine system functions…

…Meaning that you should consume lots of oysters and animal-products daily, and on top of that maybe supplement with some extra zinc to make sure that you're getting adequate amounts of the mineral (zinc (as well as magnesium) evaporates through sweat, so in athletes, supplementation is almost mandatory).

There's plenty of clinical research backing up the benefits of zinc supplementation.

During strenuous exercise, elite wrestlers who supplemented with 3mg/kg of zinc daily for a month, were found of having significantly higher testosterone and thyroid hormone levels (309) when compared to placebo group which saw steady decreases in both of the hormones due to excessive workload, the likely explanation being that the placebo group lost plenty of zinc through sweating on a daily basis, and their diets weren't sufficient enough to replace the lost mineral in their bodies. On the supplementation group however, the trend was not only to preserve testosterone, but also to increase both free and total testosterone levels from the baseline at both states; rest and exhaustion.

The same researchers went and reproduced the study with 10 young "sedentary male volunteers" in 2007 (310) using the same dosage of zinc for the same duration of time. The men were subjected to *"fatiguing bicycle exercise"* during those 4-weeks and as in their previous study, zinc supplementation was able to maintain and increase total and free testosterone levels, as well as thyroid hormones when compared to placebo pill. These two studies suggest that at least in exercising population, supplementation with zinc is beneficial for hormonal health. Since both of the studies saw improvements in free-testosterone levels, it's also plausible that zinc can inhibit serum SHBG levels and leave more testosterone bio-available for the androgen receptors.

In patients suffering from chronic renal failure (a condition linked to significantly depleted zinc levels) mega-dosing with 250mg/day of zinc was – as to be expected – able to significantly increase serum zinc, testosterone, and LH levels. (311)

Another study consisting of 37 infertile-subjects (312) had the men take an undisclosed amount of zinc for 6-months and noted that the men who had testosterone levels on the lower end (less than 480 ng/dL) noticed significant improvements in testosterone and DHT levels, whereas the men on the higher levels of testosterone (more than 480 ng/dL) noted no increases in testosterone, but still significant increases in DHT levels. On an even more positive note, Nine of the subjects were able to conceive a child during the study period.

When it comes to animal and cell-culture studies, zinc administration has been noted to significantly increase testosterone, LH, and DHT levels (313, 314) while reducing the activity of the female-hormone estrogen towards it receptors by 57%. (315) Surprisingly enough, one in-vitro study done on isolated cells (316) noted that zinc can inhibit DHT production, however this doesn't seem to happen when humans take it orally as you can see from the above studies…

So does zinc increase testosterone levels?

Answer: Yes. At least if you're deficient in the mineral and/or exercise a lot. In the fortunate case where your zinc levels are already saturated, you'll probably just see increases in DHT, which isn't a bad thing at all.

Does it block estrogen?

Answer: Yes, this seems to happen in isolated cells at least.

How much zinc can I take?

Answer: Mega-dosing with 100 mg's of zinc daily has been shown to be safe in long term studies (2-4 months).

However if you megadose with the mineral, make sure that you're also supplementing with copper as too much zinc will deplete the body from it.

A good rule of thumb is to take them at 10:1 ratio (that means that you take 1mg of copper for every 10mg's of zinc).

What's the most bio-available form of zinc to supplement with?

Answer: We at Anabolic Men recommend and use the high quality zinc picolinate from Thorne Research. Other quality choices would be citrate and orotate.

I've heard that calcium should be avoided when taking zinc?

Answer: Calcium, zinc, magnesium, and iron all bind to the same receptors inside the body, however the receptors can uptake around 800 mg's of minerals, so unless you're mega-dosing on all of them simultaneously, you should be fine in terms of absorption.

Conclusion

Every guy interested in natural hormone optimization should be aware of zinc.

It's the master mineral of the endocrine system. Correcting micronutrient deficiencies is one of the key factors in healthy natural testosterone production, and zinc just happens to be one of the key minerals to make sure you're getting plenty of.

In my opinion, if you're not eating a ton of oysters and meat every day, zinc supplementation would be a valid option, and since the mineral is lost via sweat the people who exercise should be extra sure to keep their zinc levels topped... And for such purposes, the well absorbing *zinc picolinate supplement from Thorne Research* should work perfectly. It's the most potent form with greatest bio-availability, and dirt cheap to supplement with.

Foods Rich In Zinc

Zinc is an extremely important mineral for testosterone and thyroid hormone production, studies constantly show how deficiency can slash the levels of total and -free testosterone, as well as T3 and T4 thyroid hormones, (317) restoration of zinc is able to rapidly restore these crucial hormones.

The RDA for zinc is set to around 15mg/day for normal sized male, this is relatively easy to get from foods, and can also be supplemented in highly bio-available form of zinc piliconate.

Athletes should definitely be consuming more zinc than the RDA as it evaporates through the sweat.

Another worthwhile mention is that correcting a zinc deficiency is much easier to do with animal based zinc rather than plant-based, as animal sources are much denser in the mineral and also because the zinc from animal sources is better assimilated by the body.

Here's your five best high-zinc foods:

1. Oysters

When it comes to zinc – and being testosterone friendly – oysters fit the bill.

They're ridiculously high in zinc, 100g of them containing a whopping 78mg's of zinc (524% of the RDA).

Oysters are also high in some other micronutrients necessary for healthy testosterone production, such as; selenium, vitamin D, and copper, and they're chock-full of high quality protein.

The legend says that the famous ladies-man, Casanova, ate 50 oysters for breakfast to enhance his libido, he obviously knew what he was doing.

2. Beef (Especially Lamb)

Red meat should be a staple in every man's diet, due to it being one of the best sources of high-quality protein for testosterone production, as well as containing the perfect T-boosting fatty-acids; palmitic acid and stearic acid.

On top of that, beef – especially the kind from lamb – is very high in bio-available zinc.

100g of lamb beef contains roughly 12mg's of zinc (82% of the RDA).

NOTE: *When you eat plenty of steak (muscle meat), be sure to also include some collagen (connective tissue protein) into the mix to get a more balanced amino acid profile. The easiest way to do this is by consuming some gelatin.*

3. Raw Cacao Products

Raw (unheated) cacao products are beneficial for erectile and vascular health. Their high antioxidant content makes them quite possibly one of the healthiest foods on this planet.

But when choosing cacao products, the key is that they're **a)** unheated **b)** have high cacao percentage.

The basic super-market "milk-chocolate" is unfortunately far from that. The kind you should look for is slightly bitter dark chocolate, if it's unheated its probably labeled as "raw".

100g of raw cacao without any processing contains up to 7mg's of zinc (45% of RDA). It's without a doubt the best source of zinc for someone who refuses to eat animal-products.

4. Egg Yolk

Eggs make for damn near perfect testosterone boosting food.

The protein is high-quality with good amino acid balance, it's chock full of micronutrients, and it also contains cholesterol and some fat to make those nutrients absorb well to the body.

One of the micronutrients found high amounts in egg yolks is zinc. *100g of egg yolks can contain up to 5mg's of the mineral (33% of RDA). This means that you'd have to eat quite a few eggs to actually get all your daily zinc from eggs, regardless, it's still one of the best food sources of the mineral.*

5. Liver

Animal liver is a nutritional powerhouse. containing some connective tissue protein, high amounts of necessary fat-soluble vitamins, and bunch of other goodies.

Beef liver also packs 4mg's of zinc per 100g, making it a decent testosterone-friendly source of zinc.

Since liver is a storage organ for many micronutrients, eating it is like consuming a naturally occurring multi-vitamin…

…Just take a look at this chart comparing liver to vegetables, fruit, and muscle-meat, (318) liver outshines them all when it comes to overall vitamin and mineral levels.

Conclusion

There you go, 5 best testosterone-friendly foods rich in zinc.

If you feel that you can't meet your daily zinc requirements (~15mg/day for sedentary people, 30-45mg/day for someone involved in exercise)…

…consider getting yourself a high quality supplement containing bioavailable zinc like Testro-X or zinc picolinate supplement.

— Chapter 21 —

Boron

There are multiple micronutrients (vitamins and minerals) that contribute to testosterone synthesis, such as: vitamins A, C, D, K2, zinc, magnesium, iodine, calcium, etc...

...But what is often left unmentioned is the trace mineral boron. When in fact it's the boron that currently holds the most impressive results on natural T production in terms of scientific evidence.

Many experts believe that we're getting significantly less boron through the diet than our ancestors did, and this is because the modern day "power farming" quickly depletes the soil in which our food is grown, leaving less boron – and less of multiple other naturally occurring micronutrients – into the end product.

But is boron something you'd want to miss from the diet? Definitely not according to the research which shows the benefits of boron:

Boron and Testosterone Levels

Boron is a rare mineral on Earth, and in this whole universe. And this is because boron is a "trace leftover" of the big bang, arriving Earth via cosmic dust and meteor materials...

...Hence why only about 0.001% of the Earths crust is boron.

Not only is boron rare in the Earth, it's also somewhat uncommon as a supplemental micronutrient. It isn't even included in the list of "essential vitamins and minerals for human survival", and there isn't a set minimum requirement for dietary boron (although it has a RDI of ~3 mg/day).

However – as unnecessary as boron may seem like – what most of the guys don't know is that boron can be easily labeled as a natural testosterone booster. This one ridiculously cheap and unpopular trace mineral is actually much more effective in raising ones natural T production than most of the "T-Booster" products flying of the shelves at your local GNC are...

Take this study from Naghii et al. (319) as an example. The researchers in this trial gave eight of their male subjects ~10 mg's of boron supplement, every morning for 7 consecutive days. After the week had passed, the scientists compared their subjects blood results from day 0 to day 7, and found out that:

- free testosterone levels had increased by 28%
- free estrogen levels had decreased by -39%
- dihydrotestosterone (DHT) levels rose by 10%
- many inflammation biomarkers (hsCRP, TNF-α) dropped significantly

NOTE: The same researchers measured testosterone levels on their subjects in a study conducted in 1997 (320) set to examine boron's effects on cardiovascular risk, in that trial 10 mg's of daily boron increased total testosterone levels by 15%, slight increases were also seen in total estrogen levels, which should be noted.

Another study from Mjilkovich et al. (321) looked how boron supplementation impacts serum vitamin D levels, but on the side they also measured free testosterone levels. After 2 months of giving their 13 subject males 6 mg's of daily boron (*calcium fructo-borate*) the levels of free testosterone had increased by 29.5% on average, a number similar to the findings of Naghii et al.

Two rodent studies (322, 323) examining boron's toxicity have also found significant dose-dependent increases in testosterone levels after boron supplementation, highest dose (500 mg/day) leading to a massive 160% increase. Though this amount – not only crazily expensive – would be highly toxic also, since dosages exceeding 25 mg/day start showing symptoms of toxicity and are not recommended.

Conclusion on Boron Testosterone Supplementation

There's good amount of scientific evidence speaking for the health benefits of boron. It has the ability to increase testosterone levels in healthy human males, and in rodents, and also in women (with boron deficiency).

That is why I recommend you take a boron testosterone supplement.

A dose range that should be able to increase testosterone levels (without becoming toxic) falls in between 3-25 mg/day.

Aside from supplementation (Testro-X contains a healthy 10mg boron per serving), some good dietary boron sources include: *raisins, gelatin, prunes, dates, avocados, almonds, Brazil nuts, and honey.*

Foods Rich In Boron

Boron might not be one of the 24 essential micronutrients for human survival, but it still has some interesting benefits in terms of testosterone production.

More specifically, boron at 10mg for 7-days was able to;

- *increase free testosterone levels by 28%*
- *decrease free estrogen levels by -39%*
- *boost DHT by 10%*

Similar results were seen in a study that used 6mg's of boron for a bit longer duration (29% increase in free testosterone levels). (324)

Supplementation is without a doubt the easiest way to get 6-10mg's of boron per day, but there are also a handful of foods loaded with the trace mineral.

1. Raisins

The densest known nutritional source of boron is raisins.

100 grams of them contain a whopping 3mg's of boron, which is 100% of the RDA and about half of the recommended amount to impact testosterone production.

Fitting in a cup or two of raisins per day is a great way to make sure you're getting enough boron on a daily basis. Raisins can also further benefit testosterone production by being a good source of resveratrol, which may also stimulate testosterone synthesis. (325)

When it comes to raisins, we recommend **organic Californian kind.**

2. Avocado

Avocados are pretty great for testosterone production. They're very dense in nutrients, and the fatty-acid profile is great for T levels.

When it comes to boron, 100 grams of avocados have 2mg's of the trace mineral, which accounts to about 65% of the RDA.

Getting the boron requirements to impact testosterone levels (6-10mg) solely from avocado might not be wise, as this would mean eating at least 300 grams of the fruit, which is pretty dense in calories and can easily aid in putting you to a caloric surplus (sure this isn't bad for skinny guys, but if you're trying to lose weight, maybe just eat raisins or get a boron supplement).

When buying avocados, remove the small stem part on the top, if you find that the stem peels of easily and there's green underneath it, you've got yourself a perfectly ripe specimen.

3. Brazil Nuts

Brazil nuts are awesome.

They're mainly praised for their very high selenium content (2 of them is actually enough to fulfill the daily need), (326) but Brazil nuts are also good source of boron.

100 grams of them contain 1.7mg's of boron, which is 55% of the RDA, making Brazil nuts a good testosterone boosting food to use for covering the daily needs of boron.

Maybe make a snack trail mix with Brazil nuts and raisins? Just remember to choose the kind with plenty of skin, as that's where most of the minerals are.

4. Prunes

Similarly to raisins, prunes (dried plums), are also loaded with boron.

100 grams of prunes provides you with 1.1mg's of boron, which is about 35% of the RDA.

Combine them into a snack mix with raisins and Brazil nuts, and you got yourself a great boron-rich testosterone boosting snack.

Prunes are also loaded with antioxidants, which is as you might know, great for testosterone production.

5. Dried Apricots

Dried apricots are not only delicious, but also a nutritional powerhouse providing decent amounts of vitamins A, C and E...

...Along with plenty of important antioxidants.

What makes apricots awesome for testosterone production, is their relatively high amount of boron, as 100 grams of dried apricots provides 2mg's of boron (66% RDA).

Add them to a trail mix of raisins, prunes, and Brazil nuts, and you got yourself boron to spare.

Conclusion

Boron is great for total and free testosterone levels, but sometimes getting it from foods can be tricky (hence why in some cases supplementation is ideal).

So stock up on raisins, avocados, prunes, Brazil nuts, and dried prunes.

— Chapter 22 —

Calcium

Calcium is the fifth most-abundant mineral in the crust of the planet Earth. In humans 99% of the calcium in our bodies is located in bones and teeth...

...The 1% that's left has a role on various processes inside the human body, such as cellular functioning, neurotransmitter release (think dopamine), muscle contraction, conducting the heart, etc.

Which is why calcium is one of the 20 essential vitamins & minerals for human survival.

The governmental recommendation for calcium is roughly 1 gram a day for normal sized adult male. In my opinion you should aim a bit higher than that, while also adding in vitamin D, magnesium, boron, and vitamin K2, which all work in a synergy with calcium.

If you're consuming plenty of products that already contain calcium (milk, cheese, yogurt, etc), extra supplementation might not be that useful. For example, here in Finland – and if I recall correctly, in the whole Scandinavia – milk consumption is so high that calcium supplementation would be somewhat just a waste of money.

The thing that got me interested in calcium however, is the fact that it seems to have a role in testosterone production.

Here's what I'm talking about:

Calcium and Testosterone

Calcium is not that often linked to testosterone production, but still, there are a few studies that show some promising results with the mineral.

The researchers aren't even sure how calcium works to increase testosterone...

...Few logical explanations could be the fact that it controls neurotransmitter release (dopamine for example rises in correlation with T), and plays a role in cellular functioning (which in theory could improve the signaling between cells and hormones).

Whatever the reason, here's what the studies say:

a) Back in 1976 a group of researchers studied the effects of calcium ions on isolated rat leydig cells. (327) They found out that in combination with luteinizing hormone (LH), calcium significantly increased testosterone synthesis. When the researchers tested LH's effects on the cells without the calcium, the increase in testosterone was significantly smaller.

b) 33 Years later, this study gets published in the Journal of Biological Trace Element Research. (328) The researchers found out that calcium supplementation (35 mg/kg) didn't really alter testosterone levels on the subjects who remained sedentary when compared to placebo. However there were also two groups on the study that did resistance training for 90 minutes, 5 days a week. The first group received 35 mg/kg of calcium, and the other group got a placebo pill.

Both of the training groups noted increases in their testosterone levels. However the group that received the extra calcium had 18% higher free testosterone levels after the workout than the placebo group did.

The researchers weren't sure why calcium was able to increase the amount of bio-available testosterone in resistance trained men, but they suspect that it increases the sensitivity of the messenger hormones LH and FSH.

Conclusion on Research

Calcium seems to increase free testosterone in men who practice resistance training. The mechanism of action is somewhat unknown, and more studies are needed to validate the claims.

All-in-all, you should probably consider a calcium supplement if you're not a big fan of dairy products, but still love to workout.

Foods Rich In Calcium

It also has a role in testosterone production, and of course, in maintaining healthy bones and teeth. If you can't get enough from your diet, it's highly recommended that you consume it daily in supplement form.

Here are five foods high in calcium that also fit a testosterone boosting diet:

1. Cheese

Cheese is a good source of high quality casein protein, along with good amount of testosterone boosting saturated fat.

Its also rich in multiple important vitamins and minerals for testosterone production, such as: vitamins K2, A, selenium, and zinc. And then there's the calcium. Cheese is the richest known natural source of calcium with 100 grams of Cheddar cheese having 721mg's of calcium, covering 72% of the RDA.

NOTE: *There is some mixed evidence towards high-fat dairy products having hormone traces which could lower testosterone levels, (329) so if you wan't to be extra sure that this doesn't affect you, opt for low-fat dairy, it still has the calcium.*

2. Eggshells

What you do with eggshells after using the insides? Throw it away?

Mistake. Eggshells are one of the best natural sources of calcium and you should eat them.

Not whole, obviously. Instead, make natural eggshell calcium supplement by:

1 Fill a stock pot with some water, bring to boil.
2 Pour the eggshells into the water (this destroys pathogens).
3 Cook for 10 minutes and then drain the pot.
4 put the eggshells on a baking tin and allow to dry for a day.
5 Use coffee grinder or pestle & mortar to grind the dry shells into powder.
6 Store the powder in a jar.

Now, you have high quality calcium supplement, with a teaspoon providing you the 1000mg's (100% RDA) of calcium.

3. Milk

Like all dairy products, milk is rich in calcium.

And just like the cheese above, it's rich in high-quality casein protein, and some key micronutrients like zinc and selenium.

100 grams of milk (1dl or 3.3oz if you're from US) contains 125mg's of calcium, which covers 12% of the RDA.

Drinking a liter (usually whole carton) of milk per day is a great way to get in that quality protein and all of your needed calcium.

4. Yogurt

Yogurt is filled with probiotics that have shown to favorably impact testosterone levels in studies.

Yogurt is also a relatively good source of protein and certain micronutrients such as zinc and iodine.

When it comes to calcium, 100 grams of yogurt provides 110mg's of calcium (11% RDA).

We at Anabolic Men recommend few servings of grass-fed yogurt daily, mostly due to its probiotic density but also to cover vitamin and mineral intake.

5. Leafy Greens

If you're not a fan of dairy products or eggshell calcium, you may find that it's really hard to cover the daily need for calcium through foods.

Which is why we recommend high-quality multivitamin supplementation for everyone not consuming plenty of dairy products.

Aside from dairy, eggshells, and calcium supplements, there is one group of foods that still ranks pretty high in calcium content...

...And that's the leafy greens, such as:

- kale (150mg/100g)
- *spinach (99mg/100g)*
- *collard greens (232mg/100g)*
- *mustard greens (115mg/100g)*

NOTE: *Another great benefit of eating lots of leafy greens is their high natural nitrate content which can beneficially impact erection quality.*

Conclusion

Calcium is essential - for life and for testosterone.

These 5 foods are the best natural testosterone-friendly sources of this very important mineral and if you can't eat enough of these (and I'd say even if you can), consider using a high-quality calcium supplement.

Chapter 23

Selenium

Selenium is mostly known for its antioxidant properties, due to the fact that its a necessary micronutrient in the creation of glutathione (the body's principal antioxidant compound).

Selenium also works in conjunction with vitamin E and C to prevent oxidative damage in the body, and with iodine to upregulate thyroid function and metabolic rate.

Multiple studies have shown that high selenium levels positively correlate with high serum testosterone levels and sperm quality in men.

Here are five foods rich in selenium:

1. Brazil Nuts

Highly intelligent Capuchin monkeys are known of loving the nutritious Brazil nuts. They like them so much that they have learned to use rocks as tools to open the thick shells protecting them. (330)

When it comes to humans, I believe that all men should be consuming few of these nutrient bombs on a daily basis.

They're incredibly rich in boron, magnesium, phosphorus, zinc, and manganese, with good fatty-acid ratios in terms of testosterone production...

...And then there is the selenium content. 100 grams of Brazil nuts contain a staggering 1917 mcg's (3485% RDA) of selenium, so much that just two of them per day is enough to meet the daily needs.

2. Grass-Fed Beef

Grass-fed beef should be one of your top protein sources if the goal is to increase testosterone levels.

The high-quality animal protein, saturated fat, several micronutrients, and carnitine make it optimal protein source for hormone production.

When it comes to selenium, there's plenty in grass-fed beef, however not quite as much as in Brazil nuts.

100 grams of grass-fed beef can contain up to 35 mcg's of selenium (63% RDA).

3. Egg Yolks

The yolk of an egg contains nearly all of the necessary vitamins and minerals for human survival.

It also has fat and cholesterol which significantly improve the absorption of the micronutrients.

And the amino-acid profile of eggs is considered optimal for human needs, making eggs "complete protein".

Not a big surprise that eggs are also a great natural source of selenium. 100 grams of the yolks provide 56 mcg's of selenium (101% RDA).

4. Wild Sardines

Sardines are one of the best seafoods to consume for a testosterone optimized diet.

They are filled with high-quality protein and several micronutrients.

Just be sure when buying sardines that you're not paying for farmed fish, which is fed with soy pellets and ridiculously high in heavy-metals.

100 grams of wild sardines contain 52 mcg of selenium (94% RDA).

5. Oysters

Oysters are a man's best friend, on a plate that is.

It has been said that the famous ladies man, Casanova, ate 50 of them every morning to keep up his libido. He might of have been on to something.

Oysters are very high in certain pro-testosterone micronutrients like zinc, magnesium, and vitamin D, and they contain high-quality animal protein that nourishes the endocrine system.

Then there's the selenium. 100 grams of oysters provide you with 71 mcg's (129% RDA).

Conclusion

There are many foods naturally high in selenium, most notable of these are Brazil nuts.

In fact, if you feel like you can't get enough selenium from the foods that you eat regularly, I would say don't buy a selenium supplement.

Instead get a bag of Brazil nuts, since two of them have all the daily selenium you need.

There's this endangered specie of monkeys, called the Chapuchin monkeys, who actively search for these nuts covered with a thick shell...

...Only the strongest and wisest monkeys are able to crack the shells open, but once they finally succeed, they're famous for the next day or two, because in the world of the Chapuchin monkeys, the male with the Brazil nuts is the ultimate alpha male.

I'm eating a handful of Brazil nuts daily, and Tim Ferriss who sports a testosterone level of 1200+ ng/dl mentions them in his quick "triple your testosterone guide"...

...But why?

Here's a low-down on why the Brazil nut is awesome:

Brazil Nuts And Testosterone

There's hardly any science backing up the use of Brazil nuts as a testosterone booster, but I think we don't even need science to crack this nut…

…You see, Brazil nuts contain so much pro-testosterone building blocks, that they simply have to increase natural testosterone production.

Here's what I'm talking about:

1. **Packed with selenium** – Brazil nuts are the richest known source for bio-active selenium in the whole planet, and selenium has been linked to elevated testosterone levels. (331) Brazil nuts are actually so rich in selenium, that even as little as 1-2 Brazil nuts can easily fill the daily requirements of selenium.

2. **Contains Natural Cholesterol** – Cholesterol gets converted into testosterone inside the leydig cells of testes, and that's the main reason why men should never underestimate the power of this wonderful nutrient which should definitely be the staple in every high testosterone diet.

The good news: Brazil nuts are filled with bio-active natural cholesterol, which will work wonders for your natural testosterone production.

3. **Strong antioxidant** – Brazil nuts are filled with antioxidants known for protecting your sensitive testosterone molecules from oxidization. Recent studies also show that certain antioxidants will stimulate the leydig cells to produce more testosterone. (332)

4. High in L-Arginine – Arginine is a substance that will significantly increase your nitric oxide production, (333) which means that your veins will dilate and relax allowing your blood to flow more freely. *The good news:* Brazil nuts are packed with the most bio-active form of Arginine.

5. Improves Sperm Quality – The 2013 Journal of Andrology reported that dietary selenium was able to significantly increase sperm quality, volume, and motility. (334) The quality of your sperm is highly linked to testosterone levels, as it's a scientific fact that men who have the highest testosterone, also tend to have the highest sperm counts.

Conclusion

These cheap nuts are amazing for your testosterone levels, and I can easily say that the Brazil nut qualifies to be a valid testosterone booster in my books.

When purchasing Brazil nuts, keep in mind that most of the selenium content is in the skin, so for maximal testosterone boosting benefits, always purchase these bad boys with as much skin as possible. Also avoid all the salted and roasted kinds, the more natural, the better.

— Chapter 24 —

Copper

Copper (Cu) is definitely not the first thing that comes to mind when we talk about testosterone boosting micronutrients, or just about plain minerals. All-in-all, it's a very unpopular mineral to supplement with, and nobody really cares about copper.

But I think we should be a little more interested in our copper intake than what we are now...

...Because chelated copper could actually increase testosterone levels, when taken at optimal dosages.

Here's what I'm talking about:

Copper and Testosterone Production

Copper is an essential trace element in both humans and animals, and the recommended daily allowance (RDA) for copper in normal sized human male is about 3mg/day.

It has multiple important functions in the human body, including: oxygen transportation, iron uptake facilitation, photosynthesis, etc.

Copper deficiency is also associated with thyroid problems, impaired growth, osteoporosis, and with abnormal glucose and cholesterol metabolism.

But is copper deficiency actually a problem for most people?

…And is there any need for supplementation in the first place?

Answer: Severe copper deficiency is not that common, and people who eat balanced whole-food diets, should be able to meet their daily copper needs from dietary sources alone (oysters, kale, mushrooms, nuts, avocados, and fermented foods are all high in copper).

However, there are two very important facts about copper that you should take under consideration. Firstly, almost all kinds of dietary copper is poorly absorbed by the human body (30-40%)… (335)

…And secondly, eating a lot of zinc depletes copper from the body (and vice versa). As zinc is known to boost testosterone levels, many men tend to supplement with high-dose zinc supplements on a daily basis, without taking in any copper to balance that zinc-induced depletion (optimal ratio of zinc and copper is considered to be between 10:1 and 10:2).

Basically if you supplement with 30 mg's of zinc per day, then you should also take 3-6 mg's of copper to balance out the zinc-induced copper depletion.

With that out of the way, we can finally get to the actual subject.

Here's why you don't want to be depleted in copper:

a) In this old in-vitro study, (336) the researchers saw that when isolated hypothalamic cells were altered to chelated copper complexes, gonadotropin releasing hormone (GnRH) increased by a nice 68%. As GnRH is basically the hormone that starts the whole cascade of events that lead to testosterone production, even a slight boost in it should increase testosterone levels. To what degree this happens when chelated copper is orally ingested? Hard to say.

b) This Indian study (337) wanted to take the above experiment further, and they decided to inject copper chloride straight into the guts of living male wistar rats for 26 consecutive days, with varying doses (1000 mcg, 2000 mcg, and 3000 mcg/kg).

They found out that the 1000 mcg dose significantly increased testosterone levels via luteinizing hormone (LH) stimulation. Which supports the findings of the first study above.

However, the 2000 mcg and 3000 mcg doses started to become toxic for the rats, and on the higher dosed groups, testosterone was actually decreased. Several human studies have also found out that when copper intake gets too high, it becomes unhealthy and toxic, but lower intake is absolutely essential for the health of the human body (338, 339, 340).

c) Then there's this other quite old in-vitro study, (341) which found out that when isolated hypothalamic neurons were altered to chelated copper, luteinizing hormone (LH) release increased by 45%. As LH is the hormone that stimulates testosterone synthesis inside the ballsack, these findings furthermore support the theory that copper should increase testosterone production.

To put that all together, there's evidence that a modest dose of chelated copper could increase testosterone levels by stimulating the release of GnRH and LH. And there seems to be a toxicity limit where everything backfires once the copper intake gets to be too high. Of course we have to also remember that these are only studies done on isolated cells and rats. To which degree these results can be seen when humans take oral copper? It will remain unknown until someone decides to study that. The mechanism exists for sure though.

Conclusion

In the view of this evidence, I would highly recommend you to keep your copper levels in check, either by eating a diet rich in whole-foods, or by supplementing with bio-available chelated copper.

What is the optimal dose for chelated copper you might ask?

Personally I take either 2x the daily RDA (2 x 3mg's) if I'm not supplementing with zinc. When I do supplement with zinc though, I take some copper with it to balance out the zinc-induced copper depletion.

For this I follow the optimal human ratio of zinc and copper (10:1-2), meaning that if I take 30 mg's of zinc, I also take 6 mg's of copper (on top of the 2 x RDA).

— Chapter 25 —

Vitamin K2

There's one vitamin that really deserves a whole lot more attention than what it's getting now, and that's the vitamin K2 (menaquinone). Heck, most people don't even know that it exists, nor that it reduces cardiovascular disease risk, (342) and greatly enhances bone formation. (343)

Actually, there are thousands of different forms of vitamin K, but the ones that we associate with the term are the K1 (phylloquinone), and K2 (menaquinone).

For some odd reason, the K1 form, which is present in almost all leafy green vegetables is getting all of the attention in media.

While nobody seems to talk about the K2 from, which can be found in foods such as: cheese, egg yolks, butter, fermented foods, and liver.

Our diets contain roughly 10 times more K1 than K2. And a common misconception is that we wouldn't need K2 since the human body would convert K1 into K2. But even though the occurrence is seen on animals, the human body doesn't seem to do it as effectively. In fact, recent studies suggests that we need to consume the actual K2 form in order to get the benefits (344, 345).

The benefits you ask? Well, aside from K2 being awesome for our cardiovascular health and bone density, especially when taken in stack with vitamin D, there's a bunch of other great effects associated with vitamin K2 supplementation…

…And one of them is the link between vitamin K2 and testosterone:

Vitamin K2 and Testosterone Synthesis

The importance of vitamin K2 is quite a new thing, even to most researchers. And that's because for a long time, it was believed that the K1 form was all that we need, and that both of the vitamins (K1 and K2) would of have had similar effects.

However a few recent studies have proved this to be not true at all. For example: in this study, (346) vitamin K2 supplementation reduced prostate cancer risk by 30%, whereas vitamin K1 had no effect. And then this study (347) where vitamin K2 significantly lowered cardiovascular disease risk by removing calcium deposits from arteries, but vitamin K1 again, had no effect.

The forms of vitamin K2 that we're most deficient in are the MK-7 and MK-4.

- MK-7 is produced inside our gastrointestinal system, we can get it from fermented foods. MK-7 is also considered to be very effective in terms of supplementation, as it lasts for roughly three days in the bloodstream.

- MK-4 is synthesized all over the body from enzymes (being exceptionally high in the brain and reproductive organs). We can get it through diet by consuming grass-fed animal meats (grain-fed doesn't contain it). You can also supplement with MK-4, but it only lasts for roughly 8 hours in the bloodstream, and therefore is considered to be worse for supplementation than MK-7.

Still there's one major reason why I consider the MK-4 form to be superior to the more long lasting MK-7. And that's because it has a mechanism to increase testosterone production:

a) In this Japanese study, (348) Asagi et al. fed 75 mg/kg of vitamin K2 (MK-4) to male Wistar rats for 5 weeks, while simultaneously measuring the testosterone content from their blood plasma and testicles. The results after the fifth week showed a nice, more than 70% increase in plasma testosterone levels, and an even bigger increase was seen inside the testes (nearly 90%). And as you can see from the pictures below, luteinizing hormone (LH) levels didn't budge, which probably means that the K2 works by stimulating testosterone production directly inside the ballsack, and not via the brain.

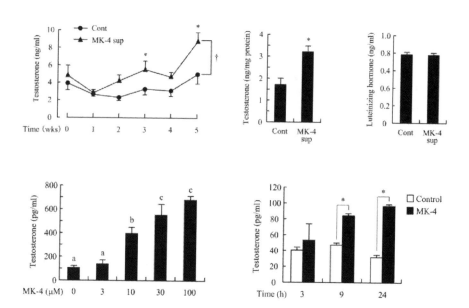

b) In the same study which is presented above, the scientists tested vitamin K2 (MK-4) incubation directly on the testicular I-10 cells inside a petri dish, and found out that the more MK-4 they exposed to the cells, the more testosterone was produced.

c) Another Japanese study (349) from different researchers found out rather similar results. They saw that in male rats, vitamin K2 deficiency reduces testosterone levels significantly, as it messes up with the genes involved in the biosynthesis of testosterone from cholesterol. When these rats were given vitamin K2 (MK-4), their testosterone levels increased rapidly. Similar results were seen in this study.

Conclusion

The studies above are somewhat solid proof of the fact that vitamin K2 (MK-4) has a mechanism of increasing testosterone levels, but so far the mechanism has only been tested on rodents and isolated testicular cells. And the dosages used in the rat studies are abnormally high.

The human equivalent of the dosage in the first study is 12mg/kg. That's a huge dose. Given that 45 mg's is considered to be the upper safe limit for humans. I doubt that you'd ever need to take that high dose of vitamin K2 to actually see the benefits, but when there's no human studies on its hormonal effects, you can't really tell...

There will be a time when K2 supplementation is tested similarly in humans, but before it happens, I have no problem supplementing with 30-45 mg's of vitamin K2 (MK-4) once every few days, just to maintain heart and bone health. And if there's a bonus testosterone boost happening in the background, I wouldn't mind at all.

— Chapter 26 —

Choline

Why do you feel so run down, exhausted, irritable, and unmotivated?

Why do you feel as if you are stuck in a persistent brain fog? Is it stress? Fatigue? Depression? It could be all of the above and this could be caused by a choline deficiency leading to lowered levels of testosterone and decreased overall brain and physical health.

Choline is one of the most important compounds our body needs.

However, most of the Western population is massively deficient in choline. And the use of cholinergic drugs, pharmaceuticals, and high stress lifestyles, coupled with a general lack of dietary choline consumption has left many of us in a state of constant brain fog and irritability. Our brain heavily relies on choline for neurotransmission so it's no wonder we feel out of whack when our choline is low.

I'd like to introduce you to the wonderful choline, and give some tips on choline food sources as well as which types you should supplement with.

The Importance of Choline

A key nutrient for the human diet is choline. Choline, commonly grouped in the B vitamin family, is integral to many human body functions some of which are brain, liver, cellular, and endocrine system.

Choline has been known to help reduce symptoms of depression, memory loss, and seizures. Endurance athletes also use choline as an aid to build and maintain muscle as well as combat fatigue throughout peak training periods.

Side effects of low levels of choline include difficulty focusing, low levels of energy, and brain fog. Deficiency in choline is no joke, it can lead to increased threat of a condition known as Fatty Liver, which results from slowed metabolizing of fat and increased accumulation of lipids in the liver.

Choline deficiency also slows the processes of the nervous system decreasing vital neurotransmission throughout the body. If the brain does not get enough choline to maintain proper neurotransmission, it may resort to cannibalizing cell walls in order to obtain additional choline... plus it lends to a higher risk of memory loss and mental disorders.

Choline as a Natural Libido-Booster

As soon as your body catches wind of choline, it processes it for expedited shipping in the form of neurotransmitters and sends the messages to...well, your package (too much?).

The arrival of choline prompts the release of nitric oxide, which is said to be the main center stage neurotransmitter and chemical mediator of erectile functioning. To put it bluntly, choline sparks the fire that helps you maintain a healthy erection. Other hormonal benefits of choline are increased mood, energy, and motivation which can lend to overall increase in sex drive. Well, I say that's a pretty good delivery.

Popular High Choline Food Sources

Now that you know the importance of choline and what it can do for your testosterone levels, the question is how can you get more choline in your life? Choline is obtained mostly through the diet.

The modern diet, which tends to be geared more towards convenience and ease rather than obtaining the key nutrients the body needs, is lacking in choline.

The increased use of microwaves (heat is a real buzz kill for choline) along with the degrading quality of food, and the fast food culture has resulted in less and less choline in the modern human's diet.

Bottom line, choline is important…really important. The next section will guide you through ways in which you can specifically supplement your diet with choline.

Dietary Choline Supplementation

Though there is no official recommended Daily Value of choline in the human diet, the National Academy of Sciences recommends **a minimum daily intake of 550 mg for adult males**. Choline is found in the form of phosphatidylcholine. Phosphatidylcholine is a lecithin and the most abundant phospholipid in all cells. This lecithin can be found in the following foods:

- **Proteins:** Egg yolks (best if consumed raw), meat livers and kidneys, veal, beef, chicken, cod, salmon, caviar, pork, and beans
- **Carbs:** Brussel sprouts, wheat germ, broccoli, spinach, bok choy, cauliflower, cabbage and mushrooms (consume with grass-fed ghee, this aids in the absorption of the nutrients)
- **Fats:** Peanut butter, almond butter, vegetable oil, and yogurt, kefir, and raw milk

The best way to obtain choline in food form is from animal products. Foods such as nuts, and legumes contain anti-nutrients that may decrease choline absorption. These foods can be consumed, but it is suggested that they are consumed in moderation.

When natural sources of choline are not enough, some may find it beneficial to seek a supplement to aid in maintaining a healthy level of choline in the body. **Cortigon**, an all-natural cortisol suppressant nootropic blend aimed at lowering cortisol levels and increasing mental clarity, focus, memory and learning, is a great supplemental source of Cortigon.

Cortigon, being a nootropic supplement, can have a positive impact on intelligence and cognitive function as well as aid in the maintaining of choline levels.

Avoiding a Choline Deficiency

Now that you know what choline is, how it can impact your testosterone, and what you can do to supplement your diet with the likes of its greatness, the choice is yours: live in a brain fog of tired moodiness and low sex drive, or get out there and be the man.

Chapter 27

Iodine

Lack of iodine makes us sick, fat, and lazy. Frankly lack of this mineral affects almost all of us and here's why:

There are 4 different halogens that we're constantly in contact with. 3 Of them are toxic to the human body which are fluoride, bromine, and chlorine.

However there's still one halogen that is extremely essential to the human body, as it's virtually needed in every single cell and gland of your body, especially in your thyroid where it's the number #1 compound that regulates almost all of your hormones and bodily functions.

This one extremely important halogen is called iodine.

Sadly our world has fucked up this halogen stuff majorly. As we shouldn't be in any contact with fluoride, bromine, or chlorine because they're more lighter than iodine, which means that these 3 halogens will flush iodine out of your body, and take its place inside your cells.

This occurrence will then lead to lowered thyroid levels, which then leads to lowered hormone levels, which then leads to low testosterone, low dopamine, low serotonin, low growth hormone, etc.

It will also cause the calcification of your glands, including: pineal gland, thyroid gland, hypothalamus, and your beloved testicles.

Sounds pretty horrible right? Well it's true and it's happening inside of your body right now as you're reading this piece of text.

There's one simple reason for that: <u>You're bombing your own body with those 3 toxic halides,</u> and you have been doing so for your whole life.

Why?

Your toothpaste is full of fluoride, our water supply has been shown to contain fluoride and chlorine, commercial bread uses bromide as a dough conditioner, and so on.

All of that shit will drive away the much needed iodine, that's what makes you sick, and that's the leading cause to hypogonadism and low testosterone. It's a cold hard fact.

Fortunately you don't have to stand for this any longer because now you know better.

<u>So here's what you need to do if you really wan't to take control of your own hormones and health</u>:

Stop consuming those 3 toxic halides. Switch to fluoride free toothpaste, drink spring water, eat organic foods, and stop swimming in chlorinated pools.

Then once you've gotten rid of the sources for your problem, start your supplementation with very strong liquid iodine which will flush out that excess fluoride, bromine and chlorine from your body so you can finally replace it with iodine that your body has been yearning for all these years.

And trust me, once you get that iodine back into your system then you will know it. You don't need to ask for any clues of if it's working, as you will see them yourself.

Frankly if you're not buying the above then that's not my problem anymore. after all it's your own body and I'm here just trying to help you out.

If you decide to flush out that shit from your body then that's great, I suggest that you start from **strong nascent iodine**.

PART 4:
NUTRITION
(MASCULINE OPTIMIZATION PYRAMID LEVEL 2)

— Chapter 28 —

Cholesterol

Diet plays an enormous role in natural testosterone production.

The most misunderstood, but vitally important, molecule in your diet is cholesterol. This chapter will set the record straight: what is it, why should you care, how can you optimize your cholesterol intake, etc.

First off, if you were one of the millions of people duped into believing that a low cholesterol diet was healthy - I'm sorry. By lowering, or even eliminating dietary cholesterol, you were robbing your body of optimal physical, psychological, and cognitive functioning.

Cholesterol plays a role in countless processes in your body, from acting as a precursor to steroid and stress hormones, to insulating neurons, building cell membranes, producing bile, and metabolizing fat soluble vitamins.

Given its crucial importance, cholesterol is highly regulated by the liver via a feedback mechanism that ensures our body gets the amount it needs. This amount is typically around 1000-1400 mg/day, which means if you consume the US' dietary recommended amount of 300 mg/day, you leave your body to pull upon other resources to synthesize the remaining 700-1100 mg it needs every day.

Eat more eggs.

And if you consume an excess of dietary cholesterol one day, your liver continues to regulate the production process by slowing endogenous production to offset the dietary increase.

So what's the deal with everybody blaming cholesterol for causing atherosclerosis?

The following passage by Mark Sisson on his blog MarksDailyApple.com summarizes the situation perfectly - so perfectly that I cannot try to put it better myself:

"Heart disease took off in the early part of the twentieth century, and doctors frantically searched for the cause throughout the next several decades. Tests in the fifties initially showed an association between early death by heart disease and fat deposits and lesions along artery walls. Because cholesterol was found to be present in those deposits (of course it would!) and because researchers had previously associated familial hypercholesterolaemia (hereditary high blood cholesterol) with heart disease, they concluded that cholesterol must be the culprit.

In fact, what happens is that in response to an inflammatory situation, the body uses cholesterol as a "band-aid" to temporarily cover any lesions in the arterial wall. In the event the inflammation is resolved, the band-aid goes away and repair takes place.

No harm, no foul. Unfortunately, in most cases, the inflammation proceeds, the cholesterol plaque is eventually acted on by macrophages and is oxidized to a point at which it takes up more space in the artery, slows arterial flow and eventually can break loose to form a clot.

And all this time the cholesterol was just trying to be the good guy. Blaming cholesterol for all this is like blaming a cut finger on all the band-aids you have lying around your house."

So what's the real cause of heart disease?

Inflammation that exacerbates LDL infiltration of the endothelium.

LDL cholesterol has been shown to rise in direct correlation with an increase in sugar-induced inflammation. It is then oxidized by the free-radicals in the inflammatory milieu. Trans fats can also play a role in this oxidation.

How do we combat free-radicals? A diet high in antioxidants.

This is grossly oversimplified, but for our purposes it's what you need to know.

Cholesterol is not bad at all - in fact, it is VITAL for life. Is dietary cholesterol the same as endogenous cholesterol? No. But the former does affect the latter, and a diet rich in dietary cholesterol from sources such as meat and eggs is going to nourish your body and brain in a way that a low cholesterol, grain & sugar rich diet will not.

Cholesterol is potentially the most complicated topic that we'll be discussing in this program. With that in mind, I want to keep it as simple and to-the-point as possible for maximum actionable takeaway.

Cholesterol, among the many other things mentioned above, acts as a precursor to testosterone. In short, it is converted to progesterone, then testosterone. What you need to know is this: a diet rich in cholesterol and low in inflammatory agents will promote testosterone production, especially when combined with resistance training. The best type of resistance training to undertake is discussed in the "training" section of this program, but according to studies, almost any type of resistance training protocol will work, you'll just see a varying degree of effectiveness along the spectrum of program design.

Examples of foods that you should consume as the best possible sources of dietary cholesterol are outlined further in this nutrition section, but in a nutshell you want to **focus on meats, eggs, and high quality dairy while also supplementing with fruits and vegetables that are high in antioxidants** to combat any free radical damage caused by inflammation.

It's a damn simple approach. And it works.

If you want more detail, read on as we discuss the role carbohydrates and intermittent fasting play in this nutrition equation...

Chapter 29

Carbohydrates

The macronutrient profile of the food you consume plays a major role in determining your hormonal balance.

And the best macro profile is probably not what you've been led to think.

Before we dive into further explanation, let's cover the basics first. What is a macronutrient? Macronutrients are the three large "macro" groups of nutrients (ie. substances needed for growth, metabolism, and other body processes) and are split into: fats, carbohydrates, and proteins, in terms of classification.

Each of the major macronutrients play a role in supporting the endocrine system and overall healthy functioning of the body.

So it should come as no surprise when we see research findings that illustrate potentially detrimental effects of eliminating an entire macronutrient group from an individual's diet.

Since this program is focused on testosterone, examining the research shows us:

1. Low carbohydrate diets are detrimental for testosterone optimization

2. Low fat diets are detrimental for testosterone optimization

3. High protein diets are detrimental for testosterone optimization

Much of the body of research on the subject of testosterone optimization and macronutrient composition of meals also focuses on adding the element of resistance training, so we can rest assured that a lot of the findings are pretty relevant to our goals and not just isolated, sterile results.

The Role of Carbohydrates

Your body's natural hormone levels are affected by the availability of certain macronutrients. When it comes to carbohydrates, a low blood glucose concentration stimulates a compensatory response from hormones like epinephrine, glucagon, and cortisol - known in this context as "fuel mobilizing hormones."

For example, one study found drastically higher levels of these hormones in subjects after consuming a low carbohydrate diet (11% CHO) compared to subject consuming a high carbohydrate diet (77% CHO).

Low carbohydrate (CHO) diets tend to have direct effect on the testosterone:cortisol ratio in humans.

Especially when undergoing athletic or fitness training (resistance or endurance), the body needs adequate carbohydrate to support glycogen synthesis and maintain blood glucose levels without putting extra stress on the body in the form of chronically elevated epinephrine and cortisol levels. This cortisol secretion occurs in an effort to maintain blood glucose through muscle proteolysis and amino acid oxidation, and has been found to increase similarly in response to a high protein diet as well due to neglecting adequate carbohydrate consumption on that regimen, which we will discuss further momentarily.

SHBG and cortisol binding protein levels are shown to decrease with moderate to high levels of carbohydrate consumption.

In one study that measured the effects of CHO consumption on the free testosterone:cortisol ratio over repeated days of training (as opposed to most studies which only look at acute bouts of training), the researchers found that the ratio substantially decreased in the low carbohydrate group, while the control group saw no drop or rise.

This is pretty telling for a couple reasons...

1. Remember, the fact that the ratio in high carbohydrate control subjects did not change in response to 3 consecutive days of hard training is important. This means that while overall acute levels of the hormones in the blood may fluctuate over time, their proportion to one another did not change, and that appears to be a direct result of the amount of carbohydrate in their diet (in this case 60%).

2. The low carbohydrate group was consuming 30% of their daily calories from CHO. In 'low carb' circles this would still be considered very high carb, yet even 30% saw a drastic decrease in the fTC ratio. This is telling. Imagine what a similar bout of training would do to an individual on a 10-15% carbohydrate diet (rough estimate of around 100g per day, the classic cut-off for being "low carb").

3. In the low carbohydrate test group, resting levels (tested three days post-training) found an additional 36.1% decrease in free testosterone and 14.8% increase in cortisol, indicating that not only do the effects of the training stimulus negatively impact the

individual immediately following training, but they seem to accentuate over time, even in the absence of the stimulus, due to an inability of the diet to support the training and the increased effort of "fuel mobilizing hormones" to compensate.

So adequate carbohydrate consumption is necessary to support training, and in supporting training it is also supporting a healthy hormonal profile by preventing the chronic rise in cortisol, glucagon, and epinephrine.

However, processing this information on carbohydrates in isolation doesn't do us any good either. We need to be sure and view it in the context of a complete macronutrient profile, including fats and proteins in the mix.

Only then can we make an educated hypothesis about what the optimal "testosterone-supporting" macronutrient profile should be.

It's trendy right now to omit from certain macro nutrients. Some years ago it was the low-fat craze, and not a big surprise, people got sicker than ever because of it. The mass media always needs something to demonize, and currently carbohydrates are considered to be the "root of all evil".

You may have read the *"10 Ways to Boost Testosterone"* and such lists from other websites, which often claim that you should avoid carbs to boost testosterone, but that just goes completely against the current scientific evidence.

To be honest, carbs are not bad, carbohydrates are pretty fucking important for testosterone optimization if you ask me.

Let's take a closer look:

People often claim that low-carb diets are superior to anything else, simply because they would be better for losing weight.

Fortunately the above is a load of bullshit, because weight loss is all about energy balance. If you consume more calories than you burn, you gain weight. If you consume less calories than you burn, you lose weight.

There's a mounting pile of scientific evidence to prove this fact, (360) and anyone who tells you that you could bend this law of physics by tricking around with macro nutrients, is a nutcracker.

Heck, Professor Mark Kraub lost 27 pounds (361) by eating only Twinkies, little Debbie snacks, Oreos, sugary cereals, and Doritos chips. Why? Because he simply ate less calories than what his body used.

You simply cannot escape the law of thermodynamics with fad diets.

The only time when you could actually benefit from low-carb diets, is if you have some serious issues with insulin-resistance, or leptin-resistance, or if you're prepping up for a bodybuilding show. If you don't, then there's really no need to omit from carbohydrates.

Now that I've gotten that out of the way, let's get to the meaty part of this chapter... the studies.

...Here's why carbohydrates are essentially important for testosterone production:

a) In this study, (362) the researchers divided their subjects into 2 groups. The other group ate a high-carb low-protein diet, whereas the other group ate a high-protein low-carb diet. Fat intake and calories were identical. Ten days into the study, the results showed that the high-carb group had significantly higher free testosterone levels (+36%), lower SHBG levels, and lower cortisol levels when compared to the high-protein low-carb group.

b) In this study, (363) the researchers found out that in exercising men, the stress hormone cortisol increases rapidly when they're put on low-carb diets. Needless to say that this is pretty bad thing for testosterone production. (364)

c) Gonadotropin-releasing hormone (GnRH), which is the hormone that basically starts the whole cascade of events that eventually leads to testosterone synthesis, adjusts its pulsation rate according to the glucose levels of the body. When there's high amount of glucose present, the hypothalamus inside our brains releases more GnRH, and thus your body synthesizes more testosterone. And when there's low amounts of glucose present in the body, the brain releases less GnRH, which slows down testosterone synthesis (365).

As glucose is mainly generated from carbohydrates, it's quite obvious that low-carb diets also mean lowered blood, muscle, and brain glucose levels, leading to slower release of GnRH, and therefore also lower testosterone.

d) In this study, (366) the researchers had 2 groups of men who performed three consecutive days of intensive training, the only thing different between these groups was the carbohydrate consumption. The other group ate 60% of their daily calories from carbs, whereas the other group ate only 30% (note that this isn't even low-carb anymore). The final post-study measurements which were taken in the third day, showed that the group which got the lower amount of carbs, had significantly lower free testosterone levels, and higher cortisol levels (this is one of the reasons why I recommend more carbs on training days). Similar results were observed in this study too. (367)

See? That's why we don't recommend low-carb diets.

But are all carbs created equal? Should you just slam your face with spaghetti, sugar, and hamburger buns?

Answer: There's differences between carbs, and when it comes to boosting testosterone, I usually divide them into 2 groups.

1. <u>Starchy tubers and veggies</u>: potatoes, yam, pumpkins, beets, carrots, turnips, squash, etc.
2. <u>Grains</u>: wheat, rice, cereals, pasta, corn, bread, etc.

If your goal is to eat the testosterone boosting carbs, you should eat most of your carbs from the group 1, and less from the group 2.

Here's why:

a) Most grains contain a lot of gluten, and gluten is known for its prolactin increasing effects (368, 369). Prolactin on the other hand is known for reducing testosterone levels. (370)

b) Grains (at least the refined kind) are known for causing systemic inflammation in the body, (371) and inflammation promotes cortisol, which reduces testosterone. (372)

It doesn't kill you or wipe away your testosterone tank if you have bread or pasta once in a while, but eating mostly from the group 1 is a good staple to follow if you want to increase your natural testosterone production.

Personally I like to eat a lot of potatoes, I consider them to be the god-tier when it comes to carbs, and if I have some grains, I try to have some that contains no gluten and preferably has some androgenic effects (read: sorghum).

Conclusion

Carbohydrates are essential for testosterone, and they're not unhealthy at all. Just stop believing the mass media craze, they'll always need some food group to demonize, and currently it's carbohydrates.

Be aware of this especially if you exercise a lot.

— Chapter 30 —

Protein

In the aforementioned study at the beginning of the carbohydrate chapter, researchers who examined two subject groups, one on a high carbohydrate diet and one on a high protein diet, with total calories and fat intake the same, found that the high CHO group had considerably lower cortisol levels, higher testosterone, lower SHBG levels, and lower cortisol binding protein levels, than the high protein group.

With fat intake and calorie levels being equal in both groups, this demonstrates not only the necessity of adequate carbohydrate intake to support testosterone, but also the potentially detrimental effects of neglecting one macronutrient group in pursuit of consuming an abnormally high amount of another.

Protein, especially in fitness-minded individuals, is almost always this macronutrient.

With the protein obsession prevalent in the fitness community today, it's entirely possible that the main reason many men, who are otherwise fit and appear healthy, still suffer from symptoms of low testosterone and chronic stress is that the constant pursuit of more protein in their diet (usually out of fear of muscle catabolism) is actually inadvertently sabotaging their endocrine health.

This is because the increase in protein consumption will always accompany a decrease in consumption of both fats and carbohydrates, arguably the two more important macronutrients for endocrine support.

As we'll see when we look at the research on fat intake and testosterone levels, dietary protein is possibly the least important macronutrient in terms of testosterone support. Therefore, it should be consumed at the absolute minimum level required for muscle support in training, and the remainder of the diet should consist of carbohydrate and fat - if testosterone optimization is your goal.

Luckily, at the end of this chapter, I propose a novel way to consume all of the adequate macronutrient levels while still maintaining a high training load and a lean, muscular body, as well as facilitating fat loss.

Protein is by far the least demonized macronutrient at the moment, and it's considered to be the holy grail of nutrition. It's not uncommon to see gym rats and bodybuilding websites recommending to cut down on fat and carb intake, just for the sake of getting in more of the god given protein.

Protein might be the most important nutrient for maintaining lean mass, but for testosterone production? It's the least important.

That's right, more protein is not cool for your balls, no matter what the bodybuilding sites (the guys who try to sell you their powders) say.

Here's why:

How Dietary Protein Impacts Testosterone Production

I have personally never enjoyed high protein diets. Many guys swear by them, but they're often the guys who sell the powders too (and they're usually on hormone replacement therapy, SARMS, or anabolic steroids).

For these 6 or so years that I've been hitting the gym, I have been mostly focusing on fats, carbohydrates, and total caloric intake.

Surely I do eat protein, but I eat a lot less than the bodybuilding sites recommend for a guy of my size. To give you a hint of numbers, I eat probably around half of that.

Yet I have never had any problems building muscle, EVEN when I didn't have freakishly high testosterone levels.

The reasoning behind me not eating a high protein diet is simple. I want to maintain high testosterone levels naturally, and high protein diets are detrimental for T production. The more protein you eat, the more you have to cut out from your carbohydrates and fats, and the more you cut from those two, the lower your testosterone production will be.

And that's because fats and carbs are superior to protein when it comes to natural testosterone optimization.

This is obvious when you take a look at the research:

- In this study, (373) the researchers divided their subjects into 2 groups. The other group ate a high-carb low-protein diet, whereas the other group ate a high-protein low-carb diet. Fat intake and calories were identical. Ten days into the study, the results showed that the high protein group had significantly lower free testosterone levels (-36%), higher SHBG levels, and higher cortisol levels.

- In this study (374) which had 1552 men as test subjects (aged 40-70), Longcope et al. found out that when men eat low amounts of protein, their levels of sex hormone binding globulin (SHBG) increase. This occurrence is believed to lead to reductions in free testosterone levels (SHBG is a protein which binds to free testosterone molecules in blood, making them 'unavailable' for direct use of the body). So at least in older men, low-protein intake might be a bad idea. What is low-protein according to these researchers though? Much lower than the amount recommended below in this article.

- In this study, (375) the researchers found out that diets high in protein, lower testosterone levels in men who practice strength training.

- In this Finnish study, (376) Hulmi et al. found out that consuming a drink with 25 grams protein (whey and casein) right before a strength training workout, significantly lowered testosterone and growth hormone levels in human subjects.

So as you can see, protein truly is the least important macronutrient when it comes to boosting testosterone.

I wouldn't say that it's necessarily a bad nutrient or anything like that, but eating a high protein diet leaves room for less carbs and fat, which are superior when optimizing natural T production.

The source of protein also seems to be important. For testosterone optimization, animal sources are superior to plant sources, (377) especially if your goal is to build muscle.

If you're actively lifting weights, I would recommend that about 25-30% of your daily calories come from animal proteins. This is easily enough for muscle building purposes (if, for some weird reason, you would still want to consume more protein than that, it would be best to consume more protein in your workout days, and less in your rest days, in a way that your total weekly protein intake would still be about 25-30% of your calories).

What about protein powders like whey and casein?

Answer: I honestly wouldn't even recommend protein powders. The way I see it, it's just that the companies which sell them are making some big time bank of off people who believe that they need to have that protein drink after a lifting session, if they don't, the whole workout was useless.

Just get your protein from fatty cuts of meat, and if you absolutely can't meet your daily goal from animal sources, then maybe take a sip of casein before bed, or whey after a workout.

Chapter 31

Dietary Fat

Three main dietary factors influence resting testosterone levels:

- Monounsaturated fat intake (MUFA)
- Polyunsaturated:Saturated fat ratio (PUFA:SFA)
- And protein:carbohydrate ratio

Since we've already discussed the protein:carbohydrate ratio, let's take a look at the fats, namely the impact of MUFAs, PUFAs, and SFA.

Research focused on the overall percentage of fat intake in the macronutrient profile has found lower fat diets to correlate with a decrease in testosterone levels. For example, in groups of test subjects, those on a 20% fat diet had significantly lower testosterone levels than those on a 40% fat diet, over the course of the study.

Studies in vegetarians, who are known to consume less SFA and have a higher PUFA:SFA ratio, also find similar results.

While the importance of overall dietary fat intake has been widely studied in terms of testosterone production, the breakdown of individual types of fats has become a potentially more important burgeoning sub-field, and one that can shed additional light on the specific breakdown of types of fats necessary in the diet.

One major study analyzing specific lipid profiles and their impact on testosterone in men (before, during, and after a resistance training protocol) found that the amount of MUFA intake and the PUFA:SFA ratio were reliable indicators of resting T concentration, along with overall dietary fat intake levels. Several other studies have reinforced their findings.

Researchers found a significant negative correlation between the PUFA:SFA and T levels, meaning higher amounts of polyunsaturated fats in the diet relative to saturated fats had a negative impact on testosterone levels.

PUFAs include sources from both omega-3 and omega-6s (it's favorable to have a higher ratio of omega-3:6), including processed oils like soybean, corn, and safflower oil, walnuts, canola oil, flaxseeds, and fish.

The best sources of saturated fats are fresh animal products, such as meats, butters, and cheeses, which also happen to be rich in dietary cholesterol as well as monounsaturated fats, both favorable for testosterone production.

Researchers found that MUFA intake was positively correlated with testosterone levels as well. Most nuts and even fruits such as avocados and olives are outstanding sources of monounsaturated fats that will support testosterone production.

We can see from the research on fats, carbohydrates, and protein that the macronutrient profile of your diet plays an incredibly important role in mediating your testosterone production. Aside from training, diet manipulation is one of the simplest, and fast-acting manipulations you can take to increase your testosterone levels naturally.

Most people, seeing that the overall trend of the research places a heavy emphasis on consuming more fats and carbohydrates, and putting less focus on protein consumption in order to support an optimal endocrine balance may be somewhat dismayed or confused.

According the popular paradigm, fat + carbohydrate intake together = body fat accumulation.

However, this is simply not true, and also depends highly on the type of fats consumed and the type of carbohydrates consumed.

PUFAs + processed sugar, for example in a donut or piece of birthday cake, will obviously encourage fat gain if consumed regularly and in hypercaloric quantities. But that's because it is shitty food, devoid of nutrients and high in calories. These types of foods, when consumed over time, encourage appetitive behaviors and have even been shown to have addictive qualities, similar to illicit drug- taking.

Carbohydrates and saturated and monounsaturated fats consumed via real, whole food sources, rich in micronutrients and vitamins and minerals, will nourish the endocrine system, especially when consumed together (ie. not neglecting one macronutrient group in pursuit of another).

On the surface, however, this type of diet may appear as though it does not necessarily encourage "getting ripped" - a state that most men would like to achieve. This assumption is partly correct, especially considering the fact that reaching abnormally low body fat levels typically requires considerable caloric restriction which decreases testosterone levels, and testosterone levels are also known to drop off in men below a certain level of body fat (see the chapter on body fat).

The first thing you must understand is that when proposing an ideal macronutrient breakdown for a testosterone- supporting diet, such as 30% protein, 35% carbohydrate, 35% fat, or 20% protein, 40% carbohydrate, 40% fat, that this does not necessarily have to be consumed daily.

You can spread this intake out over an entire week, and cycle the intake of certain macronutrients to better support training and rest cycles.

For example, I specifically began consuming high proportions of carbohydrate and moderate protein on my training days, with fat coming in small, trace amounts, which fully supported my training and endocrine balance, from both the carbohydrate and protein standpoints.

Then, on my rest days, I would consume very low amounts of carbohydrates (under 50g) and get my nutrition from mostly high quality fats and proteins from animal meats and products.

Over the course of the week the entire macronutrient breakdown still averaged out to moderate levels of fat and carbohydrate intake and enough protein to support my muscles in training. Intermittent fasting on this protocol enhances the experience (see chapter on intermittent fasting).

Simple.
Plus, this type of macronutrient cycling protocol *encourages fat loss*, in some cases drastically (if calories and food source quality are controlled).

It also supported much of my own fat loss back into the single digit range after reaching healthy male body fat levels of 12-14% mostly just through keeping a moderate amount of fats and carbohydrates in the diet and training correctly multiple times per week.

Some years ago, dietary fat was considered to be the utmost evil thing that you could ever put near your body, but luckily things have gotten slowly better and new research is constantly proving how important it is to eat enough dietary fat each and every day.

This is a good thing, especially for men, as dietary fat intake is one of the most crucial factors to take under consideration when optimizing natural testosterone production.

So let's dive into the fats-testosterone research:

Dietary Fats-Testosterone Benefits

There are two crucial factors to look for when focusing on dietary fat intake to optimize T.

1. The actual amount of dietary fat you eat is important. This should be pretty high, but there's an upper limit from where things start going to the opposite direction.
2. The ratio between different types of fatty acids plays a crucial role. Not all of them are equally as effective, and one of the groups actually decreases testosterone.

I'm assuming that most of you already know the difference between fats, but for the sake of simplicity, these are the three types of fat you need to know, like we mentioned earlier, along with some examples:

- **Polyunsaturated fatty-acids (PUFAs)** – omega fatty-acids (3,6,7,9), sunflower oil, canola oil, soybean oil, safflower oil, flaxseed oil, walnut oil, margarine, light spreads, etc.

- **Monounsaturated fatty-acids (MUFAs)** – olive oil, almond oil, avocado oil, hazelnut oil, macadamia nut oil, peanut butter, etc.

- **Saturated fatty-acids (SFAs)** – red meat, butter, coconut oil, palm oil, dark chocolate, egg yolks, cheese, whole milk, etc.

Here's what science tells us about polyunsaturated, monounsaturated, and saturated fats and testosterone production:

a) In this study, (378) the researchers tested several nutritional factors to see how they correlate with pre-exercise testosterone levels in healthy men.

What they saw was that the diets high in saturated fat and the diets high in monounsaturated fat, significantly increased testosterone levels. Whereas the diets high in protein, or the diets high in polyunsaturated fats, both reduced testosterone levels in a pretty much dose dependent manner.

The researchers also saw that the higher the dietary fat intake, the higher the testosterone (diet containing mixed fats).

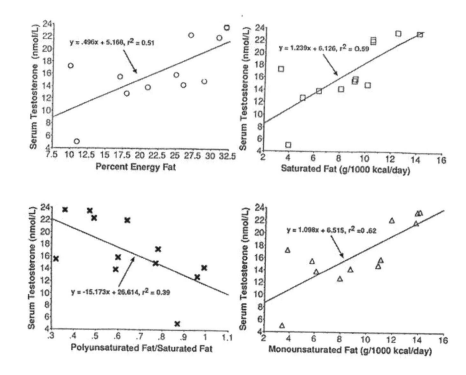

b) The data of the study above is consistent with the results that are seen in vegan/vegetarian studies. Vegetarians eat lower amounts of dietary fat, and their PUFA/SFA ratio is higher than what is seen in most omnivores. That's more than likely the main reason why vegans/vegetarians have noticeably lower testosterone levels than meat eaters do (379, 380, 381, 382, 383).

c) Several studies have also shown that when diets lower in total fat intake (~20%), are compared to diets higher in total fat intake (~40%). The higher fat intake groups always have more testosterone, and less SHBG in their blood serum (384, 385, 386).

d) In this study (387) two elite ice hockey teams were put on different diets for a period of 7 months. The other team received a diet containing 40% fat and 45% carbs, whereas the other team ate a diet with 30% fat and 55% carbs (protein intake was identical). Both during and after the study, the researchers saw that the higher fat intake group had higher free testosterone levels, along with lower sex hormone binding globulin (SHBG) levels.

At this point it becomes quite obvious that you need to eat plenty of fat to increase testosterone levels, and that the types of fat you need to focus on are the saturated fats and monounsaturated fats. Whereas the consumption of polyunsaturated fats should be kept low.

Eating 35-40% of your daily calories from mostly SFAs and MUFAs would be my recommendation for optimal testosterone production. No more than that because you have to leave some room for carbohydrates and protein too. Also, avoid trans-fat like it would be the plague.

"But what the heck? I've heard that saturated fat causes heart conditions?!"

Answer: Don't fret over such nonsense. Recent research has shown (388) multiple times that the correlation between dietary fat intake and cardiovascular disease risk is pretty much non-existent. Saturated fat and testosterone production go hand in hand. Brett from the Art of Manliness actually has a post here, (389) which shows how he ate a high-fat diet that doubled his testosterone levels, while his blood profile stayed optimal the whole time.

Conclusion on the Fats-Testosterone Benefits

It is well known that eating a diet high in healthy fats increase testosterone levels. In fact it's one of the easiest ways to do so.

Research has also shown that the higher intake of saturated fats and monounsaturated fats leads to higher testosterone levels, whereas a higher intake of polyunsaturated fats leads to lower testosterone.

— Chapter 32 —

Soy

For past decade all we've heard trumpeted through the fitness industry when it comes to male nutrition is to stop eating soy. It's true: soy is composed of two potent isoflavone phytoestrogens, diadzen and genistein.

Should you go chomping down edamame and soy burgers?

Hell no. Here's why.

First, an estimated 25-35% of Westerners do not have the intestinal bacteria required to properly metabolize the phytoestrogen diadzen. In a 10-week study on diadzen metabolism, metabolic measurements varied 1000-fold between test subjects. And this was 38 people.

In a handful of people, variation was 1000-fold. Just imagine the metabolic variation in a population of individuals the size of the United States.

Secondly, soy protein is an inferior protein when compared to animal-derived proteins. Soy proteins have been shown to metabolize quickly in the gut before reaching muscle tissue, with a significant proportion of amino acid oxidation occurring in the liver.

Animal proteins have been shown to be superior for encouraging testosterone synthesis when compared to plant-based proteins.

Third, soy interferes with proper thyroid functioning. Genistein antagonizes thyroid peroxidase, the enzyme responsible for thyroid hormone production. Soy contains goitrogens, which interfere with iodine metabolism as well. Your thyroid cannot function properly without sufficient iodine.

And oh yeah, it's also one of the most heavily genetically modified foods on the planet.

Soy is not worth your time or money, and it's definitely not worth your health.

The risks that come with consuming unfermented soy products far outweigh any potential benefits.

Note: there is a fundamental difference between fermented and unfermented soy products. Asian populations have been consuming fermented soy products for centuries, and these foods (such as natto, miso, and tempeh) are apparently benign at the very least. The fermentation process, coupled with healthier growing practices in Asian countries, mitigate much of the risk associated with the otherwise deleterious compounds in soy itself.

A massive campaign has been raging across the Western world over the last few decades, pushing GMO unfermented soy products on the general population under the guise of 'health.'

The cold truth that this is a money-making machine, and not a health movement, shouldn't surprise anybody reading this program.

95% of the soy produced in the United States is genetically modified, with production owned and regulated by Monsanto, the creators of the insecticide RoundUp and the genetically-modified soy plant with the RoundUp-resistant gene.

The massive body of independent research on GMO soy implicates it in brain damage, breast cancer, thyroid disorders, infant abnormalities, infertility, kidney stones, immune dysfunction, and food allergies.

Unfortunately, due to the multi-billion dollar advertising push in the last decade, most Americans still believe it to be a 'health food.'

While many men purposefully avoid it because of the aforementioned buzz about its estrogenic qualities, its effects are especially deleterious on women, with soy milk consumption accounting for a potent effect on thyroid dysfunction and hypothyroidism.
In rat populations, GMO soy has been linked to infertility in future generations (third generation), demonstrating that the epigenetic effects of soy on the animal's body can be passed down through the bloodline.

Many informed health professionals have been calling for complete ban on GMO soy in the Western world, however they're fighting an iron giant with deep pockets.

The debate about men eating soy and its hormonal effects has been going on for years, and there are 2 groups in particular who fuel the debate year after year...

1. The group that often contains a lot of vegans and vegetarians, who claim that soy is in fact, a really healthy superfood, and that there's no science backing up its testosterone lowering effects.

2. The group that usually contains a lot of bodybuilders and gym rats, who claim that soy is the equivalent of eating birth control pills and that it has very powerful testosterone lowering effects in the human body.

But which group is right? Or could it be that both of them are wrong? Let's find out:

Eating Soy and Male Testosterone Levels

There is really a need for debate like this, because soy is one of the most consumed foods in the world. It's literally hidden in almost everything that we stick into our mouths.

Just start reading the labels of foods at your house, and you'll soon see that almost everything has soy in it. The marinade in your meats often contains soy. See that word "vegetable oil?", that's more than likely processed soybean oil.

It's so funny how blind we are to the fact that we're eating a shitload of soy everyday, without actually eating soy. It's just hidden in everything.

Back in 1999 more than 7% of all dietary fats in America, came from soybeans. Over a quarter of all American baby-formulas are made with soy as the base ingredient. And school lunch programs across the country are even adding soy to hamburger patties. That's just crazy.

Why is soy put into everything then?

1. About 93% of the soy in the U.S is now officially GMO'd (390)(genetically modified). This means that soy is extremely cheap. And cheap is what most of the food manufacturers like.

2. SOYJOY® is one of the leading sponsors of AND (Academy of Nutrition and Dietetics), which is an agency that pretty much dictates how the Americans should eat. No wonder why the governmental food recommendations state that men should eat at least two servings of soy per day...

Well what about the claim of soy reducing male testosterone levels? What is the basis for that?

Answer: Soy contains these compounds called isoflavones (genistein, daidzein and glycitein) which act as phytoestrogens (plant estrogens) in the human body. They're structurally similar to the principal female hormone, estrogen, and are believed to have similar effects in the body.

As high estrogen level in men are almost always a direct route to low testosterone levels, eating soy – which contains estrogenic compounds – is often blamed for lowering testosterone.

But is that really what happens in the human body?

Let's see what science says:

a) Dr. Kenneth D.R. Setchell from Colorado State University, discovered this small molecule called equol from humans back in 1982. Since then he has been researching the molecule. He has already proven that the compound is formed in the gut when we eat isoflavones, and that men who eat a lot of soy have high amounts of equol present in their blood stream. (391) Back in 2004, Dr. Setchell found out that equol is a strong anti-androgen, which can almost completely shut down the activity of dihydrotestosterone (392) (the most potent androgen).

b) This study (393) followed one 19 year old man who started consuming hefty amounts of soy in his diet. Suddenly the guy lost all interest to sex and suffered from erectile dysfunction. His blood DHEA, testosterone, and DHT levels also plummeted significantly. 1 year after stopping the soy consumption, his erectile health and hormonal profile was fully regained

c) In this human study, (394) from 99 infertile men, the men that ate the most soy had the lowest sperm count.

d) In this study, (395) soy protein increased the number of epithelial cells in the breast tissue by 29% (this is a sign of overblown estrogen).

h) These three animal studies [396, 397, 398] found out that the isoflavones in soy can cause breast cancer (another sign of overblown estrogen).

i) In this study (399) the researchers found out that male infant rats who received soybean feed when they were still in womb, had problems in sexual organ development. This study (400) also found out similar effects.

j) In this study, (401) soy protein decreased testosterone and DHT levels in healthy young men.

NOTE: There are few studies which show no major differences in testosterone levels after soy consumption. However they're quite often sponsored by SOYJOY® or other large soy producers. Meaning that the results are of no use and often completely biased.

Another thing to note is that dihydrotestosterone is made when an enzyme called 5-alpha reductase converts testosterone into DHT, and as soy lowers DHT, there is actually less testosterone being converted too. Meaning that the reduction in DHT can mask the testosterone lowering effects.

— Chapter 33 —

Avoid These T-Lowering Foods

Just like there are many foodstuffs which can increase testosterone levels, there are also many foods that lower testosterone in men.

In this chapter, we're looking at 7 possible foods and/or food groups that can have a negative effect on your androgen levels.

Without further ramblings, let's check out the seven dietary foods that lower testosterone:

1. Flaxseed Products

Flaxseed products are incredibly popular at the moment, and this is due to their high omega-3 fatty-acid content, which in itself, can be ruled as a positive benefit of flax consumption.

However, when it comes to flaxseed products, I believe that the negative effects outweigh the benefits, especially if you're a guy.

You see, flax products are incredibly dense in compounds called "lignans". In fact, flaxseeds are known of having dietary lignan levels 800-fold over that of most other foods. (402)

Why would this be a problem?

Well, not only are the lignans highly estrogenic, (403) there's some evidence suggesting that they reduce total and free testosterone levels, while also suppressing the enzyme 5-a reductase (404) which converts testosterone into its more potent form of dihydrotestosterone (DHT). Lignans work by increasing the levels of SHBG (sex hormone binding globulin), which binds into free-testosterone molecules and renders them "inactive" for the direct use of the androgen receptors.

The studies on the subject point heavily towards the conclusion that flaxseed products and androgens are not exactly a match made in heaven.

Firstly, there's a case-study of this 31-year old woman (405) who had high testosterone levels which caused her to develop a condition called hirsutism (excessive facial hair growth). In an effort to control the hirsutism and drive down her high T-levels, the researchers told her to eat 30g/day of flaxseeds for 4 months. The results? Serum total testosterone dropped by a whopping 70%, and free-testosterone went down by a staggering 89%.

Well, you're probably not a woman with hirsutism, so how would flaxseed consumption affect men's hormone levels?

Turns out there's a study where the same dose (30g/day) was given to 40 male subjects for a month. (406) The decrease in total testosterone was not nearly as significant as in the case-study above (only a mere ~10% decrease), but still, it's evidence pointing towards the fact that flaxseeds can have a T-suppressing effect, even at such low dosages (2 tablespoons/day).

The same researchers had done a study with similar design (25 male subjects, 30g/day flaxseeds) 7 years earlier. (407) In that study, the average total testosterone levels dropped by ~15%, whereas free testosterone went down by ~20%. The difference in this previous study was that the subjects were told not to consume more than 20% of daily calories from dietary fat.

Few older in-vitro/animal studies have also shown that the lignans in flaxseed can increase SHBG count, thus resulting in lower bio-availability of testosterone for the receptors (408, 409).

So unless you're a woman who battles with hirsutism, flaxseed is a food that lowers testosterone and I wouldn't recommend eating too much of it.

2. Licorice

I'm not sure how popular licorice is in the US, but here in Finland, and in many surrounding European countries, it's regularly used in tobacco, teas, sweets, and chewing gums.

Even though it tastes amazing, and some alt-medicine "guru's" claim that it would actually be super-healthy, the evidence points to one big problem.

The main compound in licorice – *glycyrrhizic acid* – which gives licorice root its phenomenal taste, has negative side effects and makes licorice a food that decreases testosterone.

And this reduction in testosterone (although easily reversible) is not insignificantly small either.

The negative effects of glycyrrhizic acid on T-production were first seen in this test-tube study, (410) where the researchers found out that a very modest dose of glycyrrhetinic acid (hydrogenated version of glycyrrhizic acid), was able to significantly block testosterone production in isolated rat leydig cells, through inhibiting the activity of *17β-HSD* enzyme, which is needed as a catalyst in testosterone production.

11 years later, glycyrrhizic acid was tested on human subjects. In a study (411) where seven healthy male subjects were given 7g/day of licorice through a commercially available candy tablets (containing 0,5 grams of glycyrrhizic acid). Four days into the study and the subjects total testosterone levels had decreased from 740 ng/dL to 484 ng/dL.

In other words, their testosterone levels were almost half of what they were before popping the licorice pills.

Good news are that 4 days after discontinuation of the licorice-habit, their testosterone levels had returned back to baseline.

3. High-PUFA Vegetable Oils

The majority of the cooking oils used all around the world in this 20th century, are refined vegetable oils, aka. liquid oils extracted from plant sources, which are then processed in various ways.

To begin with, most of the vegetable oils are incredibly shitty choices for cooking, due to their low smoke point, and the often used refining process (bleaching, deodorizing, degumming, etc) which strips them of micronutrients and can leave traces of sulfates.

Even if not used for cooking, but just as is, high-PUFA (polyunsaturated fatty-acid) vegetable oils are a disaster for your testosterone production.

There's a well-done study from 1997, (412) which clearly demonstrates in human male subjects, how:

- increased total fat intake boosts testosterone levels
- increased intake of saturated fatty-acids (SFA) boost testosterone levels
- increased intake of monounsaturated fatty-acids boosts testosterone levels
- and increased intake of polyunsaturated fatty-acids (PUFA) reduces testosterone levels

Nearly all vegetable oils are LOADED with PUFAs (with the exceptions of coconut oil, palm oil, avocado oil, and olive oil).

What can make a high-PUFA vegetable oil worse, is if the polyunsaturated fatty-acids are mainly comprised of the dreaded omega-6 fatty-acids.

This is because the human body operates best if we keep the omega-3 (ω3) to omega-6 (ω6) ratio somewhere close to 1:1 or 1:2, which is near of that of the paleolithic human (the average American now has this ratio at 1:16, which is sixteen times more of the omega-6).

When the ratio of ω3:ω6 shifts more and more towards higher amounts of omega-6, the systemic inflammation and oxidative stress of the body keep on creeping higher and higher, this in turn DRAMATICALLY increasing your risk of multiple chronic diseases prevalent in Western societies. (413)

It's very much likely that one of the end-results of high omega-6 intake would also be lowered testosterone production, and even though I didn't find any studies about the subject, I did stumble upon a study (414) which shows that when the ω6 content of sperm is high (and conversely ω3 is low), men are likely to be infertile. Whereas, when the ratio is more in favor of the omega-3's, the subjects are more likely to be fertile and have high-quality sperm.

Bottom line: Dietary fat intake should be moderate-high for optimal testosterone production, and the amount of saturated fatty-acids (SFA), and monounsaturated fatty-acids (MUFA) should be prioritized. High-PUFA vegetable oils on the other hand, are a food that decreases testosterone levels and production. High-PUFA high-ω6 vegetable oils are a fucking disaster.

4. Mint, Peppermint, Spearmint

Many of the herbs from the "mentha", or "mint" -family, including spearmint, peppermint, and various other hybrids, are somewhat known of having testosterone reducing effects.

For the sake of clarity, let's focus on the two most common plants of the mint family; peppermint (*Mentha spicata*) and spearmint (*Mentha piperita*).

Both are heavily used for culinary and food manufacturing purposes, though they can also be found in many soaps, shampoos, cough-relievers, lip-balms, and in toothpaste. Most herbal teas also tend to contain plants or plant extracts from the mint family…

And even though mint-products tend to taste and smell pretty great, their effect on testosterone levels may not be that awesome.

Much of the research about peppermint and spearmint on male testosterone levels comes from studies using male wistar rats as test subjects.

In a study conducted 11 years ago, (415) 48 rats were divided into 4 groups:

- Group one received commercial drinking water (control).
- Group two received 20g/L peppermint tea.
- Group three got 20g/L spearmint tea.
- Group four got 40g/L spearmint tea.

When compared to the control group, the peppermint tea at 20g/L reduced total testosterone levels by 23%, whereas the spearmint tea at 20g/L reduced total T by a whopping 51%. If you translate this into human dosages, 20g/L is the equivalent of steeping a cup of tea from 5 grams of tea leaves.

A study from 2008, (416) showed that spearmint suppressed testosterone production and acted as anti-androgen in male rats. The researchers theorized that spearmint works by inducing oxidative stress in hypothalamus resulting in down-regulation of T synthesis in testicles.

Another rodent study conducted in 2014, (417) found out that at 10-40mg/kg spearmint showed no significant toxic effects on the reproductive system, but still, a trend towards lowered testosterone levels was noted.

What about human studies?

Unfortunately, there aren't any trials done on human males.

BUT... Spearmint has been shown to significantly reduce testosterone levels in women.

Much like in the case of flaxseeds (see number #1 above), spearmint has been studied on women with high androgen levels, and whom battle with the main cause of that; hirsutism (excessive facial hair growth).

In this study, (418) the researchers gave 21 women subjects a cup of spearmint tea, 2 times a day, for 5 consecutive days. Surprisingly, total testosterone levels didn't change much, but the bio-available free-testosterone levels did drop by ~30% on average. This study was replicated with 42 subjects in 2009, (419) only the duration of the trial was changed to 30 days. The results showed that free and total testosterone levels were significantly reduced over the 30 day period in the women who drank spearmint tea.

Are you a woman battling with hirsutism or a male wistarian rat? Probably not, so this isn't direct proof that similar effects would be seen in human males. However, the studies above are still quite heavy evidence towards the fact that the herbs from the mint family and mint foods reduce testosterone levels in men.

5. Alcohol

Drinking alcohol of any kind has a significant trend of lowering testosterone levels. However, as it often is the case with alcohol, the dosage makes the poison.

In rodent studies, it's often shown that alcohol has a dose-dependent testosterone suppressing effect (420, 421, 422, 423). One alarming study shows that when the rats are fed a diet where 5% of the calories come from alcohol, testicle size is reduced by 50%. (428)

In humans, heavy alcohol consumption is strongly correlated with lowered testosterone levels (424, 425, 426, 427), and chronic alcoholics tend to have much higher estrogen levels and much lower testosterone levels when compared to their non-alcoholic peers (429, 430, 431, 432).

It might come as a relief to some that lower amounts of alcohol are really not that bad for T production. Actually, In this study, (433) 0,5g/kg of alcohol slightly increased testosterone levels, whereas an intake equivalent to ~2 glasses of red wine has been shown to only reduce T levels by a mere 7%. (434)

The most surprising results come from this Finnish study, (435) where it was noted that 1g/kg of alcohol (equivalent to ½ glass of vodka) taken immediately after a resistance training session, increased testosterone levels by ~100%! It's uncertain why this happens, but the study at-hand is an excellent example of the fact that Finnish people tend to drink too much.

Alcohol tends to lower testosterone levels, but the dose really makes the poison, and few drinks are not going to turn you into an eunuch.

NOTE: More about alcohol and why it lowers testosterone can be found in this post. (436)

6. Soy Products

There are many controversial topics around soy consumption, one of them which is the beans effect on testosterone levels.

Because of the high amount of phyto-estrogenic isoflavones (*genistein, daidzein, glycitein*) present in soybeans, it's often claimed that soy would elicit similar effects in the body as the principal female sex hormone; estrogen. In-vitro research has shown (437) that although having a significantly lower affinity for the receptors than that of estrogen itself, isoflavones can still activate the estrogen receptors (438) and downregulate the androgen receptors. (439)

Aside from isoflavones, soy is considered to be highly *"goitrogenic"*, (440) meaning that it can disrupt the production of thyroid hormones by interfering with iodine uptake in the thyroid gland.

Suppressed activity of the thyroid is considered to be one of the leading causes of low testosterone levels in men. (441)

The third possible "hormonal problem" with soy consumption is an anti-androgenic compound called *equol*, (442) which forms in the gut when the gut bacteria metabolizes the isoflavone; daidzen.

According to research, (443) this only happens in 30-50% of men, due to the fact that not everyone has the *"right"* intestinal bacteria to create *equol*.

It's also worth mentioning that soybeans have – from a testosterone boosting point of view – quite shitty fatty-acid ratios. out of the 20 grams of fat that can found in 100 grams of regular soybeans, more than 50% comes from the testosterone lowering PUFAs. Not to mention the fact that most of the PUFAs consist of the inflammatory omega-6 fatty-acids.

So at least on paper, soy seems to be a hormonal disaster, but what does the research say?

a) On multiple human and animal studies, it has been shown that high intake of soy (even if it's coming through a low-isoflavone soy protein extract) can suppress both; testosterone and DHT (444, 445, 446, 447, 448, 449, 450).

b) Surprisingly enough, many studies also show that increased soy consumption does not correlate with lowered testosterone levels (451, 452, 453, 454).

Bottom line: Even though the research is relatively inconclusive, I see no point in consuming high amounts of soy products (that is, at least if you're a carnivore). There are many theoretical reasons for soy being a food that lowers testosterone levels, and the possible negative effects greatly outweigh the positive effects. In fact, the only positive effect of soy consumption seems to be the fact that it's quite high in protein, and since being a plant, vegans/vegetarians could cover their dietary protein needs by eating a lot of soy products (though it's worth mentioning that according to this study, (455) animal protein is superior to plant protein when it comes to testosterone production).

7. Trans-Fats

Trans-fats are a common byproduct of a process called *"hydrogenation"*. In a nutshell, this is what happens:

Raw oils (usually soybean, cottonseed, safflower, corn, or canola) are hardened by passing hydrogen atoms through the oil in high pressure with the presence of nickel (which acts as an alkaline catalyst for the process).

As an end result, some of the unsaturated molecules in the raw oils become fully saturated (and therefore also solid at room temperature). However, due to the demonization of saturated fat in mass-media, the hydrogenation process is often continued only to the point where the required texture is reached.

Now, the hydrogenation process flips some of the molecular "carbon-carbon" bonds into "trans" bonds, effectively creating trans-fatty acids. And when the hydrogenation process is completed only to the point where the optimal texture is reached (but not full hydrogenation), high amounts of trans-fatty-acids will remain in the end product.

So, if you're wondering what foods are high in trans-fats, the most common ones would be the kind that includes the use of "hydrogenated" or "partially hydrogenated" vegetable oils:

- industrial vegetable oil shortenings for baking and confections
- margarine and vegetable oil spreads
- fast-foods, especially: Burger King, McDonald's, and KFC
- potato chips (not all, but some)
- muffins and doughnuts
- cookies, cakes, cake mixes, and frostings

NOTE: There are many of the products above that are labeled "trans-fat free", but this doesn't automatically mean that they don't include the stuff, since the FDA allows them to contain up to 0,5 grams of trans-fatty acids while still being "trans-fat free".

It's also worth mentioning that during the summer, FDA announced a complete ban on all man-made partially hydrogenated fats from American foods by 2018. (456)

But why are trans-fats bad for your health and testosterone production?

Firstly: Trans-fats promote systemic inflammation in the body, (457) and a recently published large review study (458) concluded that each 2% increase in calories from trans-fats was associated with 23% increase in cardiovascular disease risk.

Secondly: trans-fats are high in testosterone lowering PUFAs. They lower the amount of "good" HDL cholesterol (459) (a crucial building block in testosterone synthesis). And a high intake of trans-fatty-acids is associated with lowered sperm counts and testosterone levels in male rodents (460) and humans (461, 462, 463).

PART 5:
LIFESTYLE
(MASCULINE OPTIMIZATION PYRAMID LEVEL 3)

— Chapter 34 —

Erectile Dysfunction

I remember having ED issues (as a teenager, nonetheless) when I had problems with low T. This was well before I had ever done any research on testosterone – let alone was even aware of how important it was in men.

The ED was humiliating and emasculating.

When I finally figured out my issue with the tumor, and went on to use this protocol to naturally increase my T up to 1200 ng/dL, my ED also completely disappeared. That was many years ago and I have now learned how to cure erectile dysfunction fast doing a handful of simple things. I'm confident I'll never have ED issues again.

We're going to flesh out that handful of things in this chapter on how to cure erectile dysfunction permanently. I'm going to go out on a limb here and guess that you are here for two reasons:

1. You are having problems with erectile dysfunction.

First let's go a little bit into what erectile dysfunction is. Erectile Dysfunction is when a man has a continuous problem getting an erection sufficient enough to penetrate in sexual intercourse. (464) NOW if you have erectile dysfunction, most men have been in a situation where they have had a hard time "getting it up." This can be for a bunch of different reasons.

If you are here because you have had this problem once or twice, you can't assume that you have erectile dysfunction.

If this is a regular thing for you and you have not been able to achieve satisfactory sexual performance due to lack of an erection for multiple occasions over some time, then you are in the right place. You are experiencing symptoms of erectile dysfunction, NOT just symptoms of drunkenness or lack of attraction.

2. You want to learn how to cure erectile dysfunction naturally.

Learning how to cure erectile dysfunction "naturally" means not taking any pharmaceuticals that are advertised in commercials along with a couple holding hands in a bath tub on the beach. We're talking about Viagra, Cialis, Levitra…

Random fact about Viagra: Viagra has saved the lives of many tigers. Asian poachers harvest tiger bones and sell them for use in medicines. One function of tiger bones in medicine is curing erectile dysfunction. Since Viagra was invented, tigers have been less used for this issue. (465)

Let's take a look at what we're going to discuss in this chapter on how to cure erectile dysfunction:

NATURAL CURES FOR ED
- Naturally Optimize Your Testosterone
- Train For Erections (Yes, there's a way…)
- Eat for Erections
- Stay on the Same Sleep Schedule
- Quit Smoking
- Be Smart About Your Alcohol Consumption
- Check Your Medications

- Try Some Acupuncture
- Ingest These Potent Natural Remedies
- Drink These Two Juices – Pomegranate & Watermelon

1. Raise Your Testosterone

This is VITAL to increasing your sex drive. You may be thinking, "My sex drive is strong, I just can't fulfill the wishes caused by my sex drive." Although normal testosterone levels are not required to maintain a normal erection, if testosterone levels dip low enough, they could be the cause of your erectile dysfunction.

You will notice as you read on in this article, that many of the natural cures for erectile dysfunction are also ways to raise your testosterone levels naturally.

2. Exercise for Erections

Exercise gets the blood flow moving, which is clearly important for getting blood into your nether regions. (466)

Exercise is a good way to prevent the onset of erectile dysfunction, but can also reverse the effects after you are experiencing the symptoms. Exercise is an amazing natural cure for ED. It is advised to walk – not run – to get the blood flow moving. Running lowers your testosterone levels and can raise cortisol levels and stress on your body. The last thing you need when you are experiencing the struggles of ED is MORE stress. (467)

Weight training (using the THOR Protocol) is a good way to get the blood flow moving while also raising your testosterone levels naturally.

Also, moving your pelvic regions around your penis is a great way to increase continence. (467) According to this study, doing kegel exercises can help with erectile dysfunction.

3. Eat for Erections

Maintaining a healthy and balanced diet is important in reversing the effects of your erectile dysfunction. A diet rich in micronutrients, the right macronutrients, and using most of the foods on this grocery list can help with the symptoms. (466)

Both exercise and diet have been proven important for preventing erectile dysfunction because studies show that a man with a 42-inch waist is 50 percent more likely to have erectile dysfunction than a man with a 32-inch waist. (467)

4. Stay on the Same Sleep Schedule

In a study published by Brainresearch in 2011, results showed that men who do not have a consistent sleep schedule have problems maintaining normal or high testosterone levels. (466) The results also showed that hormonal depletion is a cause of sexual dysfunction.

If you do not have a bed time, then you need to get one. Go to sleep and wake up at the same time on a consistent basis.

The amount of quality sleep you get is important as well. Not sure whether or not you are getting enough sleep?

A good way to know is to simply stop using an alarm. Do a week or two of testing where you can find the amount of sleep you need so that you can wake up without an alarm every morning. This is when you know you got enough sleep in the night.

If you are still tired after your normal waking time, do not go back to sleep. Make up for the lost sleeping time by taking short under 30 minute naps in the day. This is the best kind of sleep you can get in order to maintain solid testosterone levels.

5. Quit Smoking

Erectile dysfunction can be a result of vascular disease. The process occurs when the blood that is supposed to go to the penis is restricted due to narrowing arteries. (466)

Not only smoking tobacco, but also smokeless tobacco, can narrow the arteries and restrict the blood vessels necessary to get an erection.

If you smoke, this is possibly the cause of your erectile dysfunction. If the dysfunction is bothering you, consider quitting the habit to get your erections back.

6. Stop Drinking So Much

Everyone who has heard the term "Whiskey Dick" knows that alcohol can cause temporary sexual dysfunction. But alcohol is a powerful depressant and high exposure to alcohol can result in full blown erectile dysfunction. (466)

To add to the concerns, alcohol does a great job at lowering testosterone levels. So maybe cut back on the drinks if you feel this may be the cause of your erectile dysfunction.

7. Check Your Medications

Erectile dysfunction can be a common side effect of certain medications.

Medications that have been known to cause erectile dysfunction are medications for high blood pressure, antidepressants, diuretics, beta-blockers, heart medications, cholesterol medications, anti-psychotic drugs, hormone drugs, corticosteroids, chemotherapy, and medications for male pattern baldness. (466)

Look up your specific medication or ask your doctor if your erectile dysfunction could be a result of the medication you are taking.

8. Acupuncture

Acupuncture is a possible natural cure for erectile dysfunction. According to this study, acupuncture can improve the quality of your erection and it cured erectile dysfunction in 39% of its participants. (467)

So go get poked with some needles if you're having troubles poking with your needle.

9. Ingest These Natural Remedies

There are plenty of non-pharmaceutical natural remedies you can ingest in order to cure erectile dysfunction. (468)

Like previously stated, you should avoid using synthetic pharmaceutical drugs to cure your ED. While that route may lead to results in the short term, you will never address the underlying health deficiencies causing your erectile dysfunction.

What's worse is that these synthetic drugs like sildenafil citrate (generic name for Viagra) have a host of negative side effects including:

- Headache
- Diarrhea
- Urinary tract infection
- Painful erections (lasting for several hours)
- Lowering of blood pressure to unsafe levels (if taken with other blood-related drugs)

Luckily, there are natural alternatives for improving ED that have been proven to be scientifically effective through peer-reviewed research and trials. Even better, these safe, natural alternatives don't share the negative side effects of their medically-prescribed counterparts.

Here are a few of them:

- **Horse Chestnut Extract** (also known as Aesculus hippocastanum) – **actively works to improve venous circulation** which in turn results in better blood flow to the penis.

- **Pine Bark Extract (Pycnogenol) – has a plethora of science backing up its effects as a blood flow enhancer.** It works to increase natural levels of nitrogen oxide and induce cardioprotective effects that help to improve erectile dysfunction.
- **Vitamin C – increases nitric oxide production in the body, and that it also protects the molecules.** In fact, there is evidence showing that the combination of Garlic and Vitamin C can reduce diastolic and systolic blood pressure and increase nitric oxide output up to 200%!

The BEST way to effectively improve ED forever is through naturally fixing deficiencies causing the problem.

The only way to get the benefits that these herbal alternatives have to offer is by using a supplement with SCIENTIFICALLY PROVEN Ingredients at the scientifically effective dosages (like the dosages in Redwood by Truth Nutraceuticals).

Ginseng is known as "Herbal Viagra" and has been used to improve sexual function in men. It can also be used to help with premature ejaculation.

Taking high doses of L-Arginine has been known to widen the blood vessels in the penis which can stimulate the blood flow and cure erectile dysfunction.

Yohimbe taken from the bark of an African tree has been known to cure erectile dysfunction. BEWARE the side effects of yohimbe are more risky than previously mentioned remedies. This should not be used without doctor's supervision.

Vitamin C & Garlic Extract are incredible together as a natural erectile dysfunction remedy, mainly because they boost N.O. production by over 200% when combined as they work synergistically.

10. Drink These Juices – Pomegranate, Watermelon

There are two juices that you can drink to help with erectile dysfunction: Watermelon and Pomegranate. A component of watermelon called citrulline, when eaten in high amounts, can increase blood flow to the penis. (466) Although no proof exists that pomegranate juice helps with erectile dysfunction, results of a 2007 study testing the relationship were promising.

Researchers are confident that larger-scale studies will prove its legitimacy in aiding men in getting over their erectile dysfunction. (469)

Not only are these juices easy and good-tasting, natural treatments for erectile dysfunction, they also have alternative health benefits. I would recommend that anybody drink these juices regardless.

— Chapter 35 —

Sex

Sexual function and sexual desire are two different, independent things. However, they are both influenced by your testosterone levels. Let's break them down.

It may seem like common sense as to why you, as a man, would want to maintain both healthy sexual function and healthy sexual desire far into your old age.

However, most men confuse one for the other, and oftentimes find themselves neglecting to take care of their health in these areas.

Sexual Function

Sexual function refers to your ability to execute the biological act of sexual intercourse. Can you get and maintain an erection? Is it soft, or rock hard? Do you ejaculate optimally, as opposed to prematurely These are all important questions.

Sexual dysfunction occurs when biologically, your sexual ability has been compromised. Low testosterone is one of the main culprits in male sexual dysfunction. Do you have a problem with physical arousal? Do you have problems ejaculating? Do you experience pain during intercourse?

These are all signs of sexual dysfunction, characterized by one or more problems occurring at any time during the sexual response cycle.

The sexual response cycle traditionally includes:
- Excitement
- Plateau
- Orgasm
- Resolution

Desire and biological arousal both play important roles in the excitement phase of the sexual response cycle.

Sexual dysfunction is historically most common in men ages 40-60 years old, but with the recent widespread decline in testosterone levels - as much as 20% lower across entire populations according to some sources, compared to just 20 years ago - we are starting to see a disturbing trend even in men in their 20's and 30's, when most men are considered in the prime of their sexual health.

You may be one of these men.

If you are, worry no more. The fact that you're reading this guidebook is a big step in the right direction.

What Causes Sexual Dysfunction?

Sexual dysfunction can be caused by myriad things, but almost all of them boil down to a common source... the endocrine system.

Whether it's psychological stress from work or performance anxiety, causing a spike in circulating cortisol which will naturally suppress testosterone production, or alcohol and drug abuse, high levels of body fat, or depression, all of the common causes of sexual dysfunction can be resolved merely by optimizing your endocrine functioning via proper nutrition, training, and lifestyle.

And that should be quite comforting. Because the fix is rather simple.

Sexual Desire

Sexual desire is a motivational state... an innate drive. An appetite. It is commonly referred to as libido, sexual drive, and lust.

On one level, it is the main element of an individual's sexual personality. For our purposes, it is a motivational state caused by both internal and external factors, one of which is your testosterone level.

The biological component of sexual desire is commonly referred to as 'drive' and has neurophysiological underpinnings.

Individuals with acute or chronic illnesses tend to have far lower sex drive than their healthy age-matched counterparts. This makes sense, as the body allocates attention from less important processes like appetitive sexual behavior toward more important processes such as survival.

However, chronically elevated stress hormones, even when undetectable to most, can have a profound impact on a man's sex drive, especially if they're elevated for prolonged periods of time... months and years.

Stress hormones (glucocorticoids) act as an androgen suppressant so as your chronic stress levels creep upward, your testosterone production will naturally decline.

While desire and function are inherently different processes, they are intricately intertwined. And testosterone heavily influences the overall system.

Is More Sex Better?

1. More sex is indeed better for testosterone production.
2. However, more testosterone is NOT correlated with increased sexual desire or activity, with the exception of in men with abnormally low amounts.
3. The testosterone threshold is between 300-400 ng/dL, beyond which little to no increase in sexual desire or activity is noted.
4. There is a lot of individual variance in terms of the threshold's exact value.

Steroid Hormones and Behavior

The relationship between steroid hormones and behavior is complicated. Endogenous hormone levels influence behavior, while behavior also influences hormone levels. So which comes first? And which exerts the most influence?

The answer: there is no right answer; it all depends on individual variance.

A quick story: a man works on an island. The man leaves the island to travel to the mainland, and while there he visits his girlfriend. The man has sex with his girlfriend, then returns to the island.

His beard grows thicker and faster than before. As he periodically returns to the mainland to visit his girlfriend, he begins to notice that his beard is growing more rapidly immediately prior to, and during, the visits.

This is a true story, and part of a publication that, in 1970, sparked a flurry of new investigation into the exploration of the relationship between testosterone and sexual behavior. It would appear as though both the anticipation of sex and the act of intercourse itself were increasing his androgen levels (evidenced by the enhanced secondary characteristic beard growth).

Testosterone can in fact rise due to psychological stimulation, such as that from sexual anticipation. It has also been found to positively correlate with orgasm frequency: in free testosterone, serum testosterone, and DHT.

So it would appear as though more sex is indeed better.

However, there are some caveats to consider. First, if the psychological guilt associated with the act of sex is high enough, the body's stress response will negate any potential benefits, or at least have a negative impact on them.

Also, saying that more sex is better for increasing your testosterone is not the same as saying that more testosterone is better for having more sex.

The Testosterone Threshold

A threshold exists, beyond which an increase in testosterone levels has been shown to have a negligible effect on increasing sexual desire, arousal, and performance.

This level appears to be between 300-400 ng/dL in men and should be taken as the baseline level of testosterone that men need in order to operate with "normal" sexual drive (provided their free testosterone is not compromised).

Beyond this point, even in men with three times the amount of T, researchers see insignificant differences, or inconsistent enough differences, in terms of sexual activity traits to warrant the need for any additional T when it comes to sexual activity.

However, this is not to say that more testosterone is not beneficial for other things in a man's life such as support of his secondary characteristics like hair growth, vocal tone, muscle development, and well-being. But it is an interesting, and hopefully encouraging piece of information to note.

Most men reading this, even with low testosterone in the 200's, should be able to restore baseline sexual functioning naturally by merely increasing their T into the 300-400 ng/dL range.

And my recommendation, obviously, is to do this without gels or medications. Testosterone production is based on feedback loops so with a small natural increase from behavioral, nutritional, and training changes you should be able to first restore baseline functioning, then positively reinforce that production so it increases steadily in time.

Another important thing to note is this: an increase in testosterone, even at or beyond the threshold required for baseline sexual activity, does not correlate with an increase in sexual activity. And that's because testosterone levels have nothing to do with a man's ability to hold a healthy relationship with a partner.

That involves psychosocial skills, empathy, and a million other things, obviously all of which vary greatly from one individual to the next.

So yeah, just because you're a raging T-gorilla* doesn't mean you'll be able to close the deal. Sorry.

So all in all, androgens are only beneficial in terms of sexual activity and desire for men who currently have abnormally low T. But increasing your T is good for most guys, even beyond sex.

*There are inconsistent findings between testosterone levels and aggression.

Masturbation

1. The brain is able to distinguish between interpersonal touch and intrapersonal touch quite well via mechanoreceptors in the skin
2. Hormonal response to interpersonal touch, along with the psychological elements involved and the increased capacity to regulate stress hormone reactivity would seem to indicate that sexual intercourse with a partner is indeed superior to masturbation for testosterone production
3. Prolactin secretion is orgasm dependent in the sexual response cycle, and acts directly back on dopaminergic neurons in the brain to regulate sexual satiety
   Excess prolactin contributes to testosterone deficiency and erectile dysfunction, and is chiefly caused by pituitary tumors and a handful of common medications (if you're on meds, check this out)

4. Erotic film viewing linked with masturbation has been shown to increase circulating cortisol, possibly for psychological reasons, and is therefore potentially detrimental for short-term testosterone production at the neural level (and for long-term if performed chronically)

5. However, orgasm frequency, whether due to intercourse or masturbation is found to increase circulating levels of free testosterone, serum testosterone, and DHT

Author's Interpretation: Sexual intercourse is better than masturbation for enhancing testosterone production. However, there is a lot of individual variance that can occur from psychosocial variables.

For example, if the guilt associated with intercourse or masturbation is high enough, the subsequent stress response will negate any potential physiological benefits.

The Sexual Response Cycle

When considering sexual intercourse and masturbation, we can't focus merely on the physical act, and in doing so limit our scope to the genitals and ejaculation and/or orgasm; we need to understand the sexual response cycle in terms of the cerebral, spinal, and peripheral aspects, getting the full view.

Then, in that context we are able to understand the fundamental differences between having sex with a partner and masturbating alone, and subsequently posit testosterone's role as well as how it is affected.

The concept of sexual arousal implicates far more than just genital arousal. The "arousal cycle" involves a chain of events, both psychologically and physiologically: information processing, general arousal, incentive motivation, genital response, then coital (intercourse) or autoerotic (masturbation) action, followed (hopefully) by orgasm (and including all neuroendocrine events and cascades associated with these steps).

This process appears to be motivated by dopaminergic activation (dopamine being the neurotransmitter commonly associated with reward-motivation behavior) and proposed to be regulated by the prolactinergic system (prolactin being a peptide hormone associated with a huge number of things, one of them being feedback regulation on dopaminergic neurons post-orgasm, which implies a primary role in a possible negative feedback sexual-satiation mechanism).

This prolactinergic feedback occurs in response to ALL forms of orgasm, regardless of whether it is coital or autoerotic. However, the same response does not seem to occur in men who masturbate without orgasm. With those things in mind, it wouldn't seem to matter whether or not prolactin feedback is an important distinguishing factor or a "lead" in this testosterone investigation, right?

Wrong. Kind of.

Hyperprolactinemia is associated with two things (in men): impaired sexual desire (makes sense, seeing as we just learned about the negative feedback system, though it is only one small piece to the puzzle), and testosterone deficiency.

What?

Is this a chicken-egg issue? If so, how does excessive prolactin production inhibit testosterone production? This is where it gets complicated: should we assume that the PRL is inhibiting T production and not that excessive PRL is a by-product of less testosterone production in the first place?

Let's take a look.

Hyperprolactinemia induces hypogonadism (ie. low testosterone) by interfering with the secretion of gonadotropin releasing hormone (GnRH). Luckily, most forms of hyperprolactinemia are rare, and usually involve a prolactin-secreting pituitary tumor.

However, for the general population of men reading this program, you need to be aware of a handful of drugs (that you may be taking) that can induce hyperprolactinemia, and therefore inhibit testosterone production and cause sexual and/or erectile dysfunction.

Some common medications are:
- Dopamine antagonists (antidepressants, anti-emetics)
- Amphetamines
- Estrogens
- Methyldopa and levodopa (L-DOPA)
- Opiates; morphine
- Metoclopramide
- Prochlorperazine, Chlorpromazine (antipsychotic drugs)

Medically, hyperprolactinemia is managed with dopamine agonists, like bromocriptine.

Remember, after orgasm prolactin generally acts upon the brain's dopaminergic neurons. If we administer a dopamine agonist (opposite to an antagonist) then it will have a positive effect on the normally negative-feedback cycle, which is especially helpful with an excess of PRL.

Long story short, if you suffer from ED, low libido, gynecomastia (man boobs), and also have some intermittent vision impairment and/or unexplained headaches, go to your doctor and get your prolactin levels screened.

Anything further on prolactin is beyond the scope of this book. Just know that addressing an issue with it (if you have one) will increase your testosterone levels back to normal.

Anyways, let's let a handful of questions guide us in this chapter with regards to masturbation:

1. What effect does autoerotic film viewing have (in real time) on steroid hormones (and is it any different than the coital sexual response)?
2. What effect does physical (non-autoerotic) touch have on stress and/or steroid hormones?
3. Before we get to those questions, however, I must make one important point: the body of research with regards to sexual activity and arousal relative to steroid hormones, pituitary hormones, and psychology is inconclusive, at best.
4. This is due to the incomprehensibly complex interplay between all the variables involved, including but not limited to testing paradigms and study design, circadian rhythms in subjects, sleep, diet, and subjectability.

Autoerotic Film Viewing (Porn)

We begin an investigation into masturbation with the usual culprit - porn. This, in my mind, is a logical place to begin because of the pervasively of porn as a sexual arousal, and subsequently masturbation-encouraging, stimulus.

A group of scientists from the University of New England in Australia were curious about whether autoerotic film viewing could induce similar blood hormone concentrations as masturbation and sexual intercourse. They found a significant rise in blood pressure in test subjects while viewing the pornography, compared with the control group, but little else other than slightly increased transient prolactin levels throughout the viewing. Cortisol and adrenaline were unaffected, while noradrenaline levels increased slightly.

None of the test subjects reached orgasm, and prolactin levels were therefore nowhere close to other studies that showed similar prolactin increase post-orgasm between masturbation and intercourse.

This reinforces the idea that the prolactin increase is entirely orgasm-dependent, regardless of stimulus, and that autoerotic film alone does little other than stimulate routine sexual arousal. In terms of hormonal effects, it has little negative impact on stress hormones.

However, autoerotic film linked with masturbatory orgasm specifically was found to significantly increase plasma cortisol levels following orgasm, which is likely a by- product of the normal experience of psychological guilt that stems from this sequence of activity.

Following sexual intercourse with a partner, plasma cortisol is unaffected.

Plasma testosterone levels have also been found to be unchanged following masturbation, even with a rise in FSH during the orgasm phase, while plasma T levels have been found to be either unaffected or increased leading up to and following sexual intercourse (see how inconclusive this all is?)

In summary, masturbation-induced orgasm has been found to have little effect on GH, T, B-endorphin, and LH levels with only slight variance in FSH and prolactin levels during/post-orgasm and a transient increase in noradrenaline levels throughout.

In terms of testosterone and visual erotic stimuli, it's been found to either increase or be unchanged - but not negatively affected with viewing. Use that knowledge as you will.

The Science of Interpersonal Touch

The skin is the oldest and largest of human sensory organs. Therefore, it would make sense that we examine the relationship between interpersonal touch and steroid hormones so we can extrapolate those findings into a logical conclusion with regards to advantages or disadvantages to one form of orgasm-induction over another.

The big question we need to answer is, "Is there any clear advantage with relation to the element of interpersonal touch during intercourse over the solitary action of masturbation in terms of steroid hormones?"

The brain distinguishes between interpersonal and intrapersonal touch, and elicits separate hormonal responses accordingly.

The importance of touch in romantic relationships is almost unanimously agreed upon. So much so, in fact, that some researchers even go so far as to assert that love and interpersonal touch are indivisible.

This would lead us to believe that touch plays a rather large role in eliciting an oxytocin (OT) response in both genders, which is a major player in the sexual arousal cycle. In animal studies, centrally administered OT induced erection, an effect that was apparently testosterone dependent. And OT-blockers stopped all noncontact erections.

Direct sexual contact from a partner has been found to induce the highest OT response.

Researchers also believe that the apparent ability of dopamine agonists to enhance sexual response is due to dopamine's relationship with oxytocin in this respect.

Also, in studies done on stress responsiveness, subjects who were exposed to massage from their partner (who they were either married to or had been cohabiting with for at least 12 months prior to testing) demonstrated significantly less cortisol responsiveness to the controlled laboratory stressor than the other groups.

In males, lower cortisol generally correlates with healthy testosterone levels.

Sexual intercourse is favorable over masturbation in terms of both testosterone production and stress hormone regulation. And not just for reasons discussed so far.

Another important consideration is the psychological assertion of dominance in a situation, which has been shown to increase male testosterone considerably, and is something that cannot be achieved in masturbation.

Even if masturbation and intercourse with a partner were comparable in terms of hormonal responsiveness, I'd still argue that the psychological act of sex itself for the male is more likely to elicit its own hormonal response, dependent on performance.

For example, if the male experiences anxiety during intercourse (an unlikely scenario during masturbation) and subsequently underperforms during sex, his testosterone is likely to be lower than if he were to just masturbate. However, if the male performs well (to his own judgement) and subsequently feels dominant and like intercourse was a successful endeavor, then his testosterone levels post- intercourse are likely to be considerably higher.

Sex and Testosterone Levels

Luckily, there's plenty of research about sex and how the act of lovemaking affects testosterone levels.

And why wouldn't there be? Testosterone is the principal male sex-hormone.

Researchers are not exactly sure why sex boosts the big T production, but they suspect that it has to do with dopamine, pheromones, feelings of domination and power, and even winning.

Here's some studies that I managed to find:

a) In this study (470) the researchers took saliva samples of testosterone from their 44 subject males before they entered a sex club, and then waited outside for them to return to take another sample. They found out that the men who had sex inside with a woman, experienced 72% increase in testosterone, whereas the men who only watched the act, noticed a 11% increase in the hormone.

b) In this 1992 study, (471) the researchers examined four couples and their sexual activity. They found out that on the nights when the couples had sex, both the male the female subjects had significantly higher testosterone levels than on the nights when there was no sexual activity.

c) The scientists in this study, (472) found out that older men who have more sex, also have more testosterone in their serum.

d) In this animal study, (473) researchers found out that even the anticipation of sex increases testosterone levels quite significantly, most likely due to the elevations in the motivation/pleasure hormone, dopamine.

e) This study (474) found out that the lack of sexual activity (caused by erectile dysfunction in most subjects), lowered testosterone levels a lot. The researchers conclude that this happens through a central effect on the hypothalamic-pituitary axis.

f) Not only does sex increase testosterone, but higher testosterone levels will also make you want to have more sex (475, 476). So this clearly creates a positive feedback loop where the sex stimulates testosterone production and that testosterone then makes you want to have more sex.

So clearly, testosterone and sex are deeply tied together. More sex = more testosterone, whereas more testosterone = more sex.

But this seems to be the case only when you're with a real person.

One of the more frequently asked questions I get is around the topic of ejaculation and testosterone. Does masturbation and/or ejaculation lower testosterone levels? Honestly, that's a valid question surrounding the topic of ejaculation and testosterone, since the internet is loaded on opinions about the topic.

Obviously, it makes a lot of sense that ejaculation, masturbation, and having sex could all lower T levels, since 95% of the good stuff is made in the ballsack, and during an ejaculation you're basically dumping the contents away, but even if something "makes sense", doesn't always mean it's correct.

The topic of refraining from ejaculations itself has been talked about for years, and many athletes are known for their habit of abstaining from sex before big events, such as: Mike Tyson, who abstained because he felt like having sex before fights made him a "weaker boxer". Or another boxing legend – Muhammad Ali – who wouldn't have sex for 6 weeks before his big fights.

Athletes aren't the only ones who avoid ejaculations for a "greater cause". Many highly successful men of the past have also abstained in order to use the sexual energy as a fuel for other things, these guys include: Napoleon Bonaparte, Thomas Jefferson, George Washington, Oscar Wilde, William Shakespeare, Abraham Lincoln, and many more.

But does any of the above have to do with testosterone? Or is it just a mental thing? And do ejaculations even lower testosterone levels in the first place?

Ejaculation and Testosterone

It's almost taboo to even talk about this very topic, and it's funny to see how some men get all angry when they don't like what they see.

With that in mind, I'm going to just go through some of the actual scientific research about masturbation, sex, ejaculations, and testosterone – in animal and human subjects – leaving all opinions aside...

...If something below doesn't justify your porn addictions, or if it just makes you get all hot and bothered, please leave the site and never come back I'm not here to instruct you how often to have sex or masturbate, this post is just here to show you the real evidence behind busting a nut and testosterone levels.

So, here's some of the research:

a) It's known that short-term abstinence of 3 weeks can slightly increases testosterone levels in healthy human subjects, (477) and one interesting study shows a significant 145% spike in T at the 7th day of abstinence (478) (probably an evolutionary trigger to reproduce). However, long-term abstinence of 3 months has been shown to significantly reduce testosterone levels (479) (note that this is only researched in men with erectile dysfunction, so the low T can be caused by something completely different).

b) In multiple human and animal studies, it has been noted that ejaculation does not acutely change serum testosterone levels, busting the common myth that ejaculation would rapidly deplete the body from testosterone (480, 481, 482, 483).

c) Even though ejaculations seemingly have no significant effects on serum testosterone levels, they can (at least according to rodent studies) alter the body's ability to utilize testosterone. It has been seen that after multiple ejaculations a sharp decline in androgen receptors takes place inside the hypothalamus, (484) and not only that, but a sharp increase in estrogen receptors follows as well. (485) One rodent study (486) also found out that 1 or 2 ejaculations in short span of time increased androgen receptor activity in the body, while 4 or more ejaculations caused a significant drop in the activity of AR, suggesting that ejaculating yourself to "sexual exhaustion" might lower your body's ability to utilize androgens.

d) While masturbation induced ejaculations don't seem to have that big of an effect on serum testosterone levels, sex with a real person does. For example: In a study of 44 men visiting a sex club, (487) it was noted that the men who actually had sex in the club with a woman, noted a nice 72% average increase in their testosterone levels, while the men who only watched the act, got a boost of 11%. In another study, (488) it was seen that on couples, testosterone levels increase on the nights that they have sexual intercourse, but not on the nights that they don't. One study also saw that older men who have more sex, have higher T levels. (489) What causes this if ejaculations don't? It could be the interpersonal touch, the female pheromones, the feelings of dominance, power, and even success.

Conclusion on Sex, Ejaculation, and Testosterone

Ejaculations and their effects on testosterone is quite an understudied topic on humans, but from the current evidence, we can draw the following assumptions on testosterone and ejaculation:

- Short-term abstinence from ejaculations can slightly increase testosterone levels.
- Long-term abstinence can reduce serum T.
- Having an ejaculation does not acutely affect testosterone levels.
- Ejaculating to the point of "sexual exhaustion" can make it harder for your body to utilize testosterone.
- Masturbation doesn't seem to affect testosterone levels in any significant manner.
- Sex with a real person can boost testosterone levels significantly.

— Chapter 36 —

Stress

It's hard to pinpoint exactly what the term stress means, but an explanation that comes rather close, goes something like this: *"stress is the body's principal method of reacting to a challenge"*. To open up the term a bit more, this *"reaction to challenge"* can be divided into two categories.

Short-term stress, where a quick challenge (a fight for example) arises and the body reacts to that with a burst of stress hormones (glucocorticoids), which makes you more alert and focused to tackle the stressor. This kind of stress is often not detrimental to health and has no long-term effects in the body. Many experts believe that short bouts of manageable stress (ie: small daily challenges) can in fact be a healthy thing to have.

Long-term stress, where the challenge is something that goes on for a long period of time (for example: a demanding boss that gives you work related tasks that feel unbearable, or a debt that you simply can't pay, etc). It's this kind of chronic stress that keeps stress hormone levels high for extended periods of time, often leading to detrimental effects on health of the body and mind. It's also this kind of stress that wrecks havoc in the endocrine system, and the kind we will be covering in this article.

So, short-term stress can be a good thing to have.

Long-term stress on the other hand, why it's so unhealthy? And how does it affect your hormonal health?

Long-Term Stress and Testosterone

There are two major reasons as to why chronic long-term stress hammers testosterone production.

Firstly, the principal stress steroid hormone; cortisol, which is released from the adrenal cortex during times of prolonged stress, has a direct testosterone suppressing effect inside the hypothalamus and testicular leydig cells.

Secondly, the synthesis of cortisol requires cholesterol, a molecule that is also needed in the biosynthesis of testosterone. When cortisol levels skyrocket during stress, more of this essential building block goes towards creating cortisol.

Obviously those are not the only reasons that can cause fucked-up T levels during prolonged stress. As a guy who battled with some serious work-related stress few years ago, I can guarantee you that increased alcohol consumption, messed up sleep quality, poor diet, lack of exercise, and depression can (and more than likely will) contribute to the stress induced reduction in testosterone.

The research on how long-term stress (both physical and mental) alters testosterone levels is rather cruel:

a) In multiple animal studies, it has been noted that nearly all kinds of long-term stressors (surgical stress, noise stress, immobilization stress, oxidative stress, chronic stress, etc) can significantly lower testosterone levels in various species (489, 490, 491, 492, 493, 494, 495, 496, 497, 498, 499, 500, 501). In pretty much all of these studies, the suppression of testosterone goes hand-in-hand with the increase in cortisol, and the reduction in testosterone is not caused by increased exertion, but through decreased production.

b) In military studies, psychological stressors (such as the fear of combat or death) have been linked to significant reductions in testosterone. (502) Same goes for stressful military training courses, such as: the officer school, ranger school, and survival training (503, 504, 505, 506, 507, 508, 509). One study (510) also showed that refugees who experience physiological stress, have low testosterone and luteinizing hormone levels, coupled with very high cortisol levels.

c) In non-military men, chronic stress, and stress-related depression has been linked to low testosterone production and elevated cortisol levels (511, 512, 513, 514, 515).

d) Surgical stress is no different (be this physical or psychological), it lowers testosterone levels too, usually the magnitude of the suppression is directly correlated with the severity of the surgery (516, 517, 518, 519).

Bottom line: Chronic stress (be it physical or psychological) has a tendency to lower testosterone levels, and this suppressive effect is nearly always caused by elevated cortisol production. (520)

How can you combat this chronically high stress then? Try some of the tricks below.

Meditation and relaxation exercises have been very effective at lowering cortisol and increasing testosterone levels in multiple human studies (521, 522, 523)

Just simply walking in nature (forest walking, hiking, etc), has been linked to significantly lowered cortisol levels in Japanese test subjects. (524)

Adaptogenic herbs (Rhodiola Rosea, Ashwagandha, Shilajit, etc) have a really good track-record at lowering cortisol, while simultaneously increasing testosterone.

Vitamin C has been shown to reduce the secretion of cortisol during stress, and it also has the ability to relieve the damaging effects of the stress hormone.

Increased duration of sleep has a significant cortisol suppressing effect in stressed subjects. (525) However, restful sleep is not always that easy to achieve during chronic stress.

Exercise is often recommended as a "stress-reliever" but it's important to remember that high-intensity exercise can also skyrocket the already elevated cortisol levels. (526) So stick to something light if you're under chronic stress.

Just a simple posture-hack can increase testosterone levels by 20%, while lowering cortisol by -25%, in less than two minutes. This has been proven in a human study conducted by the Harvard University. (527) We will discuss this technique in this book, in the chapter on body language.

Carbohydrate consumption has been shown to significantly reduce cortisol levels (528, 529, 530), whereas low-carb dieters often have high serum cortisol. The take home message? Don't eat low-carb when you're under stress.

Chronic stress is a real testosterone killer, and if you're under "real stress" (as in something that truly fucking crumbles you) I don't even have to tell you that, you can feel it yourself.

As a guy who has been under that kind of stress few years ago, I know that it doesn't help shit when someone just tells you to *"stop thinking about it"* or gives you some tips such as: *"try to sleep more"*, *"exercise"*, *"drink more water"*, etc.

But just so you know, chronic stress really hammers your testosterone production, the quicker you can get rid of it, the better.

— Chapter 37 —

Lower Your Body Fat

What does your body fat percentage have to do with your testosterone levels?

It is, in fact, one of the more important variables in the testosterone equation. Below a certain level of body fat, which in men tends to be sub 8-9% (but there is some variability, depending on age, training maturity, genetics) testosterone levels drop.

In competitive bodybuilders we see a drastic decrease in testosterone levels (even when many of them are on drugs) in the final weeks before the show as they reach sub-7% body fat levels.

This is the body's natural response to attempt to handle the stress associated with unnaturally low body fat levels by reallocating energy away from less vital processes like reproductive capabilities and over toward baseline functioning of vital organs and processes.

Ultra low body fat levels also tend to take a considerable amount of calorie restriction to reach, and low calorie diets hit testosterone levels hard as the body struggles to leech the necessary nutrients from the limited food source.

However, I'd be curious to see n=1 tests run on men who have reached sub-7-8% body fat levels slowly over the course of many years via a slight caloric deficit, as opposed to most data we have that measures less longitudinally, looking mostly at test groups over the course of a mere 12- 16 weeks of intense calorie restriction, or bodybuilders who in fact, only drop ultra low in calories and spike their training intensity in the final 12 weeks before competing in a show.

Longitudinal data over the course of many years in experienced trainees who do not yo-yo in body fat levels but instead either maintain or slightly decrease body fat every year would be a far more interesting look at the human body's capabilities in terms of endocrine function adaptability.

I would posit a guess that guys who train for years and very slowly decrease body fat through calorie and carbohydrate cycling and/or small deficits of 10-20% over time would develop the capacity to support normal testosterone levels naturally, at 5-8% body fat.

Low body fat is only one side of the coin when it comes to adipose and testosterone. The other side is far meatier (or flabbier), and far more relevant to most people reading this guide.

Body Fat & Testosterone Production

To put it simply, testosterone (both free and SHBG and albumin-bound) levels correlate inversely with measures of insulin resistance (insulin, C-peptide, and HOMA-IR) and body fat levels.

And the inverse association between testosterone and insulin resistance is mediated by adipose tissue, and independent of SHBG.

To put it in even simpler terms, the more body fat you have, the less testosterone you will naturally be able to produce.

So if you are overweight (or skinny fat, with >15% body fat in men), the single best thing you can do for yourself in terms of naturally optimizing your testosterone production is lose body fat. It really is that simple.

However, dropping that body fat may not be an easy task. You need to train correctly and eat the foods that will nourish your endocrine system, as opposed to crash dieting down, which will also lower your T levels considerably.

Do the correct training and eat in a moderate deficit of around 10-20% to allow for minor, non-stress-inducing endocrine adjustments over time.

If you have high levels of body fat, your endocrine system is suffering. It is nowhere near as healthy as it could be. However, you must realize that this took time to achieve. You didn't screw it up overnight so don't expect to fix it overnight either.

In terms of regional versus total body fat (i.e. belly fat versus full body fat), the research is somewhat conflicting and inconclusive. Some studies find total body fat levels to be a better inverse correlate to testosterone levels, and some find regional abdominal fat levels to be better. However, the overall body of knowledge on the subject would indicate that they are both decent correlates.

So while abdominal body fat is a noticeable warning indication of compromised ability to produce natural testosterone, so is total body fat percentage.

Moral of the story: lose body fat to increase testosterone, regardless of where the fat tissue is concentrated.

Let's talk about cortisol here for a second.

Low levels of androgens are linked to central adiposity in men, and a high risk marker for Type-2 diabetes. Testosterone administration has been shown time and again to decrease intra-abdominal adiposity and increase insulin sensitivity over time.

Another important thing to note: an overall and predictable increase in cortisol levels occurs in overweight and obese individuals, as well as an increased sensitivity to cortisol. This means you'll be more stress-reactive the fatter you get, which is a bad thing.

The decrease in insulin sensitivity and glucose tolerance associated with an increase in cortisol levels is well- established. Muscle tissue rapidly becomes insulin resistant, especially the insulin-sensitive red muscle fibers (i.e. glycogen synthesis becomes insulin resistant). And increased activity in the CRF-ACTH-Cortisol axis will inhibit hypothalamic secretion of gonadotropins (ie. testosterone precursors).

So to paint the doom-and-gloom picture for you in laymen's terms, increased cortisol makes it easier to gain fat, and as you gain fat you become more insulin-resistant which perpetuates cortisol circulation so you gain more fat. You also compromise your ability to properly use and store muscle glycogen, giving you further issues with glucose and insulin regulation.

You also increasingly compromise your brain's ability to secrete the hormones that trigger testosterone production.

Long story short, the more you reinforce stressful behaviors that increase body fat (e.g. lifestyle and job stress, overeating, insufficient exercise, psychological stress, processed shit diet, etc) the worse your life is going to get.

The good news (especially if you're frequently stressed out, especially after reading that): lowering your body fat will increase your ability to handle stress and decrease the amount of circulating cortisol in your system, which will in turn make it easier to continue losing body fat. It's a positive feedback cycle.

I repeat: lowering your body fat percentage is the single most important thing you must do to naturally optimize testosterone production (not to mention nurture well-being in general).

— Chapter 38 —

Intermittent Fasting

Special thanks to two men in particular, Martin Berkhan and Brad Pilon, for laying the foundation of much of the information in this chapter in terms of reviewing the literature on intermittent fasting, especially with respect to its effects on the endocrine system. You can find their work at http://leangains.com and http://eatstopeat.com, respectively.

I would like to begin this very important chapter by saying that intermittent fasting has been, hands down, the most useful tool in my tool box over the past couple years when both dropping body fat and increasing testosterone levels naturally.

Even in the absence of perfect nutrition (nobody can, or should, eat squeaky clean all the time) and less-than-ideal sleeping conditions and lifestyle stress situations (living in NYC and sleeping on a couch for a year on noisy 14th street, for example, while under extreme stress with a venture-funded mobile tech startup = stress to the max), intermittent fasting became my go-to daily form of hitting the reset button with my physiology.

And over time, I truly believe that IF played a major role in bringing my health from mediocre, to very solid.

What is intermittent fasting?

Intermittent fasting is quite simply abstinence from caloric consumption for a short period of time.

During this fasting period, an individual can consume non- caloric beverages without negatively impacting the fast, but no foods or caloric liquids should be consumed, or the individual leaves the fasted state.

Fasting has been used for centuries as a medicinal exercise in humans, and is a natural response for many animals during times of sickness or healing.

Arguing for or against the nature of fasting is not within the scope of this program. I will instead assume that you are reading this in order to learn more about how to increase your testosterone naturally, and therefore I'll lay out the myriad benefits of IF for doing so.

Not only does intermittent fasting provide a means to decreasing body fat, either by easily facilitating a caloric deficit without the negative hormonal side effects of calorie restriction or by facilitating some of its own fat-burning influence in the absence of a calorie deficit, making body recomposition more effortless, but it also boosts testosterone by influencing expression of key pituitary and satiety hormones including GnRH, LH, insulin, and leptin.

The research on intermittent fasting in the scientific literature is either, or both: 1. woefully nascent 2. non- applicable to both humans and/or us, fitness-conscious individuals.

Most short-term fasting studies are conducted in animals like monkeys, rats, or cows, and are carried out with methodological 48 - 72 hour fasts. For our purposes, this is considered a long-term fast, especially because most humans will never undergo a fast over 48 hours. And the results are non-applicable to us.

Almost all of these studies find the suppression of testosterone and an increase in circulating cortisol, as if that was a surprise. Between 24-48 hours of fasting, depending on individual variance, most humans will have an acute stress response to the lack of feeding. Hormones such as cortisol, insulin, growth hormone, and testosterone will likely be affected.

However, for fasts under 24 hours, the benefits are myriad, and this acute stress response is less likely.

For example, in obese men short-term fasting was shown to increase LH production after just an overnight fast. While the LH increase in this case did not directly lead to a noticeable increase in testosterone levels in these men (it was, remember, a mere overnight fast) the increase in LH was promising enough for the same researchers to perform tests in non-obese men.

In the non-obese men, the results of a mere overnight short-term fast were staggering: a 67% increase in LH response and a 180% increase in testosterone. With this in mind, doing a short-term fast daily may have profound, almost immediate effects on your endocrine balance, especially because LH pulsing needs to spike regularly in order to have a noticeable effect on your overall T levels, something that regular daily intermittent fasts can have a positive effect on.

In terms of these results, short-term fasting appears to affect men differently based on their level of body fat, with normal, nonobese men seeing a rapid rise in LH, then testosterone following a short fast.

However, in obese men, the rise in LH does not seem to affect testosterone levels, which may be an indication that IF induces a strong enough stress response in this subgroup of men to effectively negate the LH increase before it triggers testosterone production or because it is not strong enough to overcome the powerful estrogenic influence exerted by the excessive levels of body fat.

Testosterone has been found to be positively correlated with insulin sensitivity, which also reinforces the idea that body fat levels matter in terms of healthy testosterone levels, with normal and fit body fat levels exhibiting improved insulin sensitivity over overweight and obese individuals.

This fact also sheds a bit of light on when we should fast during the day.

For years I've been a proponent of skipping breakfast. Since reading Martin Berkhan's work and realizing that breakfast was not a physiologically necessary, but more a socially expected ritual, I began experimenting with life, sans my morning sustenance. And boy did dieting get easier.

In Martin's article on Leangains.com entitled, "Why Does Breakfast Make Me Hungry?" he sheds a little light on why most semi-fit individuals experience hunger relatively soon after eating breakfast, and why skipping breakfast is indeed preferable for your hormonal functioning, not to mention diet adherence.

The body's circadian cycle has a natural cortisol spike shortly after waking, and this happens to be the time most individuals eat breakfast as well. With fit, or somewhat fit, individuals, the insulin spike with the food intake, along with an already high insulin sensitivity, and the high levels of circulating cortisol at this time of day leads to a rapid drop in blood glucose shortly after consumption. The quick and possibly lower-than-normal blood glucose drop triggers the feeling of that "false hunger" within minutes to hours after that meal, so by mid-morning for most people.

By skipping breakfast, you are regulating your blood glucose levels, insulin, and cortisol during the period of the day in which they are most sensitive, and can have profound immediate effects on your body.

You are also allowing your body time to burn additional fat for fuel and rid itself of minor toxins before it needs to allocate energy to focus on things like digestion and glycogen synthesis.

The hormone leptin is also effectively regulated by intermittent fasting, and has been shown to be inversely correlated with testosterone levels and BMI in men, which means with a regular IF regimen, individuals can control yet another hormone that could potentially exert an influence over testosterone production.

Leptin is more popularly known for its major role in regulation of appetite and energy balance, but it is also involved with linking energy stores to the reproductive system.

Leptin is secreted by the fat cells and plays an important role in reducing food intake and increasing energy expenditure.

Recent rodent studies have also linked it to providing metabolic information to the reproductive system, both in females and males. In male mice, leptin treatment elevated FSH levels and increased seminal volume.

Leptin and testosterone levels are inversely correlated, with a rise in leptin resulting in a fall in testosterone and vice versa. Because of this, males have naturally lower levels of leptin than females. This gender difference suggests that gonadal steroid hormones may be potent regulators of leptin levels.

Because of the added variable of body fat levels being so intricately tied to both leptin and testosterone levels, it's very difficult to make conclusive statements about the dance between the three. Lean men have lower leptin levels, naturally, than overweight men (because leptin is secreted from adipocytes). We also know that lowering your body fat, in general, is one of the easiest ways to naturally increase your testosterone. These are all intricately tied together.

Intermittent fasting decreases leptin levels during the fast in men, and boosts them at re-feeding, operating in a peaks and valleys fashion. During the fast, leptin also has less power over regulation of the catecholamines epinephrine and norepinephrine which has positive implications for fat loss during the fast.

Intermittent fasting also increases levels of a hormone called adiponectin, which, along with leptin, is regulated by adipocytes, though adiponectin levels are inversely correlated with body fat levels, unlike leptin. This increase in adiponectin during the fast helps improve insulin sensitivity. Adiponectin is so powerful, in fact, that it's been shown to reverse insulin resistance in mice.

There are three popular methods for intermittent fasting that I recommend:

1. The Leangains Method
2. The Eat Stop Eat Method
3. The "Just Skip Breakfast" Method

Yes, other protocols exist. However, these three are the most realistic in terms of developing healthy lifestyle habits. Very few people can, or should, do things like alternate day fasting or 48 hour fasts. For the modern man or woman, with a job, kids, a family, social obligations, a sane mind, etc these are just not viable options.
So in this program, I recommend you fast on one of the above three protocols.

1. Leangains: Leangains is Martin Berkhan's style of intermittent fasting, and arguably the most popular and well-respected intermittent fasting protocol in the fitness world. He backs up his advice not only with solid research, but also with outstanding results from both his clients and himself.

He maintains low body fat year-round by eating and training on his protocol.

Any summary of Leangains is bound to do it an injustice if you haven't yet read the site itself. But in a nutshell, LG style of IF revolves around the 16/8 eating schedule.

- 16 hours fasting
- 8 hour feeding window

It's quite simple. For more information on DIY solutions in terms of macronutrient cycling and training protocols, which are unrelated to this program but very well-done nonetheless, you can look here at Andy Morgan's great site (rippedbody.jp).

2. Eat Stop Eat: ESE is the brainchild of Brad Pilon, a proponent of flexible dieting and using intermittent fasting as a tool to make reaching low body fat levels both easy to attain and maintain.

The ESE method is also quite simple, but at the risk of not doing it justice in this concise summary, I highly suggest you check it out for yourself at Eatstopeat.com.

In a nutshell, ESE involves two 24-hour fasts per week as metabolic resets and fat-burning stimuli.

For example, during a normal week, an individual could eat regularly every day except Wednesday and Saturday, electing instead to undergo a 24-hour fast.

If this protocol suits your personality or work/life schedule I recommend giving it a shot. Even one 24-hour fast per week will give you benefits.

3. The "Just Skip Breakfast" Method: This is the lazy man's method, and my protocol of choice.

Just skip breakfast.

Then resume eating around noon for lunch then have a dinner and possibly a night time meal, depending on your caloric goals for the day. It's very simple and doesn't require counting hours.

Most of the time you will end up on a schedule similar to the Leangains 16/8 protocol, but this includes a bit more flexibility, possibly at the expense of results (ie. lower body fat), but that makes it a great lifestyle option.

To wrap things up on IF: use it as a tool to give you both lifestyle flexibility and a boost in your testosterone levels, especially when integrated into a solid training and nutrition strategy. You can train fasted or fed, they both work.

Regular fasting will also provide your body with a nice reset and potent fat-burning potential, which will, once again, aid in testosterone production and regulation of satiety hormones over time.

Chapter 39

Sleep and Testosterone

We don't sleep enough. We're so seduced by the modern day electronic marvels that instead of hitting the sack, we can do thousands of other things instead.

And unfortunately that's what usually happens. When the sun sets and your body is ready to shut down and recharge itself, your brain tells you that its OK to watch one more episode of Breaking Bad instead.

Sure you'll be bit more tired the next day but that's about it right?

A Few Extra Hours of Sleep Can Double Your Testosterone

There are three major things that lay the foundation for your testosterone levels. They're sleep, diet, and exercise. The utmost important of them all, is sleep.

After all, your testosterone levels follow a circadian rhythm. They peak in the morning and slowly plummet towards the evening.

And when you're in the REM stages of your sleep, the endocrine system comes to life. Your brain starts sending signals down to your balls, telling them to produce massive amounts of testosterone, preparing you for the day ahead.

But how much testosterone is actually secreted during the night?

That's where science might help us:

a) Take this study (531) from Penev et al. for example. Where the researchers gathered up a group of healthy men to test their testosterone levels first thing in the morning when they had just woken up. They also gave these men a wrist band that showed how long each guy had slept.

The results showed that the guys who had slept for 4 hours, had testosterone levels hovering around 200-300 ng/dl.

Compare that to the guys who slept for 8 hours, they had their levels at around 500-700 ng/dl.

The results showed that the more you sleep, the more testosterone your body produces. It's just that simple.

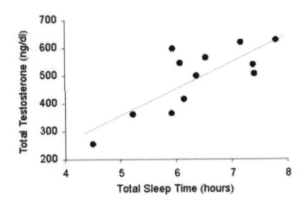

b) This study from Gov et al. (532) found out similar results. They had 531 healthy men as test subjects, and they examined how the amount of sleep correlated with their testosterone level.

The results again show that the men who slept more also had significantly higher testosterone levels. In fact the guys who slept for 4 hours had about 60% less testosterone in their serum, than the men who slept for 8 hours.

The researchers in both studies concluded that men with low T are probably put on hormone replacement therapies far too quickly, as just one night with lack of sleep can more than halve serum testosterone levels.

Aside from sleeping longer, you can also supercharge the nightly testosterone production by improving the quality of your sleep.

How to Improve Sleep Quality

How many hours you sleep is completely up to you. However you can get more out of those hours by incorporating some simple sleep quality improving tips to your daily life.

You've probably heard the age old useless tips like drinking warm milk or counting sheep. But here's a list of ways that will actually work:

1. Sleep in complete darkness. By this I mean that there should be not a single led light visible in the room where you're sleeping in. As even a single dot of light in your night clock or mobile phone is enough to disturb the pineal gland's ability to secrete the sleep hormone melatonin.

2. Close all the mobile-networks and wi-fi hotspots. This Saudi-Arabian study (533) found out that the electromagnetic frequencies decrease sleep quality.

3. Exercise during the day, as research has shown (534) that just a simple exercise session incorporated in your daily life, can dramatically improve sleep quality.

4. Melatonin. This is the hormone that your pineal gland secretes to make you sleep, thus it's called the "sleep hormone". You can supplement with it, and few studies also show that it may boost testosterone levels via inhibiting the aromatase enzyme.

5. Sleep in a cold room and be naked if you can. Firstly because cold room will mimic the natural sleeping habitat of the human body (we were meant to sleep outside), and secondly because the testicles need to be a tad bit colder than the basal body temperature is, for optimal functioning (that's why they hang in a pouch outside the body and that's also why cold showers and loose boxers increase testosterone).

6. Don't watch bright electronic displays before you hit the sack, as the "blue light" in most electronic screens will impair pineal gland's ability to produce melatonin (I use a software called f.lux, which automatically dims the screen and reduces "blue light" when its getting close to bedtime).

7. Supplement with Ashwagandha, as several studies have found that it positively influences sleep quality, which is likely due to the fact that it lowers the stress hormone cortisol (it's also a potent testosterone booster).

8. Consume some simple carbs a hour or two before hitting the bed, as this will skyrocket your insulin production, making you energetic for a brief moment, but then your insulin will crash which makes you fall into sleep more easily.

9. Consume some high quality protein before hitting the bed, as certain amino acid's such as L-tryptophan will increase melatonin production in the brain, thus also improves sleep quality.

Sleep quality and timing are of utmost importance when it comes to optimizing your natural testosterone production.

You may be thinking, "Obviously I just need to sleep more - everybody always says to sleep more, but I still have trouble finding the time, or I just cannot fall asleep in the first place anyways."

Here's the deal: most people miss the point with an overly simplistic view of sleep, and the role it plays in optimizing testosterone production.

It is true, however. You do need to sleep more.

That study conducted in young men found a significant drop in testosterone levels with even just the reduction from 8 hours of sleep per night to 5 hours.

In the Western world, a 5 hour night is commonplace. Most people live like that for the majority of their lives. No wonder we're all having issues with this.

Sleep is especially important for those of us who lead hectic, busy, hard-charging lifestyles. You might work a challenging job in a big city, study around the clock as a student, or sit on the highway for a 2 hour commute every day.

Most of us lead lives and have careers that are inherently stressful in the first place, so high levels of circulating cortisol put us at major risk for low testosterone... even if we're doing everything else right in terms of training and nutrition.

So adequate sleep should be a priority.

What exactly happens in the body when just a couple fewer hours of sleep causes such drastic drops in testosterone?

Quite simply, less sleeps means less activity in the pituitary- gonadal axis during the prime part of your body's natural circadian cycle. This reduction in activity comes in the form of less LH secretion, with the limited LH leading to a reduction in testosterone production.

Studies have found this reduced activity to take effect with as little as 3 hours reduction in total sleep time and to become increasingly more pronounced up to 48 hours of sleep deprivation.

While the exact determinants have not been examined as to precisely how this happens, scientists do know that it has a lot to do with the body's circadian rhythms and the pulsatile manner in which pituitary hormones are secreted.

Because of this vitally important rhythmic cycle in the body, however, like I hinted at before, quantity of sleep is not the only important part of this equation, timing of wakefulness appears to be just as important.

In a 2012 study published in the Journal Of Clinical Endocrinology, researchers decided to look deeper into the matter of sleep timing and the role it plays on hormonal secretion. They split test subjects into two groups: one group had sleep restricted early in the night but awoke at normal times (i.e. they basically just stayed up late and woke up at a normal time in the morning) and the other subjects were forced to wake up unnaturally early.

What did they find?

The group that stayed up late over two nights showed no significant change in LH, T, or PRL secretion following the trials.

The group that was forced to wake up early showed significantly reduced pituitary activity which resulted in markedly lower LH, testosterone, and PRL levels in the morning.

So if you ever needed a good excuse to hit the snooze button on the alarm clock - now you have it. Waking up too early can have a notably adverse effect on your testosterone production.

And although this particular study did not examine the relationship between cortisol and these parameters as well, these findings make perfect sense in the context of natural cortisol secretion being higher in the early mornings.

So, long story short, if you intermittently need to sacrifice sleep in the name of getting extra work done, I advise you to stay up late and not to get up early in order to finish that project in time.

However, this study was only conducted over two days. Remember, other studies show a significant reduction in testosterone levels with just slightly limited sleep quantity over time. So you must take measures to aim for the recommended full 8 hours of sleep per night, and not take this as a free-pass to stay up late every night.

Use this knowledge to make better decisions when the time calls for it. Staying up later is better than getting up earlier.

Chronically staying up late, and sacrificing overall sleep in the process, will still lead to chronic reduction in pituitary- gonadal activity and a chronic increase in circulating cortisol - so don't do it often.

4 Evidence-Based Sleep Supplements

But what about supplements? Surely there's some over-the-counter options that can significantly improve sleep quality? And, Well, yes there is:

1. Magnesium

Perhaps one of the most well-known and dirt cheap natural sleep aids there is, is a high-quality magnesium supplement.

Magnesium is a mineral that can be found in all of bodily tissues, and it regulates over 300 enzyme functions. It's safe to say that it's one of the most important dietary micronutrients for our health. Heck, there's even research showing how magnesium supplementation can increase testosterone levels.

According to this study, (535) 68% of Americans are deficient in magnesium. The National Health and Nutrition Examination Survey (NHANES), sets this number to 60%. (536)

When it comes to improving sleep, magnesium is superb. It's involved in muscle relaxation, and works as an agonist to the brain GABA-β receptors (the receptors which after activation, produce sedative-like effects in the body).

The evidence on the effectiveness of magnesium for sleep parameters is very interesting. A double-blind randomized clinical trial with 46 elderly subjects, (537) found that 500 mg's of daily magnesium taken for 8 weeks, significantly increased sleep time, sleep efficiency, and melatonin production, while simultaneously reducing cortisol levels and sleep onset latency.

In another study, (538) increasing dosages (10mmol-30mmol) of effervescent magnesium tablets were given to 12 elderly subjects 3 times a day for 20 days, resulting in: significantly lower cortisol levels and improved sleep parameters (measured by brain EEG).

One study consisting of 100 subjects (539) also showed improved sleep quality with a daily dose of 320mg magnesium citrate (this is roughly the RDA of magnesium).

Bottom line: There's good amount of evidence suggesting that magnesium can be particularly effective at increasing sleep quality in humans. A dose range of 300-900 mg/day seems to be effective, and magnesium glycinate is considered to be the best OTC supplement form with highest bio-availibity in the body.

2. Ashwagandha

Ashwagandha (Withania Somnifera) is a herbal supplement (commonly root powder or extract) widely used in the Indian herbal medicine, aka. Ayurveda.

It has some good research behind its back and apart from being able to increase testosterone levels (big article about that coming this week), there's evidence that ashwagandha supplementation could also promote optimal sleep by serving as an agonist to the brain GABA-receptors which promote sedative effects and relaxation in the body. Ashwagandha can also suppress the stress-hormone cortisol and reduces symptoms of anxiety & stress. (540)

It's one of the "better" supplemental herbs out there and one of my all-time favorites. I take few caps of this KSM-66 extract before hitting the sack almost on a nightly basis, and I can honestly feel the difference in my sleep quality (additionally you can dissolve some ashwagandha root liquid to chamomile tea for similar effect.)

Anyhow, don't take my word for it, there's research on this too. For instance, in mice, 100-200 mg/kg of ashwagandha is as effective as 500 mg's of Diazepam (powerful prescription sedative and sleep drug) in inducing sedation (541, 542). Few other studies on mice (543) and rats (544) have found that ashwagandha increases sleep quality relative to placebo.

As for human studies, combined with few other herbs, 2000 mg's of ashwagandha was able to improve sleep quality. (545)
In a study that used a fairly high dose (up to 1250mg) of KSM-66 ashwagandha (546) (water extract) improved sleep quality was also reported.

A study of women who underwent chemotherapy for cancer, noted a significant trend of self-reported improvements in sleep quality with ashwagandha supplementation. (547)

Bottom line: If you count out the rodent studies, ashwagandha doesn't have as good scientific evidence behind its back as magnesium does, but still, the evidence is there and ashwagandha should deepen your sleep to some extent. I have used the herb (both extract and pure root powder) for years now, and my personal experiences are in line with the research. Without a doubt, the best kind of ashwagandha you can find, is high-quality standardized KSM-66 extract.

3. Gelatin

Short on cash but still would like a little something that helps you sleep like a baby? Then consider gelatin.

Gelatin is the odorless, colorless, brittle stuff that is used when you make jelly. It's in fact the connective tissue that is derived from collagen of various meat industry by-products (animal hearts, brains, skin, etc).

Why would gelatin be good for sleep you ask? Well, let me explain:
In our modern society, we tend to consume only the muscle-meat of animals, which gives us plenty of the amino acids tryptophan and methionine, but very little of glycine. We could use more of that glycine though, since it's an important amino-acid needed for the synthesis of various bodily enzymes, along with being a sedative (kind of like a "downer") neurotransmitter in the body.

The last part of that sentence is the reason behind glycine's ability to improve sleep quality. It's a sedative neurotransmitter.

And what would be the best source for glycine then? That would be, connective tissue. And besides eating bones and organs, the simplest way of getting more of that connective tissue would be gelatin (which is 22% glycine by weight).

NOTE: you could also buy pure glycine powder, which is extremely cheap too ($24 for a kilo if you live in the states).

Besides the many theories of the importance of glycine and the warnings about not getting enough of it in our modern diets, there's actually some research on its ability to improve sleep.

For instance, 3 grams of glycine taken 1-hour before hitting the sack, was able to reduce morning fatigue and improve self-reported sleep quality in this human study. (548)

In another study, (549) 3 grams of glycine taken before bed-time, not only increased self-reported sleep quality and day-time cognitive abilities, but also resulted in reduced onset sleep latency and faster time to reach slow wave sleep when tested with EEG apparatus (the kind of machine that senses brain activity via scalp electrodes).

The same dose of 3 grams glycine taken 1-hour before bed was also tested successfully in subjects which suffered from mild sleep problems (the day-time cognitive improvements were also noted in the study). (550)

Bottom line: Glycine seems to be very effective at improving sleep quality and day-time cognitive abilities. It's also cheap and easily accessible in the form or gelatin or pure glycine powder.

4. Melatonin

Melatonin is the neurohormone that causes and also regulates your sleep. It's naturally secreted from the pineal gland in your brain at evening and when you're in a dark room, and conversely light suppresses the synthesis of melatonin (which is why sleeping in a completely dark room improves sleep quality, and why hitting the sack when the sun goes down and waking up at sunrise would be a good idea).

If you're doing shift work, supplemental melatonin can be extremely effective, due to the fact that the natural production of the hormone is suppressed during day-time (which is when most shift-workers tend to sleep).

The research on melatonin is solid, which is not a surprise since its usually used as a go-to treatment for insomnia and many sleep related conditions.

Firstly, taking supplemental melatonin is able to increase blood melatonin levels, both at day-time and night-time. (551) Also, supplemental melatonin at doses ranging from 2 to 10 mg's is fairly effective at reducing insomnia (552, 553, 554).

In few studies, melatonin at 2-3 mg doses has improved sleep quality and morning-alertness without any noted withdrawal symptoms or side-effects (555, 556).

NOTE: It's common sense to think that more melatonin would be better for deeper sleep. However this isn't the case, and high dosages might actually cause drowsiness in the day-time. It's recommended that you work the dose up from small amounts first to see what is effective for you.

Bottom line: Melatonin is very effective, especially for reducing the time it takes for the user to fall a sleep, aka. at reducing onset sleep latency. For shift-workers, it's almost a must have supplement. Opt for non-time released form of melatonin. If you're already following a reasonably normal sleep-awake rhythm and have no problems falling to sleep, then there's always a change that melatonin might not do much for you. I personally only use melatonin at nights when I hit the sack "too late."

— Chapter 40 —

Avoid These Disruptive Chemicals

Plastic. The savior of the modern day human, and the solution to all of our daily problems.

What could we do without it, now that we have gone and invented it already?

The answer is, that we couldn't do much. I once tried living a day without touching anything that's made from plastic, and I lasted 2 hours. A challenge that sounded extremely easy to accomplish, but once you try, seems impossible.

I mean just think about it. You wake up, maybe you brush your teeth? Well there you go, the toothpaste comes out of a plastic tube, and the brush is made out of plastic. What's next? Maybe you have some bacon and eggs for breakfast and then you realize that the bacon is wrapped in plastic. And what we're you going to cook the bacon and eggs with? Let me guess, a pan, and some plastic cooking utensils.

Maybe you want to hit the gym after the breakfast, which means that you're going to need some water, and where does that water go into? That's right, straight into a plastic bottle. Oh, and after the gym, what about the recovery drink? Maybe mix some whey powder and milk together in a plastic shaker bottle.

To put it mildly, we are surrounded by plastics.

Some might argue that it's a good thing, and surely, plastics are extremely useful in multiple daily tasks, but they also have a flip side.

They're like poison to your balls and testosterone production, and likely the main cause to this global decrease in testosterone levels.

Let's take a closer look.

Why Plastics Lower Testosterone Levels

I know what many of you guys are now wondering the exact same thing as I was years ago.

How the fuck could plastics do anything for the human body? And what makes plastics so bad?

I mean the whole idea of plastics being harmful sounds like some tinfoil-ufo-controversy-BS at first. But once you understand the idea behind the harmful effects, you also understand what makes plastics unhealthy.

1. The first problem is a chemical group called phthalates. They're used to make plastics soft and flexible, and as you might guess, they're found in nearly all kinds of flexible plastics ranging from soda bottles to plastic bags. Phthalates are linked to delayed puberty, low testosterone, and feminine characteristics in various human and animal studies (explained more in detail below).

2. The second problem is a chemical called Bisphenol A or BPA. It's also linked to low testosterone, increased estrogen, delayed puberty, and feminine characteristics in various human and animal studies (also explained in more detail below).

3. The third problem is that a huge list of chemicals used in the manufacturing process of plastic products are labeled as xenoestrogens, meaning that they mimic the effects of exogenous estrogen (female hormone) in the body. This includes the phthalates and BPA that I mentioned above, and also: PCBs, Bisphenol S (BPS), dioxin, vinyl chloride, styrene, phenolix, epoxy resin, PMMA, PTFE, and many many others.

In short, the toxic load of xenoestrogens and endocrine system toxins that gets into your body through the usage of plastic products, is easily enough to cause massive damage in your endocrine system and testosterone production.

Here's some science about the matter:

a) This Swedish study (557) had 196 boys as subjects. The researchers measured phthalate levels from their mothers when they were still pregnant, and once the kids were 21 months old, their "anogenital distance" – which is a pretty solid physical measurement of testosterone – was measured, to see if the phthalates had effect on the hormonal health of these 196 subject boys. The results were clear, the more phthalates the mother had in her system during pregnancy, the shorter the anogenital distance in the baby (the shorter the distance the lower the testosterone).

b) This study (558) compared the men who worked at a chemical plant which manufactures BPA, to men who worked at a tap water factory. The results show that the men who worked in contact with BPA had significantly lower serum testosterone levels, and especially free testosterone levels, when compared to the tap water factory fellows.

c) This human study (559) found out that Bisphenol A causes sexual dysfunction in men. Several animal studies have also found that BPA is estrogenic, lowers testosterone, and causes sexual dysfunction (560, 561, 562, 563, 564).

d) This study (565) saw that Bisphenol A inhibited the enzyme 5-alpha reductase, thus blocked dihydrotestosterone (DHT) production. Same study also found that BPA increased the activity of aromatase enzyme, which converts testosterone into estrogen.

e) This study (566) found out that the phthalates used in the manufacturing process of flexible plastics can be considered xenoestrogens, due to the fact that they bind into estrogen receptors and induce feminizing effects in the body.

f) In this study, (567) the researches analyzed 18 different samples of bottled water. Eleven of the samples showed significant estrogenic response.

g) This rat study, (568) found out that a mixture containing 5 different phthalate esters, strongly inhibits testicular testosterone production.

h) The researchers in this study (569) concluded that phthalates can be straight on labeled as anti-androgens, and that they contribute to testicular dysgenesis syndrome (TDS)

i) In this study, (570) the researched tested 445 common plastic products to see if there was any estrogenic activity in them. 70% of the products induced significant estrogenic activity, and the number jumped to 95% when the products were altered to "real life" conditions, such as the microwave heat and putting them to dishwasher. Also note that many of the products in this study were labeled as BPA-free, yet they still induced estrogenic effects similar to BPA plastics.

There's hundreds of similar studies on the internet, and if you're interested in seeing more of them, Google is your friend.

How come these chemicals can be found inside the human body? I don't eat plastics!

Answer: We get most of the chemicals mentioned above through foods and drinks. For example: most of the meat products, fish, processed foods, and certain oils, and spreads are all packed in plastic wraps/packs. Bottled water is also loaded with phthalates (this study (571) found that out of the 18 analyzed samples, 11 induced significant estrogenic response).

Microwaving plastic is also one extremely efficient and quick way to load up your body with phthalates and BPA, as is drinking soda (just think about all that acidic drink sitting in those freshly produced soft plastic bottles for months).

Is there any proof that humans are altered to these chemicals, or is it just a theory?

Answer: It's not a theory, just take a look at the studies presented above. Also take a look at these studies with similar conclusions (572, 573, 574, 575). It's a simple fact. The chemicals leech from various products straight into our bodies, and the levels in most people are dangerously high.

Is there a way to avoid this exposure then?

Answer: Yes of course! Just avoid plastic products as much as possible (you can't avoid them completely though). Don't drink bottled water, soda, etc. If there's a relatively useful alternative to plastic products, made from wood, metal, or ceramic, etc. use it instead.

Let me give you some quick examples: Switch plastic cooking utensils to wood or metal alternatives, use a metal flask as a workout bottle, never microwave anything in plastic, don't use tupperware to store your foods (instead use something like these)(576), and so forth. Basically just use your brain.

BPA

Bisphenol A (BPA) is a man made chemical that was first synthesized back in 1891. It's heavily used in the manufacturing processes of polycarbonate plastics and epoxy resins, and it's often hailed as one of the most conventional chemicals.

Bisphenol A is also the most tested chemical in the world, and through that testing, some rather alarming evidence has been found.

The thing that we're interested in here, is BPA's effects on the endocrine system, and mainly how it affects male testosterone levels, estrogen levels, and sexual function.

Some Science About BPA and the Endocrine System:

a) This study (577) compared the men who worked at a chemical plant which manufactures BPA to the men who worked at a tap water factory. The results show that the men who worked in contact with BPA had significantly lower serum testosterone levels, and especially free testosterone levels, when compared to the tap water factory fellows.

b) This study (578) found out that phthalates and BPA from plastics caused delayed puberty, lower free and total testosterone, increased serum estrogen, and increased SHBG count, in boys between the ages of 8-14.

c) Several animal studies have found that BPA is estrogenic, lowers testosterone, and causes sexual dysfunction (579, 580, 581, 582, 583).

d) This study (584) found out that BPA causes sexual dysfunction in human males.

e) This study (585) saw that Bisphenol A inhibited the enzyme 5-alpha reductase, thus blocked dihydrotestosterone (DHT) production. Same study also found that BPA increased the activity of aromatase enzyme, which converts testosterone into estrogen.

What's even more troubling is the fact that in all of the studies I've seen, 95-99% of the test subjects had detectable levels of BPA in their system. So BPA affects nearly everyone.

That's why I created this list of 5 hidden sources of BPA, so that you can avoid the things that are slowly crushing the life out of your testicles.

Let's get to it.

1. All Kinds of Receipts

Grocery store receipts, bus tickets, air plane tickets, and basically everything that's "instantly printed" after your purchase, contain huge amounts of Bisphenol A.

This is because the thermal paper on which the receipt is printed on contains alarmingly high levels of BPA as seen in this study. (586)

When you handle those receipts or even worse, store them in your wallet, you're constantly exposed to BPA. This study (587) actually found out that you can experience a five-fold increase in your BPA levels, few hours after fiddling around with thermal paper.

You can avoid this by not taking the receipts that you don't actually need, or if you do, don't fiddle around with them and wash your hands as soon as you can.

NOTE: The ink also contains BPA, the same ink is also used to print newspapers (588).

2. Toilet Paper

This is a relatively new and one hell of an annoying discovery to me. But the truth is that our toilet paper is laden with BPA.

That's due to the fact that toilet paper is mostly recycled paper, which contains the BPA laden thermal paper discussed above.

The fact that toilet papers usually contain alarmingly high levels of BPA was first seen in this study. (589)

This is probably one of those things that we have to just live with, because as far as I know there's no BPA free toilet paper around, mainly because people don't know that we wipe our asses with the estrogen mimic daily.

3. Plastics

Plastics are probably one of the biggest reasons behind the fact that our global average on male testosterone levels is so rapidly decreasing.

They're just filled with estrogen mimics and testosterone lowering chemicals, such as the notorious phthalates and Bisphenol A.

And yes there's a lot of BPA-free labeled plastics out there. However this excellent report (590) found out that nearly all of the them still contain a chemical called Bisphenol S (BPS) which is basically the same thing but with a different name, and if they don't, then they're laden with other estrogen mimics.

Every type of plastic commonly used in food packaging tested positive in some cases, which suggested there was no surefire way to avoid exposure to estrogen mimics.

And that's the reason why I've been as plastic free as I can for the past few years.

Obviously no one can fully avoid plastics, as they're literally everywhere, but this doesn't mean that we have to expose ourselves to all of them constantly.

I'm personally using this metal bottle in the gym, (591) I have thrown away all the plastic Tupperware containers and only use metal, glass, or wood based containers, I don't drink from plastic cups, I use wooden cooking utensils, a cast iron pan, etc.

There's a lot of easy switches that can be made to reduce our exposure to BPA and phthalates, you just have to start making them.

4. Canned Foods

The epoxy lining in nearly all aluminum cans is made with BPA.
And if the content of the can is something acidic, like tomatoes or soda for example, then you can be sure that the foods are also laden with the chemical.

Stainless steel cans however are much more safer alternatives. In general there's no BPA used in the linings, as there's in aluminum alternatives.

Few companies have also switched to BPA-free aluminum cans, such as Trader Joe's, Eden Foods, and Muir Glen. Campbell's has also said that they will switch to BPA free cans but they haven't said when. In other words they probably won't.

Obviously, your best bet is to make your own foods instead of eating canned goods and processed junk.

5. Some Old Water Pipes

Some old water pipes were also coated with BPA in order to extend their life.

And it's not a big co-incidence that traces of BPA, phthalates, and all kinds of endocrine disruptors have been found in the U.S tap water in numerous studies.

Even the cleanest tap waters in the world are contaminated with a wide variety of estrogen mimics.

If you're from U.S (where the water supply is in much worse condition), I would highly recommend you to get a filter of some kind.

Personal Care Products

This might be a weird topic, but it's a fact that you will likely increase your testosterone levels, while slashing estrogen, by changing your everyday personal care items (toothpaste, shampoos, soaps, deodorants, etc) to chemical-free and natural alternatives. This effect is largely due to lower exposure to endocrine disruptors.

That's right, there can be an absolutely ridiculous amount of estrogen mimics and anti-androgenic endocrine system disrupting chemicals in your everyday convenience-store bought personal care items. These include (but are not limited to):

Parabens (methyl-, butyl-, ethyl-, propyl-, heptyl-, etc) which are preservatives used in nearly all kinds of cosmetics, such as; sun lotions, moisturizers, personal-lubricants, shampoos, shaving gels, toothpaste, and even as food additives. They're classified as xenoestrogens, and can have a weak affinity to estrogen receptors in the body. (592)

Phthalates which are commonly used to make plastics more flexible, but they are also used as stabilizers and emulsifying agents in many personal care items. Increased urinary phthalate traces have been strongly correlated with decreased testosterone in men, women, and children. (593)

Benzophenones (BP-1, BP-2, BP-3...) which are permeability enhancing UV-stabilizers are used in a wide range of personal care items, but most commonly in sunscreens. Concerns have been raised of their effect in reducing the activity of enzymes needed in testosterone production. This has been studied for BP-1, (594) BP-2, (595) and BP-3. (596)

Triclosan and Triclocarban, both of which are antibacterial agents found in many antibacterial soaps, lotions, hand sanitizers, etc. Not only are they highly ineffective at reducing bacteria, they also have direct mechanism in lowering testicular testosterone production. (597)

Those and many more man-made chemicals that can act as hormone disruptors, are generously used in the manufacturing process and as ingredients of many personal care items.

Not good thing considering that you're constantly in touch with them on a daily basis, and your skin is very permeable to most of the chemicals applied. Since many of the endocrine disrupting chemicals are completely unnecessary for the consumer, it's really easy to just change the brand and buy something that does not contain them.

Below are some brands & products that I recommend and use.

- Duke Cannon Big American Brick of Soap (only for bad-asses)
- Acure Organics Natural Shampoo (argan stem + oil)
- Himalaya Herbal Healthcare Neem & Pomegranate Toothpaste
- North Coast Organic All Natural Deodorant
- Lather & Wood's Luxurious Sophisticated Mens Moisturizer for the Man's Man
- Pacific Shaving Company All Natural Shaving Cream

Fluoride and Testosterone

Everyone knows fluoride. It's the naturally occurring inorganic chemical used heavily in toothpastes, salts, and tap water supply for the prevention of tooth decay. And even though some hippie "alternate medicine" people like to claim that it doesn't work and is "pure evil conspiracy", there's plenty of evidence to show that it does protect the teeth by reinforcing the enamel shield. (598)

With that being said, I have been actively avoiding fluoride for roughly 3 years now. That's right, I use fluoride-free toothpaste, I have a tap water filtration system that filters away fluoride under my sink, and I try to avoid fluoridated foods and/or foods high in naturally occurring fluoride (as a side note, my teeth are still in great condition without any extra fluoride use).

The reason behind my - as some might say "crazy" - fluoride avoidance?

It's a well documented fact that fluoride can disrupt normal testosterone and thyroid hormone production. This is due to the facts that fluoride is toxic at low levels in the human body and causes oxidative stress, it can displace iodine from androgen receptors and thyroid gland, and it can adversely impact testicular cells and enzymes needed for healthy testosterone production.

There's a good reason why every toothpaste package has a warning that states how small children should never swallow the contents.

And that "just a pea sized portion is enough". This is so that the fluoride would only go topically to your teeth (where it protects the enamel), but not so much into your digestion and circulation (where it acts as a neuroendocrine toxin).

Much like the other light halides (chlorine and bromine), fluoride can displace iodine from human cells, (599) when that happens inside testicular leydig cells, sertoli cells, androgen receptors, and at the thyroid gland, you're in for a hormonal disaster.

However, the displacement of iodine is nowhere near the only negative side effect of ingested iodine. It can also increase oxidative damage in testicles, (600) reducing the protective antioxidants and impairing enzyme signaling needed for healthy testosterone production.

In case you need some research to believe it, here's what a quick search gets you:

a) Fluoride anions that come in contact with calcium ions in the body, form a compound called calcium fluoride, which can mess up with the function of many neuroendocrine glands, causing calcification and impaired protein signaling (601, 602, 603).

b) In multiple rodent studies, it has been seen that fluoride has a dose-dependent negative impact on testicular testosterone production, (604) due to impaired enzyme functions, oxidative damage, impaired cholesterol transportation, blocking androgen receptors, and direct cell damage (605, 606, 607, 608, 609, 610, 611).

c) In a human study (612) where males from a high-fluoride water area were compared against males from an area with low-fluoride water, the males who were exposed to higher amounts of fluoride had 40% lower serum T levels on average. This study was replicated with larger amount of subjects in 2010, (613) with similar conclusions: "the serum level of T in men of fluoride polluted district was significantly less than that of control group".

d) In this human study, (614) it was noted that people who suffer from skeletal fluorosis (too high intake of fluoride, aka. fluoride toxicity), have significantly lower testosterone levels when compared to control subjects.

e) In this 2003 human study, (615) it was seen that even lower doses of 2-13 mg/day of fluoride are capable of significantly lowering free testosterone levels.

NOTE: Fluoride also accumulates in the body, so the problem is not only caused by high acute exposure to fluoride, but also because we're constantly exposed to it at lower doses. Major sources of fluoride being; unfiltered tap water, fluoridated salt, toothpaste, and certain foods naturally high in fluoride (black tea being the worst offender). (616)

Pesticides

The global average on male testosterone levels is crashing down rapidly, year after year. In a 17 year study (617) with 1,700 men as subjects, the researchers found out that since the late 80's, the average US men's testosterone levels have dropped by 1% every year.

In a Finnish study (618) with somewhat similar design, it was seen that men born in the 70's have roughly 20% less testosterone at age 35 than their father's generation had at the same age.

Even when the researchers adjust the results according to age, obesity, smoking status, etc. the drop in testosterone still shows up, and there hasn't really been a conclusion about what is causing this decline that seems to just speed up as years go by.

While the scientifically proven conclusion to the above has yet to be found, many endocrinologists believe that there's a clear reason behind the global decline in T.

Increased exposure to man-made chemicals. Many of which act as xenoestrogens and endocrine disruptors in the body.

We're constantly exposed to them on a daily basis, as they're hidden in soaps, shampoos, deodorants, house cleaning products, car care products, air fresheners, plastics, preservatives, and so forth.

The worst offenders though? Pesticides sprayed to conventionally raised foodstuffs, which tend to end up and accumulate in our bodies after consuming the foods laden with such chemicals.

Pesticides and Testosterone Production

Whenever I mention to someone that I'm mainly consuming organic foods, the response is often as follows:

"Whaaat? Why the fuck, that's more expensive and it's not at all different or more nutritious than eating conventional produce."
It's true that eating organic is significantly more expensive, one doesn't have to be a genius to see it. Also, the taste is rather similar to conventional stuff. Heck, they are not even that much more nutritious than the conventional produce is.

Yet, I still do spend my money on organic foods, rather than the cheaper conventionally grown kind.

It's because of the stuff that I don't want into my body; the pesticides, herbicides, insecticides, and fungicides. You know, those man-made chemicals that are sprayed into the crops by people in breathing masks and moon suits.

Some say that there's no evidence of these chemicals being harmful to hormones or general health as a whole, but that's where I have to disagree. At least on the hormonal part.

And here's why:

Pesticides and Testosterone Research:

a) In this study, (619) the researchers tested 37 widely used pesticides to see if any of them had any anti-androgenic effects in-vitro. Out of the 37 tested chemicals, 30 were shown to be anti-androgenic. 14 of the tested chemicals were previously known for having a hormone disrupting effect, but the researchers were shocked to find out sixteen more that had no known hormonal activity until now.

b) In this large-scale study, (620) it was noted that 91% of the US test subjects had noticeable amounts of the insecticide; chlorpyrifos, in their bodies. In another human study, (621) TCPY (3,5,6-trichloro-2-pyridinol) which is a metabolite of chlorpyrifos, was noted of having a dose-dependent testosterone lowering effect in multiple linear regression models. Several animal studies have also shown that chlorpyrifos has a significant testosterone lowering effect (622, 623, 624).

c) In this study, (625) it was noted that RoundUp, one of the most used herbicides in the World (especially in GMO foods), has a direct testosterone suppressing effect in testicular leydig cells at very low environmental doses.

d) In this 2007 study, (626) various pesticides (some of which have been already banned) were shown to be anti-androgenic and mess up with the 5-a reductase enzyme, which is responsible for dihydrotestosterone (DHT) synthesis.

e) Atrazine, one of the most widely used herbicides in US, has been shown to decrease testosterone levels in fish, amphibians, and rodents (627, 628, 629, 630, 631, 632, 633). Also, according to this study (634) increased atrazine concentrations in water can transform male frogs into females (literally to the point where they grow ovaries). I haven't seen any human studies about atrazine's effect on testosterone levels, but I'm fairly sure, only after looking at the animal evidence, that this stuff is something I'm not going to ingest willingly.

f) Finclozolin is a common fungicide generously sprayed on fruits and vegetables. According to EPA (635) (Environmental Protection Agency), vinclozolin is a competetive antagonist to androgen receptors, and can activate the receptor similarly to testosterone. However it's suspected that the chemical doesn't activate the receptor properly, and hence just "steals" the place from the actual male hormones. Furthermore, two vinclozolin metabolites have been identified as anti-androgens and the chemical is suspected to have feminizing effects in humans. Vinclozolin is also banned in Finland, Sweden, Denmark, and Norway.

g) In this Peruvian study, (636) it was noted that men who work as organophosphate sprayers experience significantly lower testosterone levels and worse semen parameters than control subjects.

h) In Denmark, the farmers of organic produce have significantly higher sperm quality and sex hormone levels, (637) when compared to their conventional produce farming peers. Same researchers have also found out that greenhouse workers in contact with fungicides, experience suppressed testosterone levels and reduced sperm quality. (638)

i) In American men, exposure to PCB's (polychlorinated biphenyls) is strongly associated with lower serum testosterone levels. (639) PCB's were heavily used in multiple chlorinated pesticides many years ago, but they're extremely persistent in the environment, lasting for years or even decades in soil and lake sediments, which is why we still continue to get this stuff into our bodies.

Sunscreens

What puzzles me almost daily, is how and why people have seemingly lost their ability of rational thinking. This lack of common sense, is especially true when it comes to sun protection. We are told by so called "experts" that being out in the sun without some SPF 100+ lotion, would cause rapid skin cancer, and also damage our skin.

Yet our ancestors spent a lot more time out in the sun than we do, and didn't use any sun blockers. They also had significantly lower amounts of skin cancer, and if you look at old pictures, you can see that even their skin was in a much better condition than ours. Something is not right with that.

We are out in the sun for significantly shorter durations than our ancestors, and we use more "protective" lotions that block the so called "harmful" sun rays, yet the skin cancer rates have skyrocketed since the invention of sunscreen.

Recent (non-sponsored) research is even more puzzling: according to this European study (640) – which looked at 57 different studies – a continuous exposure to sun rays (note that this doesn't mean sunburn), significantly reduces the risk of skin cancer (melanoma).

The debate on if sunscreen use is necessary or not to prevent skin cancer is beyond the scope of this article. What I'm going to talk about with you, is the potential testosterone lowering effects of these so called "sun blockers".

Common Endocrine Disruptors in Sunscreens

- benzophenones (BP-1, BP-2, BP-3, – permeability enhanching UV stabilizers)
- 4-Methylbenzylidene camphor (4-MBC – UV filter).
- parabens (methyl, butyl, propyl, etc).
- octyl-dimethyl-PABA (UV filter).
- octyl-methoxycinnamate (UV-B filter).
- homosolate (UV filter)

Benzophenones

a) In this in-vitro study benzophenone-1 (641) (BP-1) reduced testosterone levels and the activity of androgen receptors.

b) Furthermore, in this study benzophenone-2 (642) (BP-2) reduced testosterone in-vitro in human testicular cells and also in male rats. BP-2 also significantly reduced thyroid hormone levels, but the researchers say that the reduction in thyroid hormones was only partly responsible for the reduction in testosterone.

c) And then, in this study (643) conducted by Dr. Peter Dingle, the application of three active ingredients commonly found in sunscreens (benzephone-3, 4-MBC, and octyl-methoxycinnamate) for one week, led to a drop in testosterone and estradiol levels in men.

d) In this study, (644) BP-3 metabolites were found to be xenoestrogenic in cultured human cells, even though BP-3 itself didn't show estrogenic activity in this previous study. (645)

e) Few more studies have also found that benzophenones are anti-androgenic and can block dihydrotestosterone from binding into the androgen receptors (646, 647, 648, 649).

f) The worst thing about benzophenones, is the fact that they're particularly penetrative. This is caused because they're the least lipophilic of the most common UV filters, meaning that they can easily absorb through the bi-layer of phospholipids of the human skin and into the bloodstream. In fact, the researchers in this study (650) tested 2,517 patients just to find out that 96.8% of urine samples tested positive for benzophenones. Similar results were seen in this study, where all the 30 adult subjects tested positive for benzophenones. (651)

4-Methylbenzylidene Camphor

a) There are few studies which have shown the UV-B filter 4-Methylbenzylidene Camphor (4-MBC) to be a potent xenoestrogen, meaning that it mimics the actions of exogenous estrogen in the human body by increasing estrogen levels and also activating its target receptors. These results have been noticed in both: in-vitro and in-vivo studies (652, 653, 654).

b) In this rodent study, (655) 4-MBC caused pituitary effects comparable to hypothyroidism (elevated TSH and lower T4 and T3 levels). Note that lowered activity of the thyroid gland is strongly associated with lowered testosterone levels in humans. (656)

c) 4-Methylbenzylidene Camphor was one of the 3 ingredients in the lotion that lowered testosterone levels in the study led by Dr. Dingle (657) (the same one as in benzophenones above).

Parabens

a) Parabens are a class of widely used preservatives in cosmetics. You can find them in most skin moisturizers, soaps, shampoos, and of course: sunscreens. They induce a very weak estrogenic response (658) in the human body, but are still considered xenoestrogens. The estrogenic activity of parabens increases with the length of the alkyl group, and their estrogenic potency, according to this study, (659) is as follows: butylparaben -> propylparaben -> ethylparaben -> methylparaben.

b) Even though parabens are only weakly estrogenic, many doctors still believe that they can cause problems in the endocrine system, due to the fact that continuous usage causes the accumulation of the compounds inside the fatty tissues (660). I'm not a chemist, nor a doctor, so I can't really say if you should avoid parabens or not, but personally I don't like the idea of lathering myself with accumulating xenoestrogens, even if they're weak.

c) Few in-vitro and in-vivo animal studies have shown that propylparaben can directly suppress testosterone synthesis via mitochondrial dysfunction in the cells responsible for testosterone production (661).

Octyl-dimethyl-PABA

a) Octyl-dimethyl-PABA (padimate-O) is an UV-B blocker which, according to few studies, is a weak endocrine disruptor with estrogenic activity being slightly less potent than what is seen on propylparaben (662, 663). Not much more is known about this chemical hormone-wise other than that, but that's still enough for me not to put it anywhere near my skin.

Octyl-Methoxycinnamate

a) Octyl-methoxycinnamate (octinoxate) is an UV-filter which caused major concerns back in 2000, when it was shown to be toxic in rats (664) with a dosage that's about identical with one that you'd get from applying sunscreen. However another study (665) rushed in to conclude that Octyl methoxycinnamate is not that effectively absorbed by the human body.

b) With that being said, the chemical has shown estrogenic activity in cultured human cells and in animal studies (666, 667).

c) And Octyl methoxycinnamate was also one of the three ingredients in the lotion used by Dr. Peter Dingle on his subjects to achieve lowered testosterone levels after just one week of application, (668) suggesting that it might disrupt the human endocrine system, even though it's weakly absorbed (there's also the possibility that the effect could of have been caused solely by the 2 other ingredients in the lotion (benzephone-3a and 4-methylbenzylidene camphor).

Homosolate

a) Homosolate is an UV-filter which has shown endocrine disrupting effects in cultured human cells and in rodents. It's chlorine byproducts also show weak estrogenic activity (669, 670).

b) And according to the good old Wikipedia: "Homosolate has been identified as an antiandrogen in vitro, as well as having estrogenic activity toward estrogen receptors, and general in vitro estrogenic activity. Homosalate has also been shown to be an antagonist toward androgen and estrogen receptors in vitro. There is also evidence that homosolate (and other UV filters) can break down into more toxic products"

c) Homosolate is also very permeable when applied to the human skin (671).

Conclusion

In the view of the mounting pile of evidence above, I made a decision to go nowhere near supermarket-sunscreens. Instead I purchased organic sunscreen, which is made from all-natural ingredients and is free from the plethora of endocrine disrupting chemicals that I can't even pronounce.

The brand that I purchased is called Biosolis, but from Amazon you can only purchase it as SPF 50+ kids version and it costs 3 times as much as it did in Finland.

You could also get some good old coconut oil, and then mix some zinc oxide powder into it, which should offer you a great non-absorbent, and all-natural shield from the sun.

As a final conclusion I would also add that using a high SPF sunscreen blocks most of the vitamin D synthesis in the skin. (672) A synthesis of a vitamin that is hugely important for testosterone production and also our natural defense system against sunburns.

Chlorine in Swimming Pools

The actual act of swimming may increase testosterone levels, but if you're swimming in one of those chlorinated pools, then you're going to experience some of the negative side effects of chlorine and do your body more harm than good.

So how do the chlorine in water side effects manifest?

In a study led by Nickmilder et al., (673) it was found out that adolescent boys who'd been "heavy users" of chlorinated swimming pools had significantly lower testosterone levels than boys who weren't that keen on swimming.

Nickmilder and his crew took serum hormone samples from 361 school male adolescents (aged between 14-18 years) who had visited swimming pools treated with chlorine.

What they found out was that the boys who had visited chlorinated pools for more than 250 hours before the age of 10, and for more than 125 hours before the age of 7, had significantly lower testosterone levels when compared to the boys who'd never visited a pool in their lives.

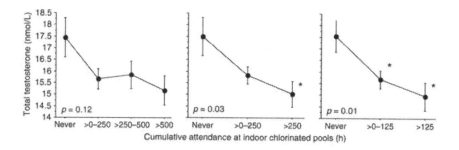

Chlorine in Water Side Effects Study Results

This is what the researchers say: "Swimming in indoor chlorinated pools during childhood is strongly associated with lower levels of serum inhibin B and total testosterone. The absorption of reprotoxic chlorination by-products across the highly permeable scrotum might explain these associations."

So do these side effects of chlorine on testosterone apply to adults? Answer: Unfortunately it does. Chlorine is easily absorbed even through the thicker skin of an adult male.

You can test this out by filling a cup with the water from your local chlorinated pool, then test the water with chlorine testing strips to see how much chlorine there is in the cup. After that wiggle your fingers in the glass for 60 seconds and test the water again with another strip.

You'll notice that there's no chlorine in the water anymore, as it's now inside your body.

Is there a way to reverse this and flush chlorine out from the body? Answer: Yes, you can supplement with strong liquid iodine which replaces the chlorine in your cells with the much needed iodine.

Conclusion on Chlorine Side Effects

There's a clear connection between the exposure to chlorine and low testosterone levels, as shown in the study about chlorinated pools. Even though the study was done in young adolescents, the results will still apply to adults too.

So if you're a keen swimmer or have spent a lot of time in those chlorinated swimming pools and don't want to experience any chlorine side effects, it could be wise to look into iodine supplementation, so you can get that much needed essential mineral back into the androgen receptors.

Excitotoxins and Testosterone

Excitotoxins are compounds added to most packaged foods, which can bypass the blood-brain barrier, and wreck havoc in certain brain receptors. They have a really shitty rep in the mass media, and some people seem to blame excitotoxins for just about any medical issue they can think about.

But is the rep justified, or are excitotoxins safe to consume?

Let's find out.

Potential Dangers of Excitotoxin Consumption

The word "excitotoxicity" describes a pathological process where nerve cells are damaged or killed because of excessive stimulation by neurotransmitters such as glutamate and similar substances.
Most common of the excitotoxins is the notorious MSG (monosodium glutamate), which binds into the NMDA and AMPA receptors of the brain, causing the receptors to uptake too much calcium ions, (674) which overexcites the receptors, and eventually damages them.

- Common Excitotoxins Added to Processed Foods
- Monosodium Glutamate (MSG)
- Monopotassium Glutamate

- Monoammonium Glutamate
- Magnesium Diglutamate
- Glycyrrhizin (in licorice)
- Aspartame
- Sucralose
- Neotame
- Carrageenan
- Alitame
- Thaumatin

The negative effects aren't only happening inside the brain. There is a legitimate concern that excitotoxins could also negatively influence testosterone production.

This happens because the oversynaptic activation of the NMDA receptors, shuts down some of the cAMP (cyclic adenosine monophospate) activity in the brain. (675) And cAMP serves as a signaling molecule between the brain and the balls.

There's also some theories about excitotoxins overexciting the androgen receptors of the brain in a similar manner than what is seen with the NMDA receptors. And few animal studies have shown a clear link between lowered testosterone levels, central nervous system damage, and excitotoxin intake in male rodents (676, 677 678).

Conclusion

The manufacturers and their lobbyists work hard to sell us the idea that excitotoxins would be perfectly safe, while the "natural-health hippies" will tell you that the compounds slowly kill you.

I believe that the truth may fall somewhere in-between.

Yes excitotoxins can be bad for your brain health and testosterone production when continuously consumed, but no, you won't get a brain seizure after drinking one bottle of aspartame sweetened soda.

I personally eat real organic foods, so I don't have to worry about man-made bullshit compounds like excitotoxins. That's what you should be doing too.

— Chapter 41 —

Body Language

Yes, a simple posture hack will have a large scale impact on your testosterone and cortisol levels.

Almost immediately.

Amy Cuddy, a social psychologist at Harvard Business School gave an eye opening TED talk in 2012 on the subject of using your body language to shape who you are, or more appropriately... who you want to become.

Body language is dependent on non-verbal cues.

However, the majority of research on non-verbals has historically focused on non-verbals as perceived by outsiders. For example, how your body language governs how other people think and feel about you.

But the really important question isn't that, but rather: do our non-verbals affect how we feel about ourselves?

We know that our brains can change our bodies, but is it also true that our bodies can change our brains? Our hormones?

Yes.

And interestingly, in the research, Cuddy and company found that the main hormonal markers that played roles in these non-verbal dynamics were testosterone and cortisol.

A hormone that influences dominance levels, and a hormone that governs stress reactivity.

In primate hierarchies, the alpha male always has high levels of testosterone and low levels of cortisol. In dominant, effective leaders, we also find - almost across the board - high levels of testosterone and low levels of cortisol.

This means the leaders are not just hard-charging testosterone juice heads, but also have low stress reactivity. They're flexible and cool under pressure.

The researchers found that with a couple quick physical manipulations, changes you can implement in mere minutes, their test subjects were able to considerably increase their testosterone levels and decrease their cortisol. Again, in minutes.

Not days, weeks, or months.

They ran a series of tests with a group of subjects, measuring testosterone and cortisol levels before and directly after the subjects made some simple changes. And the results were significantly different.

Now imagine if you were to integrate these simple physical hacks into your everyday life, eventually just making them a part of who you are. Sounds great, right? It is.

So what are the hacks?

1. Change your role
2. Change your posture

Let's look at these further.

First, change your role. What is your role in life? How do you identify yourself? Do you think of yourself as dominant, as a leader, as a power player?

Or do you think of yourself as a pawn? Are you just a cog in the machine?

It doesn't matter if you actually are just a cog in the machine, most of us are in some respect. What does matter is how you perceive your life situation and your social role in that situation.

In primate hierarchies, when a lesser male is forced to take over the role of alpha male in the society, within a matter of days his testosterone levels are significantly increased.

He's the exact same animal, the same being, he just changed his role. And his hormone levels compensated for that change. They rose to the occasion, so to speak.

So what does this mean for you?

Take a few minutes to reflect on your current role in life. If you're experiencing low testosterone, or symptoms of low T, is there a time in the recent past when you can recall a role change, and did that have an effect on your not just your outlook, but your biology? On your health?

If so, how are you going to change that? Now that you understand this, you are faced with the opportunity to alter your role to better suit your endocrine health.

Here's my recommendation: take on more responsibility. Increase the amount of risk in your life, with an equally measurable increase in potential for reward. Higher testosterone males are generally far less risk averse, and that's not just a consequence of their predetermined biology. It is possible for you to increase your testosterone and/or maintain its current level, by placing yourself in certain social and life situations. Change your role and your circumstances.

If what you're doing right now isn't working for you, what is holding you back from making the necessary changes?

And if you've always considered yourself a beta, or maybe just never considered yourself an alpha male, then give it a shot. Change your role - upgrade, in your own mind (because that is where all change begins), your role to alpha male and stop being so submissive.

Don't be one of those pseudo-alpha douches though. We've all seen them. The guys who walk into the bar with their chests puffed out, acting macho. Being an alpha male is not about acting macho to compensate for your insecurities. It's about feeling secure with who you are, and not letting anybody else threaten that security.

Cuddy et al. found some incredible results with a simple posing experiment, and that leads us to this next point... change your posture.

The researchers had a group of test subjects come into the lab, spit into a vial (for saliva testing) then assume several different posture positions for 2 minutes before spitting into another vial (for post test results).

The results: the subjects who assumed what the researchers termed "high power" positions (ie. spreading out, becoming physically bigger by standing straighter, or with hands on hips and power pose with legs) saw a whopping 20% increase in overall testosterone levels (in minutes)! They also saw a 25% decrease in cortisol.

So increase your testosterone by 20% and decrease your cortisol by 25% by just standing or sitting in a more powerful position. Assume a position of dominance with your body, and your brain will "rise to the occasion."

On the flip side, those test subjects who assumed the "low power" positions (i.e. sitting with legs crossed, arms crossed in front of themselves for protection, slouching, touching their neck, looking at the floor, etc) saw a 10% immediate decrease in testosterone and a 15% increase in cortisol!

So two minutes can literally configure your brain over the short-term to either be assertive, confident, and comfortable or stress reactive and feeling shut down and vulnerable.

So yes, your body can change your brain.

Beyond just integrating a role change and some more assertive posturing into your everyday life, I believe most guys can benefit from specifically using these quick hacks in situations where your dominance might be compromised.

Again, don't be a douchebag, but just be deliberate.

If you're giving a speech in front of an audience, or a presentation in a boardroom to a group of executives, take that opportunity to be deliberate with your non-verbal cues, not just for the sake of how your audience perceives you, but for yourself.

See it as a challenge and rise to the occasion. Be assertive and protect your inner level of security by not compromising your alpha male status.

Stand tall, deliver your speech powerfully, don't succumb to 'low power' poses, even when your body might naturally gravitate toward them.

Again, be deliberate.

Over time, with continual practice, the way you sit, stand, and move in your everyday life will transition to "high power" and away from "low power." And this will actually increase your testosterone and lower your cortisol quickly and predictably. So keep that tool in your back pocket.

— Chapter 42 —

Cold Showers

There is little evidence to directly correlate cold water immersion with testosterone increase.

There is, however, a theoretically sound hypothesis in support of it - the body of research just doesn't yet support the claims beyond anecdotal evidence.

There is a ghost study floating around on the internet that claims testosterone increase with cold water immersion, yet nobody actually links to it, and it doesn't exist in any reputable academic journal databases.

Short-term cold water therapy is very healthy for humans for its anti-depressive effects, metabolic increase, and proposed leptin enhancing effects.

So what's the deal with cold showers?

Cold water immersion gets a lot of play, both in popular books as well as internet articles and forums, for increasing testosterone production in men.

But does all the hype actually stack up with the evidence?

Unfortunately, no.

At least not in terms of direct scientific research that demonstrates convincing evidence of testosterone increase itself.

However, cold showers and/or short-term cold water exposure can be good for your health in general, for other reasons, but we'll get back to that shortly.

Here's the deal, everybody and their mother cites a 1993 study by the "Thrombosis Research Institute" as implicating cold showers with a direct increase in testosterone levels.

However, after hours of scouring the internet for this study, I could not even find the damned thing. I searched far and wide, first in reputable academic databases like Pubmed, Google Scholar, JSTOR, Science Direct, and Wiley, then in Google search, forums, and blog articles.

Nothing.

The study doesn't appear to exist, at least not online.

So what gives?

Well, at first glance this appears to be a case of he-said-she- said. One blogger or author hears about something on a forum, "cites" a study, writes an article on it, then another blogger picks it up and cites it, then the spark ignites and the unfounded information runs rampant across the internet.

While it may actually be true - short term cold water immersion may actually improve transient testosterone production - I unfortunately will not explicitly recommend it, or recommend against it, due to the fact that I have never read any evidence to support this claim. I'm not going to jump on the bandwagon just because it is popular.

However, there is evidence that points to prolonged cold water exposure as having negative stress effects on non- cold-adapted rats, with decrease in testosterone levels being one of the outcomes. And negative effects of prolonged cold exposure in non-cold-adapted humans has been reported as well.

And if we pull our heads out of the books for a second and think about it, prolonged cold exposure in a human who is not adapted to it generally leads to one thing... hypothermia.

In terms of cold water immersion, here's how things work:

- Short-term immersion (5-10minutes): positive effects (discussed below), though little to no evidence of testosterone production beyond speculation
- Proper cold-adaptation via steady habituation: adaptive responses such as increase in subcutaneous fat level (seen in many long distance pool swimmers, and especially in cold water distance swimmers - not necessarily preferable)
- Long term cold exposure in non-adapted individuals (20+ minutes): negative stress effects, potentially decreasing testosterone levels due to increase in glucocorticoids

Noradrenaline has been shown many times to increase significantly with cold exposure. This is actually the main mechanism of action that scientists credit for the perceived anti-depressive effects of cold water therapy on subjects.

The short-term cold (or cool) water exposure increases blood levels of beta-endorphin and noradrenaline, also increasing synaptic release of noradrenaline in the brain. The immersion of the palms and feet in the water, areas with very high concentration of heat sensory receptors in the skin, would theoretically send a large amount of neural impulses to the brain to accentuate this process.

However, researchers acknowledge that the body of research is quite small in terms of cold water therapy acting in this manner and they call for wider and more rigorous study before conclusive arguments can be made.

One hypothesis might be to speculate that since noradrenaline increases substantially with short term cold exposure, and since noradrenaline acts on the preoptic area of the hypothalamus, which, as we already know, is the site of excretion of GnRH, which stimulates the pituitary to release LH which leads to testosterone production, that ice baths will increase testosterone production.

Due to our knowledge of noradrenaline's regulatory nature on the GnRH secretion pathway, this may be a sound hypothesis.

It may work.

The body of research on this is minimal, at best, however. So for results, you'll need to conduct n=1 studies on yourself.

Many anecdotal reports confirm the benefits of short cold or cool water immersion on perceived libido enhancement, which may indicate a testosterone increase.

In terms of my own experience, I have intermittently used 10-minute cool water baths with 2-3 ice packs after hard training sessions for recovery, and underwent this process a significant number of times over the period of the last few years as I increased my testosterone levels so drastically.

However, I did it specifically for either muscle recovery from training or because the occasional cool bath invigorates me, and I'd be lying if I claimed to do it specifically to increase my testosterone.

I can neither deny nor confirm that the cool water baths had any impact on my overall testosterone levels, sadly. Though this is definitely an area for some direct home- testing experimentation in the future.

Other cold water benefits include an increase in metabolic rate, as well as proposed contributions to restoring homeostatic leptin levels (in Dr. Jack Kruse's "Leptin Reset"), with other promising results for chronic fatigue syndrome, chronic heart failure, and some types of cancers - even a hypothesis for anti-tumor immunity.

So it is definitely something you may be interested in trying out. Remember, short-term exposure to cold or cool water for 5-10 minutes is all you need.

— Chapter 43 —

Career & Risk Taking

Your job might be destroying your testosterone production. Symptoms of andropause (ie. depression, low libido, lack of energy, erectile difficulties) have been studied in men with relation to psychological job-related stress, and research shows some interesting findings.

This entire paradigm clearly demonstrates how important psychology is to your health.

Symptoms of andropause, according to the research, can appear independent of testosterone levels. Researchers have found men with both normal and low testosterone to experience these symptoms. The main culprit is psychological stress, much of it lifestyle and job-related.

So if you work a stressful job, this is a crucial area of your life to address. You need to learn proper psychological coping mechanisms as well as make sure the rest of your life is handled fairly well in terms of nutrition, training, lifestyle, and relationships.

However, men with lower testosterone in general are at considerably higher risk for andropause symptoms, especially with exposure to high-stress job environments, which can elicit depressive symptoms, insomnia, and musculoskeletal problems alone, in otherwise healthy men.

In a study in Japanese men working in stressful job environments, researchers found that, almost across the board, the subjects were more likely to be obese, have high cholesterol, have tension related to anxiety and depression, and suffer from chronic lower back pain. Sound familiar?

I know I've felt many of this in my own life: first in college, then during my first start-up company post-college.

Luckily, many of these symptoms can be beat with proper nutrition, training, and sleep. However, taking the correct psychological measures is vital as well, otherwise much of your progress with the other aspects will be in vain.

Unfortunately, you may have more cards stacked against you than you realize, however.

Even the building you work in could be negatively affecting your testosterone production.

Yes, researchers have actually linked "building-related sickness" and the chemical impact traditional office and school buildings have on people with negative correlations in stress-related blood hormone levels.

Another, often overlooked influence over your psychosomatic stress levels is technology, especially technology commonly found in work environments.

A Swedish study followed a large group of skilled IT workers at Ericsson Laboratories over a 6 month period of training.

They chose this group of individuals as test subjects, as opposed to "normal" office workers exposed to technology, because Ericsson engineers are highly-skilled and completely immersed in technology, both psychologically and physically.

No convincing correlations have yet to be linked between purely physical exposure to technology and negative effects other than reported eye strain from screen exposure and occasional headaches.

However, when studying a group of subjects who make a living building computer architecture, we're able to more accurately gauge the impact technological psycho-stress may have on an individual because engineers will have far less psychological stress related to routine computer handling than an average office worker with limited technological prowess, who may become highly stressed even when they need to make a spreadsheet or perform simple tasks.

In this particular study, the researchers had workers go about their normal routine over the study duration, and split them into groups. They were specifically studying how effective certain stress-management techniques were on the individuals.

Quite obviously (in my opinion) stress management techniques proved to be more successful over the course of the study in terms of regulating psychological stress as well as some biological markers such as prolactin and blood pressure. However, and this is the one result that they chose not to elaborate on in the discussion section, total testosterone levels dropped considerably in test subjects over the 6 months.

Interesting.

Because the researchers failed to comment on this (important) issue in the study, we are left to craft our own hypothesis. I think this drop may either be:

1.) Routine, and normal for these individuals and/or related to work- specific events not mentioned in the study itself, or

2.) Reflect the nature of the individuals who, normally in control of their domain and more likely to function best when left alone, felt disturbed by the presence of researchers in their life, prodding with giant questionnaires and attempting to teach stress management. It may have demasculinized them slightly. Again, just speculation.

So, can technology directly affect your testosterone levels negatively? By itself, probably not - there has been no convincing evidence to support the claim.

However, technology, especially in the work environment, may be a significant contributing factor to additional stress, both psychological and physical, which could have an adverse effect on your testosterone levels as a downstream consequence of chronically elevated glucocorticoid levels and poor lifestyle decisions such as sacrificing sleep and practicing poor posture when using the computer, for example.

Also, two things to pay specific attention to with respects to your work environment, and these are more common sense than anything but I might as well reinforce some good thinking: be wary of your nutrition habits in the office, and take positive steps to improve stress during your commute.

1. Nutrition in the office: Offices are notoriously bad places for trying to eat well. From the snack machine and extreme stress and/or boredom, to Lisa from Accounting always bringing those damn Dunkin' Donuts Munchkin donut holes in all the time, you just need to pay attention and stick to your guns when it comes to making the best decisions.

2. Commuting: Even if you don't experience road rage, which is clearly stressful for everybody involved and an unhealthy habit and personality pattern, commuting hours to and from work every day, by train, car, airplane, or bicycle, can be an additional source of chronic stress, contributing to chronically-elevated cortisol levels.

Physically, you're kind of stuck. You need to physically get to work, unless you quit jobs and find a better one that is closer to home (or even negotiate a way to work from home). It's difficult to get around the fact that physically your body is going to need to undergo this additional stress on a daily basis.

However, as we've seen so far in the program, and will continue to see, your mental attitude, posture, and actions can have direct effects on your physiological conditions.

Testosterone and Risk Taking: Why Do Men Like To Gamble?

I have to admit that I'm a bit of a sucker for gambling. Not on roulette, poker or anything like that, but on sports betting.

Is my habit of sports betting due to high testosterone, or is it just a personal trait? That I don't know, but one thing is for certain.

Nearly all of the sports bettors out there are men. Same goes for poker players, casino, etc.

And the question is, why? Why women don't bet that often, and why it's almost completely a men's game?

Testosterone And Risk Taking go Hand in Hand

As a rule of thumb: if a man likes something that women don't really care about, the reason is usually behind hormones.

That's why men often like cars, women don't. Men like action movies, women love romantic comedies. Men don't really care about their appearance, for women it's the most important thing in the world, etc.

Sure there are men who like romantic comedies and women who like to work on cars, but in general, men tend to be interested in masculine stuff, while women are more interested in feminine stuff. And the reason almost always goes back to hormones.

Risk taking and gambling just happen to be somewhat masculine testosterone driven things, and that's why men are more easily interested in such habits. Basically the more of the male hormone testosterone you have in your bloodstream, the more fascinated you will be about risk taking and gambling.

Also a man with high testosterone takes more risks than a man with low testosterone. That's a scientifically proven fact.
If you don't believe me, take a look at these studies:

a) The researchers in this study (679) placed an attractive female near male skateboarders. What they found out was that the men noted a significant jump in their testosterone levels, which led them to become more risky with their tricks, resulting in more successes, but also more crashes.

b) The researchers in this study, (680) used 98 male investors as their test subjects. They found out that the men who had highest levels of salivary testosterone, were also the ones who took most of the risks when there was a change to monetary payoffs.

c) This study (681) found out that the men with high testosterone levels were more likely to play with "risky cards" in a gambling experiment.

d) This interesting study (682) saw that when high testosterone males are given "low power" they tend to take more risks to get things into their control, but when a high testosterone male is given a high power status, they start taking fewer risks.

e) The researchers in this study (683) gave their subject males a drug called letrozole, which is a strong aromatase inhibitor that increases testosterone and blocks estrogen. The results showed that the men who received the drug without estrogen control took more risks than the men who received the drug along with estrogen control.

f) The researchers in this study (684) found out that young CEO's with high testosterone are more likely than older men or women to both initiate and kill mergers and acquisitions deals. According to the researchers it's the testosterone that drives such risk taking.

g) This is an interesting study. (685) The researchers followed 17 young future traders for eight consecutive business days and saw that whenever they made money, their testosterone levels increased. Also the men that had elevated testosterone levels in the morning, were likely to make above average profits on that day. This led the researchers to believe that testosterone might be the secret ingredient behind market bubble, BUT that it might also be the reason behind the bursting of the bubble, because testosterone feeds risk taking, and vice versa.

— Chapter 44 —

Can You Grow Taller?

With height playing a prevalent psychological (and possibly evolutionarily programmed) role of importance in many cultures around the world, it comes as no surprise that many guys focus on how tall they are, and deem it an area of their life worth attention.

Is it worth the attention?

That is an individual decision, and one made based on preferences, so only you can decide that.

However, I'd like to explore the idea a little bit and look at the realistic possibilities in terms of increasing height.

I do not want to breed any unrealistic expectations though, so this exploration will be cut-and-dry, based on facts and not outlandish marketing claims like you may see on internet marketing-based "how to grow taller" products.

Anecdotally, in my own experience, I grew 2 inches from the time of beginning my journey with testosterone optimization, switching my training, nutrition, and lifestyle around.

Beyond the training, nutrition, and lifestyle elements, I attribute this to two things:

- My age
- My genetics

Age-wise, all of the additional growth occurred before I was 25 years old (I am 24 years old at the time of publication). 25 is the proposed age around which most men will stop growing entirely, but there is probably some slight variance between individuals.

This is due to full maturation of the growth plates.

Growth plates, formally known as epiphyseal plates, are cartilage plates at the end of your long bones that are responsible for bone elongation during maturation, which for men usually ends in the mid-20's, when the epiphyseal plate becomes an epiphyseal line.

Without getting too much into the biophysiology, the constant mitotic division of cells causes an aggregation along the epiphyseal end of the cartilage, causing it to "grow" over the adolescent years, with old cells stacking up along the main shaft of the long bone (referred to as the diaphysis).

The estrogen:testosterone ratio is very important in determining growth potential, with a higher proportion of estrogen during adolescence causing increased apoptosis (cell death) of the cells that eventually would become new bone. This slows down, and eventually halts growth, so it is very important for young males to optimize this ratio by controlling their estrogen production.

Once the growth plates mature, the only known way to technically "grow taller" is to surgically elongate your long bones via a procedure known as distraction osteogenesis, which is literally a surgical fracturing of the bone and attempt to regrow new bone in the gap. Ouch.

The second powerful determinant of height is genetics.

If you are younger than 25 years old, and are wondering whether or not you even have any additional growth potential, then use the following formula to determine it:

- Mother's height (inches) + Father's height (inches)
- Add 5 inches (for men), subtract 5 inches for women
- Divide by 2

The answer is your predicted growth potential, with a standard deviation of 4 inches on either side.

For me, I've currently reached my genetic potential according to this algorithm, by adding the 4 inches standard deviation to my predicted height. Considering my current height and my age, I do not expect to grow any more.

However, like anything, this probably isn't 100% accurate for every person. Some outliers always pop up.

In terms of what you can do to optimize your potential if you are young enough and think you may still have genetic potential for additional height.

First, get your diet and training correct. Use this program.

Growth hormone production is crucial, and just following the guidelines laid out in the nutrition and training chapters will put you on your way to optimize this.

Also, sleep as much as possible.

Deep sleep is the most important time in your circadian cycle for growth hormone secretion. It's no wonder early adolescent boys have been known to sleep for up to 15 hours at a time (myself and my brother included) and eat like animals while awake.

Also, don't be a fool and take anabolic steroids in high school.
I played football and baseball with a group of guys who took steroids starting from age 16. Sure, they were strong - they could hit home runs and score touchdowns - but at what cost?

Anabolic steroids have been shown to stunt new bone growth in teens as well as lower spermatogenesis, not to mention elevate blood pressure and increase risk of heart attack. One study actually found that teens with asthma (who take oral steroids via their inhalers throughout adolescence) are, on average, half an inch shorter than kids who are treated with steroids.

Additionally, posture may play an important role.

Beyond adding a solid inch or two instantly, depending on how much you slouch currently, purposeful, powerful posture has been shown to transiently increase your testosterone production within minutes (see the chapter on body language). While this may not directly translate into bone growth, it definitely helps with confidence, and when reinforced over time, could be an important component in increasing your T levels along with nutrition, training, and lifestyle adjustments.

— Chapter 45 —

Alcohol

Alcohol is a widely used depressant that we humans most often drink in the form of ethanol. And ethanol – like everyone who has hugged a toilet seat at 4am knows – is toxic for the human body. But just how toxic? How do testosterone and alcohol interact in our bodies? And what kind of effects does it have on the endocrine system?

The magic of alcohol is fairly simple: because it's a depressant, it slows down various bodily functions, which in turn triggers the feelings of drunkenness.

Alcohol also slows down inhibitions, which is why you might get the feeling of needing to fuck everything and everyone around you after 10 shots of tequila.

Sadly, this mission of having sex with everything that moves can often become impossible, since 10 shots of tequila is enough to dramatically slow down your sexual functions (ie: the battle sword might not rise to the occasion anymore).

This negative effect on the sexual function is mainly caused by a dramatic drop in the male sex hormone: testosterone.

And here's why it takes place.

Alcohol and Testosterone Production

Let's just start by the fact that you do not have to completely give up drinking in order to have naturally high testosterone levels.

Since few drinks here and there ain't enough to cause any dramatic reductions in testosterone. When it comes to alcohol and testosterone, it's the dose that counts.

However, if you're an alcoholic, and drinking yourself to the point of passing out on several days of the week, then you can be damn sure that your testosterone production has tanked (and you probably know this yourself already because of the negative effects it has on sexual functioning).

Here are the already known mechanisms of action in how alcohol lowers testosterone:

The metabolism of ethanol lowers the amount of the coenzyme NAD+ (nicotinamide adenine dinucleotide) (686) inside liver and testes. NAD+ is essential part of the electron donor process needed in the production of testosterone and various other androgens, hence why it's believed that alcohol lowers testosterone in a dose-dependent manner.

Alcohol stimulates the brain to release beta-opioid endorphins, which are the reason why you get really relaxed after few beers. Sadly those endorphins are also notorious for their negative effect on testosterone synthesis. (687)

Alcohol consumption causes oxidative damage in the testicular leydig cells and various other bodily tissues, (688) which leads to local reduction of testosterone inside the ballsack, and also to the destruction of some testosterone molecules already in circulation, due to the effects of the stress hormone: cortisol. (689)

Chronically high alcohol consumption can significantly increase estrogen levels.

This is due to the fact that it boosts the activity of the aromatase enzyme, (690) which works by converting the male sex hormone: testosterone, into the female sex hormone: estrogen.

Here's Some Research:

a) It has been noted in several rodent studies that consumption of alcohol lowers testosterone levels significantly (691, 692, 693, 694). One study (695) in particular is rather alarming, since it showed a 50% reduction in testicle size in rats who were fed a diet with 5% of calories coming from ethanol.

b) Multiple human studies have found that heavy consumption of alcohol reduces testosterone levels (696, 697, 698, 699). It's also seen that men who suffer from alcoholism have significantly lower testosterone levels, and higher estrogen levels, than men without alcohol problems, even if they have a perfectly functioning livers (700, 701, 702, 703).

c) But how much is too much then? It might come as a relief to some that a low-dose (0.5 g/kg) of alcohol has actually been shown to slightly increase testosterone levels. (704) And a moderate-dose (equivalent to 1,5 glasses of red wine) only lowered testosterone levels by 7%. (705) Even more surprising is that in this study, (706) 1g/kg of alcohol (that's about half a glass of vodka for most men) taken post-workout, was able to increase testosterone levels by ~100%! Take that study with a grain of salt though, since another one found out that if you work out drunk or in hangover, the testosterone lowering effects of alcohol will significantly increase in duration. (707)

d) It's also worth mentioning that beer is probably one of the worst alcoholic beverages to enjoy, if you're interested in not fucking up your testosterone levels. This is because the hops of which most beers are made from contain a very potent phytoestrogen called: 8-Prenylnaringenin. In fact, hops are so estrogenic that the women who pick them up by hand, often experience menstrual problems. (708) Another not so awesome compound in beer is called xanthohumol, which can impair hormone signaling. (709)

Beer and Testosterone

Beer and male hormones aren't really a match made in heaven.

Sure it's a manly drink and all that on the surface, but deep inside of your body, all that beer is as if you'd pop one of those women's birth control pills (by that I mean that it seriously skyrockets your estrogen levels).

It can be really hard to admit this as a man, but beer is by far the worst alcoholic beverage that you could drink as a man, at least if we look at things from the hormonal point of view.

Here's why.

Beer Wasn't Always As Bad For Us As It Is Now

There's really not a drink so bad for your testosterone levels as beer, but beer wasn't always like that.

Prior to the year 1487 beer was known to be a beverage that made men more aggressive, horny, and socially dominant.
It was like this 'beverage of virility'.

This is because before the year 1487 beer wasn't made out of hops. It was actually made out of multiple herbs that quite possibly had some testosterone and virility boosting benefits.

That's where the connection between masculinity and beer is really coming from. It comes from those times prior 1487, when beer was actually a drink that made men more aggressive and dominant.

But then things took a turn for the worse, as the church wasn't really digging the idea of 'aggressive and dominant men', and they soon enrolled this new law called 'the German beer purity law', (710) which stated that all the beer sold, must be brewed using only hops, water, and malt.

The only reason for that law was to make men more feminine and sensitive, in other words the church wanted men to become more like sheep than wolves.

So that's the story of why beer really is seen as a 'masculine drink'. And to be honest, it really was a masculine drink, until the church feminized it with the Bavarian beer purity law back in 1487.

Beer Really Smacks Down Your Testosterone Levels

If that story above isn't convincing enough, there's also plenty of modern day research that shows how and why exactly does beer lower our testosterone levels.

And it's not only lowering our testosterone levels, as it also increases the levels of estrogen in the male body, which obviously is not a good thing at all.
Here are some of the studies that prove the point:

a) Back in 2009, the American Association of Cancer Research published this interesting study about this new fascinating compound called xanthohumol, (711) which was found in hops. The researchers were mesmerized about the fact that this phyto-nutrient actually had some anti-cancer benefits. The only thing they kinda didn't mention was the fact that xanthohumol is also extremely effective at lowering male testosterone levels.

b) The hops of which beer is brewed from (thanks Bavarian purity law!) are extremely estrogenic. This study (712) in particular found out that the women who pick up hops by hand, experience disturbances in their menstrual cycles due to the extremely high estrogenic activity in the hops itself. The researchers claim that it's due to this phytoestrogen called 8-Prenylnaringenin (8-PN) which contains 'extremely estrogenic activity'.

c) 100 grams of hops can contain anywhere from 30,000 to 300,000 IU's of estrogen.

d) Alcohol itself is a real testosterone killer.

e) The ethanol in beer (and multiple other alcoholic beverages) has been seen to slow down the P45 enzyme system inside your liver. (713) This isn't too great of a deal as P45 is responsible for estrogen metabolism, and if it's out of whack then your liver isn't removing any estrogen from your system.

Chapter 46

Smoking

First let's look at Tobacco, then we will examine Marijuana.

For many years I used to think that smoking would completely crush testosterone levels. I didn't even read the studies about smoking and testosterone, I just assumed that as smoking is so harsh on the human body in so many ways, and the fact that its filled with chemicals and carcinogenic smoke, that it had to have a testosterone lowering effect.

The Science Behind Smoking and Testosterone

I personally don't smoke, I only do it when I'm drunk and for the reasons that I don't even know myself.

So smoking and its adverse health effects have never really interested me on a personal level.

But now after AnabolicMen.com is visited by more than 500,000 men on a monthly basis, I have been getting a lot of emails from worried guys asking me if their habit of smoking would decrease their testosterone levels.

So for the first time ever, I decided to do a proper research on the studies about smoking and testosterone.

a) This highly respected study (714) found out that men who have smoked for several years, and men who don't smoke at all, have pretty much identical testosterone levels on average. Meaning that smokers and non-smokers don't really differ in terms of testosterone.

b) This study (715) found out similar results. Men who were heavy smokers, and men who didn't smoke, had similar levels of androgens and SHBG.

c) This study (716) featured 71 men who decided to give up the habit of smoking. In short term (few months) the men did experience a slight increase in testosterone levels after ceasing the habit, but after a year the men were back at the same levels as of which they were when they still smoked, some even had lower testosterone.

d) These studies suggest that male dogs, mice, and rats, all experience a significant reduction in testosterone levels after being exposed to tobacco smoke (717, 718, 719).

e) This study (720) examined multiple studies about smoking and testosterone, and came to a conclusion that the smokers may have higher testosterone levels because of the fact that men with higher testosterone are more prone to taking risks in all fields, such as gambling, finances, health, etc. And thus the men who have high testosterone could potentially end up smokers more likely than "safe" men with lower testosterone levels.

f) This study (721) found out that the globally decreasing testosterone after men turn 30, is not part of "normal aging process" but its due to bad lifestyle choices such as poor diet, obesity, and smoking. However they didn't prove anything about smoking and testosterone in the actual study.

g) This study (722) found out that men who smoke may actually have higher levels of free testosterone in their blood serum.

h) This study (723) found out that men who smoke metabolize more testosterone. Meaning that their liver gets rid of testosterone more easily. Weirdly enough this doesn't seem to affect total testosterone levels in all of the previous studies.

i) This study (724) found out that smokers and non-smokers had no significant differences in testosterone levels, but they did find out that smoking depletes the body from zinc which is one of the principal minerals behind healthy testosterone production. Theoretically this would mean that smoking along with poor diet could leave some men zinc deficient, and thus lower their testosterone.

j) One thing that might partially explain these effects is the facts that nicotine is a potent aromatase inhibitor (725, 726, 727).

k) As you can see from the mounting pile of evidence, it truly seems like smoking doesn't decrease testosterone levels after all, which is extremely weird to be honest. But after such a tremendous amount of evidence from the scientific world, the claim that smoking reduces testosterone levels may just be an empty one.

Marijuana and Testosterone

This is not the first time I've written about marijuana and testosterone. In fact, about 6 months ago I wrote a post showcasing all the studies about its effects on androgen production, but since some serial-stoners decided to spam the shit out of the article, claiming that I was promoting propaganda, I just got tired of that and removed the whole thing.

After the deletion of the original posts, I've received a ton of inquiries about the subject, which is why I'm finally rewriting the old article about weed and testosterone.

Weed and Testosterone Levels

I don't actively smoke weed myself, but I have nothing against pot, or against the people who use it.

Which is why I try to be as objective about the subject as I possibly can.

I'm sure most of you have already seen the alarming titles, such as: "Smoking pot causes man-boobs. Beware!" or the classics like "Marijuana using men are the worst lovers."

I also know that a lot of bro's at the gym like to claim that smoking pot would completely mess up your ability to gain muscle. When it comes to marijuana and testosterone, there is going to be a lot of crazy claims.

However, in my opinion, claims such as those above, are nothing more than fear of the unknown and unnecessary hysteria. There's plenty of guys who have smoked weed for most of their lives, who don't have man-boobs, and on top of that, some of the biggest guys in the bodybuilding scene are avid pot users.

Marijuana is just a goddamn herb. To claim that a single herb would be powerful enough to stop muscle growth, is beyond the scope of my understanding. It's unlikely that you'd grow breasts by smoking it either.

Does this mean that marijuana is harmless for hormones? Well, not entirely I suppose.

The Research Behind Marijuana and Testosterone:

a) The claim that marijuana causes man-boobs has more than likely originated from these few in-vitro studies (728, 729), where crude marijuana extract had estrogenic effects on isolated rodent cells. Now, if something acts like estrogen, it can definitely induce some man-breast growth... However, it's important to note that the studies were done on isolated cells taken from rats, and the whole experiment was conducted inside test-tubes. On top of that the effects haven't been seen in in-vivo studies (inside a living organism).

b) It has been noted in several notable studies that THC (the active ingredient in cannabis) can potentially be an endocrine disruptor in humans and animals, since it blocks GnRH secretion from the hypothalamus, which eventually leads to lowered LH and FSH production and therefore also lower testosterone production. THC has also been shown to inhibit several testicular enzymes needed in testosterone production in-vitro (730, 731, 732, 733, 734, 735). Although it's worth mentioning that in all of the studies I've seen, the effects have been reversible.

c) As weird as it is, some studies have shown that cannabis does not lower testosterone levels (736, 737), despite the fact that a pile of studies has already shown that it does. Albeit, these review studies do contain research which shows cannabis to suppress testosterone, the abstracts still cleverly state that "chronic marijuana use showed no significant effect on hormone concentrations in either men or women.".

PART 6:
TRAINING
(MASCULINE OPTIMIZATION PYRAMID LEVEL 4)

— Chapter 47 —

Training For Testosterone Production

The purpose of this section is to answer the question: how should I train to optimize natural testosterone production?

However, since the subject is exhaustive and has been written about thoroughly - with attention to detail as well as full training recommendations and workout logs in the THOR Program (our training manual for natural testosterone production) - we want to provide an overview of the subject here, but we recommend you read THOR, which is available on **store.anabolicmen.com**.

To answer this question properly, we first need to examine the biological relationship between muscle stimulus and the endocrine system. This examination will lead us to further explore the neuromuscular system.

Interestingly enough, testosterone stimulation via training and testosterone stimulation via nutrition are two totally independent paradigms.

This is great because it allows us to delve into them separately. When the optimal way to live, eat, and train are combined in an individual's lifestyle, they will compound on one another, yet remain separate systems so they can more easily be manipulated.

In this training-focused section, I want to break the analysis and prescriptions down into two main areas: how to train if you are an endurance athlete (and want to remain an endurance athlete) & how to train if you are anybody else.

The latter group will be far more successful in naturally increasing their testosterone quickly. So I recommend being, or becoming, a member of that latter group of men.

However, if you are an endurance athlete and have much of your ego and life's worth (hey, maybe it's your job to win races) tied up in your sport and you aren't ready to let it go just yet, I feel for you.

I was in your shoes once. Training 4-6 hours a day so I could race in the Pro/Open category at races. So I could run just a tad faster than last race, or drown just a little bit less during the swim as a triathlete. Hours and hours in the pool and on the road will condition you to become a bit addicted to the lifestyle, addicted to the endorphin high. So I understand.

I also understand that you have probably got insanely low testosterone, probably partly due to poor nutrition strategies and partly due to chronically elevated cortisol.

Despite being able to run/swim/bike/row super-fast over long distances, you probably still have stubborn body fat hanging around. Heck, even many pro triathletes are skinny fat.

So a part of this section will be dedicated to the road warriors.
You will not see as impressive results as men who train 3-5 hours per week, but if you implement my suggestions, you will see some results, an overall improvement from where you are right now. And that's worth the price of admission alone.

Here's how this section is going to work, so you can navigate it however you please:

- Introduction to the neuromuscular system & why it is so vital to have a basic grasp on this information
- What is currently considered the best way to train for T & GH production, and why I think this is incorrect
- The solution I propose - the exercise and style of training I think is superior to how we're currently told to train... and why
- How to train if you are a normal Joe,weightlifter, sprinter, Crossfitter, or basically any guy who isn't an endurance athlete

Exactly How To Train For Optimal Hormonal Response (Short and Long-term)

Very recent study into the dual steroid (T and Cortisol) effects on training in elite athletes (as late as 2011), as opposed to older studies that often focused on untrained or moderately trained (with loose definitions of the word 'trained', varying from study to study) has, interestingly enough, opened up a ton of insight into this new paradigm for optimal endocrine response training.

In short, studying elite athletes gave us new insight into how average (untrained & moderately trained) individuals should train to optimize testosterone up-regulation.

The idea (in the following algorithm and program later in the book) is to use certain factors (workout design, nutrition, genetics, training status and type) to modify T and C concentrations and therefore influence resistance training performance and adaptive outcomes.

Changes in the concentrations of T and C can moderate or support neuromuscular (NM) performance through various short-term mechanisms such as 2nd messenger signaling, lipid/protein pathways, neuronal activity, behavior, cognition, motor system functioning, muscle properties, and energy metabolism.

A greater understanding over the recent years of T and C has led to suggestions that, beyond the more popular applications in morphological (ie. muscle size) and functional (ie. power and strength) enhancement, these hormones also exert heavy influence over NM functioning (ie. neuronal activity, intracellular signaling, and muscle force production), which means they contribute to the adaptive responses to training by regulating long term muscle performance via short term regulation of NM performance.

In short, we need to use NM training to influence long term muscle performance and optimize hormonal response to training.

It all comes back to my original philosophy of always addressing the roots of an issue as opposed to a symptomatic approach (and in life, operating on principles as opposed to stressing over details).

What is the neuromuscular system?

When I say NM system, I am referring to the peripheral nervous system (PNS in short). This consists of motor neuron units and innervated (stimulated to action) muscle fibers.

When looking to design a training program, we want to operate on the premise that acute elevations in endogenous hormones will increase the likelihood of receptor interactions, which will mediate long term adaptive responses.

Researchers are now shifting a lot of focus onto NM research in athletes because they're recognizing that neural factors may play a role beyond that of hormones, especially in early phase adaptations. However, the specific mechanisms for action still need to be examined as this is a relatively young (and ridiculously complex) field of study.

One thing that studying elite athletes made very clear to us is this: beginners may have a distinct advantage over highly trained individuals in terms of ability to elicit a workout-dependent testosterone and growth hormone response.

While elite athletes can generally elicit higher magnitude responses to their training, the stimulus needs to be far more specific.
For untrained or average individuals, the stimuli can be far reaching in variety and still elicit a high response, but they must operate on a set of known principles for the optimal response.

This initial testosterone response in untrained individuals is thought to occur mainly as an adaptive response of the NM system to support continual training under the new stimulus, which makes a lot of sense. Your muscles need to rapidly change to support your training, and the main way for them to do so (if you do the correct type of training) is to up-regulate androgen receptors with increased content and sensitivity.

So for the majority of guys reading this right now, even those who believe themselves to be highly trained (even if you are, it is probably in a very specific sport-related style) you will experience rapidly elevated workout-dependent testosterone levels with the correct training to assist muscular adaptation.

I will extrapolate this notion and speculate that even common weightlifters, crossfitters, and gym rats (ie. people with several years experience in resistance training) will find themselves noticeably untrained in this specific capacity when first embarking on this NM-style training according the algorithm I am going to propose.

Gymnasts and street workout guys will probably not have such a difficult time. Endurance athletes, yes... it's going to be a big change.

(For example, several of my clients find they need at least one short nap per day along with a good nights' sleep to recover initially from the shift in training style during the first few weeks of the program, even though training sessions only run around 60 minutes in length – they adapt shortly thereafter).

To illustrate the advantage (I'm framing it as an advantage, but of course, it's all relative) that untrained individuals have over elite athletes when it comes to general T response to workouts (again, not magnitude, but reach and lack of specificity) I'll use an example that researchers found in elite 400m sprinters vs average individuals sprinting 400m.

In the elite 400m runners, every repetition decreased T levels post-sprint and increased LH levels (which, as you'll see in article 2, act as a precursor to stimulate T production). What this says is that they may have a decreased androgen receptor (AR) response to the training stimuli due to extensive training. Either that or an increase in glucocorticoid receptor (GR) sensitivity which would naturally suppress the T. I'd put money on the notion that it's a mix of both.

By comparison, the untrained sprinters saw a significant increase in T concentrations post-sprint with unchanged LH levels, indicating an increased AR sensitivity due to the new stimulus.

This indicates that it may be better for untrained individuals to hit harder fatigable bouts, but in low enough quantity to not elevate cortisol significantly, which introduces the idea of a training stimulus threshold.

A Formula For Optimal Testosterone Production via Training

Take what you just learned, and remember it. We're going to introduce a couple more concepts now, then mash them all together to formulate the perfect algorithm for training-induced T production.

Researchers have found that explosiveness encourages NM adaptations necessary to support the training demands (ie. indicating a long term adaptation), and that a training threshold very likely exists.

We want to up-regulate AR content in fast glycolytic muscle tissue (as opposed to slow oxidative tissue).

Resistance training is unanimously agreed upon as a potent stimulus for testosterone production and muscle growth, but the specific type is either not discussed or not agreed upon. What we do know is that resistance training promotes an increase in both AR mRNA (ie. gene transcription) and protein content and T concentrations.

So combining both of these ideas, we can come to the conclusion that explosive resistance training is the optimal form of stimulus – as long as it is performed under the performance threshold (so as to continually promote AR up-regulation without compromising due to cortisol/stress-related suppression).

But that's not the entire picture. It's also not entirely different from what the pop-fitness media promotes (though rarely practices). One more key element to the equation is often overlooked. And that's the idea of workload and its relationship to muscle volume activation (MVA) relative to intensity.

It has been demonstrated that the magnitude of the hormonal response to training is proportional to the size of the muscle volume activated. This is why we hear the old paradigm of "squat, squat, squat" to increase testosterone. Big leg muscles = more muscle tissue activated.

However, this MVA-dependent hormonal response is relative to the intensity of the movement performed.

Squatting high reps for hypertrophy training may stimulate GH and T production, but I'd argue that it won't be optimal because the intensity is not high enough, it is just drawn out over more reps. On the flip side, low rep squatting implies higher intensity, but allows for less total work done on the muscle.

Work, as a mechanical construct in physics, was originally defined by French mathematician Gaspard-Gustave Coriolis as "weight lifted through a height." The main equation you see everywhere is:

$$W = Fd$$

Where W is work, F is the magnitude of the force and d is displacement.

Researchers have found that, in terms of GH response, high amounts of work done – that is, high amounts of force related to the weight displaced – generated a significantly higher hormonal response to training than low work done.

So let's recap, and combine all of the knowledge up to this point in the article in order to formulate the idea of an optimal T-response-oriented training paradigm.

High work load, with a high proportion of muscle volume activated relative to intensity of the stimulus on said muscle volume, which should be performed via explosive resistance training done under a performance threshold (ie. self-limiting) = optimal.
Expressed algorithmically, it would look something like this in its simplest form…

W (MVA * i) < Stress Threshold

Where W is work (Fd), MVA is muscle volume activation, and i is intensity.

The stress threshold is defined as the point after which negative adaptations occur in terms of GR up-regulation and the subsequent increased sensitivity to stress-hormones, which are known to suppress androgen production.

So in short, we need to use this style of training, and walk the line under the stress threshold.

This is achieved best through explosive resistance and optimized by activating the most muscle possible over maximal displacement (at explosive intensity) while remaining just beneath the threshold.

I believe that in order to keep our training beneath the threshold, calisthenics becomes an increasingly attractive form of training due to its self-limiting nature and relationship with gravity (ie. if you can't do another muscle-up, you can't just subtract weight from your body as you could with a barbell in order to get additional reps or sets into the workout session).

This is based on the idea that in the 5-8 rep range you are able to perform an explosive set with high force and displace enough weight to keep total work high, but relative stress low. Much higher than 8 reps at the correct intensity will, I think, negatively affect your performance threshold, and any lower than 3 reps will compromise the intensity of the movement.

This is also why I advocate "enough rest between sets to recover just enough to perform another intense, slightly sub-maximal set" – no more, and no less. This will vary based on the individual but will probably fall in the 1-3 minute range based on the movement and the training level of the individual. 60 seconds rest appears to be optimal for GH output during a session.

For the exact program we recommend, go to **thorprogram.com or store.anabolicmen.com** to find the THOR Program.

PART 7:
SUPPLEMENTATION

(MASCULINE OPTIMIZATION PYRAMID LEVEL 5)

— Chapter 48 —

Intelligent Supplementation

If you're doing everything else correctly and want to get the extra edge without pharmaceuticals, then leveraging particular supplements backed by clinical research may amplify your results towards hormonal optimization.

Supplementation is one of our favorite topics here at Anabolic Men, mostly because of how interesting it is that there are so many incredible compounds out there - most of which are found either in nature or produced by the human body.

While there are many incredible supplements to use to optimize your health, there are also some bad ones, and lots of shady marketers pushing crap to the general public. Our aim is to show you the good, the bad, and the great. And to act as your advocate by only bringing you the truth.

These upcoming chapters will be divided into supplementation advice based on specific goals.

For example, if your main goal is to increase testosterone naturally, then we will recommend a list of those supplements with real research behind them for T in humans.

Or if you want to eliminate your erectile dysfunction problem, we will recommend a list of supplements proven to help with that.

So without further ado, let's get into the meat and potatoes of the wonderful world of supplements.

— Chapter 49 —

Supplementation To Increase T

This chapter will cover the top supplements we recommend for increasing testosterone naturally.

This an extremely helpful little quick-start guide on the best testosterone supplements for men.

In an industry full of crap testosterone supplements that promise the world but deliver nothing in the way of real results (ie. most traditional testosterone boosting supplements), the following 4 natural testosterone supplements not only have ample scientific research to back up their claims, but they also get results in humans.

These 4 testosterone supplements I am going to outline for you today are reliable in increasing testosterone levels (and improving other important hormonal biomarkers) and affordable. Instead of falling for the clever marketing on Amazon and in Bodybuilding mags, I suggest stocking up on these solid natural testosterone supplements.

They are:

- Ashwagandha
- Micronutrient Blends
- Boron
- Phosphatidylserine

Let's break these down one by one and expand on their benefits. First up, ashwagandha.

Four Great Testosterone Supplements That Actually Work

Natural testosterone supplements for increasing testosterone levels.

1. Ashwagandha as a Testosterone Supplement

What is Ashwagandha?

Ashwagandha (Withania Somnifera) is an Indian herb known for its stress reducing and hormone balancing qualities. It is referred to as both the "Indian Ginseng" and "Strength of the Stallion" due to its healing, rejuvenating, and strengthening effects on the human body. This herb has been used since the ancient times for a wide variety of conditions. Ashwagandha, a member of the nightshade family, is a small plump plant that produces fruit about the size of a peanut. It is widely grown in the arid regions of northern Africa, India, and the Middle East as well as in areas of the United States.

Research supports that a healthy daily dose of Ashwagandha for adult males is 300-500 mg 1-2 times daily in addition to a healthy balance of fats and protein... So how do you know if you are in need of the healing effects provided by Ashwagandha? Well here is a little checklist:

Do you experience any of these side effects?
- Stress
- Fatigue

420

- Lack of Motivation
- Lack of Energy
- Lack of Focus

If you answered yes to any or all of these...Ashwagandha may be something you want to consider taking a look at...

Note: We recommend Jarrow Formulas KSM-66 Ashwagandha, available at store.anabolicmen.com

Uses for Ashwagandha

This little beauty can really pack a healthy punch, you could say Ashwagandha has a mean right hook when it comes to protecting the body. Ashwagandha is full of numerous medicinal chemicals (withanolides, alkaloids, choline (great natural testosterone booster), and fatty amino acids), and its leaves are used in herbal remedies.

Some of the identified healing properties of Ashwagandha are:

- Improves thyroid function
- Heals adrenal fatigue
- Increases endurance
- Reduces brain cell degeneration
- Stabilizes blood sugar
- Lowers cholesterol
- Boosts immunity
- Improves mood and energy
- Reduces cortisol levels
- Offers anti-inflammatory benefits
- Improves focus
- Balances hormones

Ashwagandha not only relieves stresses on the body, but it is also protective in nature. Ashwagandha is a member of a group of Adaptogenic herbs. As the name suggests, these herbs help the body adapt to, react to, and cope with external environmental stress (toxins in the air) and internal stress (depression and anxiety). All in all, this little herb seems like a big help to balancing the body and relaxing the mind.

Ashwagandha as a Testosterone Boosting Supplement

Research points to Ashwagandha having a direct impact on testosterone balance. A specific study of interest aimed to investigate what supplementation of Ashwagandha root could do to the semen profile, oxidation, and reproductive hormone levels of 75 infertile men. (738) The results were incredible...supplementation improved sperm count and mobility and the treatment with Ashwagandha recovered seminal plasma levels of antioxidant enzymes...now that is a powerful herb.

Another study investigated the impact Ashwagandha can have in treating male sexual dysfunction and infertility. (739) The 46 person study administered Ashwagandha root extract to 21 males and a placebo to 25 males and then tested both groups after 90 days. After the 90 days, the results showed that the sperm count in the 21 males receiving the root were 167% higher, the volume of sperm was 53% greater and the mobility was 57% greater... What else does Ashwagandha impact?

Ashwagandha and Cortisol

As we know, testosterone can be impacted via multiple avenues... one key avenue is cortisol...

Cortisol is a life sustaining adrenal hormone key in the maintenance of homeostasis in the body. It is also a key player in the battle to balance testosterone levels...imbalances in cortisol = no bueno for testosterone levels. If your body is overtaxed from stress (this isn't just stress from work or relationship stress, this is any kind of stress...physical, mental, or emotional...all stress impacts the body in some way, shape, or form.)

If your cortisol boat is rocked, well this indicates stormy seas for your hormones...When stressed, your body...just like you when you are under a lot of stress...shuts down. The effects of this can lead to increased signs of aging, low libido, hair loss, and even infertility.

Studies have shown that Ashwagandha has the ability to naturally balance out your hormones, combating cortisol and returning the body to a stable state. Specifically, a study in India (740) looked into how Ashwagandha influenced chronically stresses humans in a randomized study. Participants were randomly assigned 1 of 3 amounts of Ashwagandha supplement or a placebo. Their stress levels were than assessed at study onset, 30 days, and 60 days. Results indicated that those receiving supplementation had improved wellbeing and lower stress levels by days 30 and still by day 60, while the placebo group exhibited no significant decrease in overall stress.

Cortisol is a certified buzz kill to healthy testosterone production. Seeing that Ashwagandha decreases cortisol levels, (740) it naturally leaves the road open for testosterone to get all revved up again.

Another extremely effective cortisol managing supplement is phosphatidylserine, which will we will talk about here in the chapter as well.

2. Micronutrient Blend as a Testosterone Supplement

Micronutrients can be consumed separately, or altogether from smart micronutrient blends like Vitamin Code Raw One Men's Multivitamin.

Let's talk about vitamins and minerals.

The fact I'm about to present to you is so radically simple and logical that most guys overlook it completely. They suffer from low T issues: stubborn body fat, depression, "hardgainer" syndrome, skinny fat syndrome, anxiety, insomnia, etc – and run around Amazon looking for the latest and greatest "testosterone boosting" supplements that never does anything for them in the way of results. They think natural testosterone supplements should entail flashy exotic ingredients, when in reality, most of the results you're looking for could be achieved by recognizing the following fact:

If you are deficient in the vitamins and minerals that your body needs to properly produce testosterone, then you will never have healthy T levels.

Eliminating these deficiencies will quickly and naturally bring your T back up to normal levels. So simple, yet so radical.

Let's look at 10 vitamins and minerals you need to keep "topped off" at healthy levels to support your body's testosterone production:

- Vitamin A
- Vitamin C
- Iron
- Vitamin D3
- Vitamin E

- B Vitamins
- Zinc
- Magnesium
- Selenium
- Manganese

Multivitamins Are One of the Best Testosterone Supplements

Vitamin A:

Vitamin A is considered the "lost bodybuilding nutrient" – and for good reason. It is the bodybuilder's secret weapon because it is essential for the utilization of protein as well as the production of testosterone and other growth factors.

Greater concentration of vitamin A in the testes correlates with greater T production in general. Vitamin A also decreases estrogen production in the testes, and when absent, will lead to complete atrophy of the testicles – which means it is essential for T production, not just accessory. (741)

One particular study found that supplementation of vitamin A + Iron was equivalent to supplementation of bioidentical testosterone in terms of it's effect on inducing hormonal puberty and development of male characteristics (742) which highlights the importance of taking vitamin A and iron in tandem with one another. This makes sense because levels of A in the testes are also positively correlated with an increase in transferrin levels, which is the chief iron transport protein, as well as growth factors IGF-binding protein, androgen-binding protein, transforming growth factor beta (suppresses cancer cell production), and steroidal acute regulatory protein (which transports cholesterol to be converted into androgens such as testosterone).

Vitamin C:

Vitamin C's antioxidant properties are shown to help the pancreatic cells properly modulate secretion of insulin (743). In adult humans, 2g daily vitamin C supplementation has been shown to decrease insulin spiking after meals and modulate blood glucose levels for the hour following the meal (744).

In case you're wondering why I'm talking about the pancreas and insulin, remember that insulin plays a role in modulating testosterone production.

The relationship between testosterone and insulin sensitivity is what you can probably guess. Insulin resistance correlates with lower testosterone levels, while healthy insulin sensitivity with higher testosterone levels.

Vitamin C supplementation can improve insulin sensitivity, and therefore improve endocrine markers related to testosterone levels.

Secondary to its normal antioxidant properties, vitamin C has been shown to have a specific testosterone-preservation capabilities, one of which stems from its direct protection of oxidative stress in the testes. Vitamin C has also been shown to preserve testosterone levels in the face of lead toxicity, alcohol-related stress (ie. binge drinking), and other stressors such as loud noises and serious testicular burns.

Iron:

As mentioned earlier, iron is especially useful when taken with vitamin A because vitamin A increases production of transferrin which is iron's chief transport protein, leading to increased proliferation of several key growth factors. (742) The combination of vitamin A + iron will have a profound positive effect on your endocrine health and has been shown to rival direct T application in studies.

Vitamin D:

Researchers have long known that the male reproductive tract is a target of vitamin D in the body, and that adequate D levels are positively correlated with significantly higher levels of T in men (747), so it's not surprising that vitamin D supplementation would also be shown to increase serum, bioactive, and free testosterone by over 25% in healthy males. (745)

When test subjects took vitamin D + calcium together, they not only saw a significant increase in overall T levels over years, but also a decrease in age-related testosterone decline (746) which suggests that supplementing with vitamin D + calcium can not only increase T levels but also preserve its decline in general.

Vitamin E:

If you're deficient in vitamin E, you will see a noticeable and significant drop in overall LH, FSH, and therefore T levels (LH and FSH are precursor hormones secreted by the pituitary gland which signals to the testes to produce testosterone). This study (748) shows us that simple vitamin E deficiency elimination – supplementing with vitamin E to bring levels back up to normal healthy range – is enough to massively increase T levels, along with LH and FSH. The researchers claim that vitamin E administration activates the production of these gonadotropins (LH and FSH) meaning regular vitamin E supplementation may be enough to consistently produce large increases in testosterone precursor signaling from the brain to the testes.

B Vitamins:

The B vitamins encompass 8 different water soluble vitamins that are all necessary for myriad bodily functions, including endocrine functioning. Vitamin B deficiency leads to increased estrogen levels, increased prolactin levels (suppressing T production), and lower overall T levels in healthy men. Eliminating vitamin B deficiencies will increase T production and T levels (serum and free) as well as suppress estrogen production. (749) (750) (751) (752) Note: men of Scandinavian descent are prone to have genetic B12 deficiencies and are recommended to supplement regularly to keep levels healthy. Please get a blood test to check yourself if you think you fall into this category.

Zinc:

Zinc plays a major role in the aromatization process, so it should come as no surprise – and should be a bit worrisome also – that zinc deficiency can lead to upregulation of estrogen receptors up to 57% (753) – but eliminating zinc deficiency will downregulate estrogen production and simultaneously upregulate testosterone production and get your T levels back to normal.

Magnesium:

Magnesium supplementation can also drastically increase T levels, especially in deficient men. (754) This study (755) went so far as to even recommend mineral supplementation (chiefly by looking at the profound effects of magnesium on androgen increases) as a good alternative to hormonal supplementation (like TRT). If you're really interested in reading more about Magnesium and androgens I recommend reading this review (756) on the subject.

Selenium:

Selenium – while not as widely known in popular literature like blogs – is a potent T increasing compound, especially when combined with zinc (757). It stimulates production of glutathione which is one of the body's chief antioxidants (see vitamin C article above for more information about the preservative effects of antioxidants on testosterone levels), and selenium has been shown to increase a number of positive semen parameters in adult males (758).

Manganese:

Controlled supplementation with will increase GnRH levels in the brain which leads to higher growth hormone and testosterone levels. (759)

With all of this in mind, it becomes pretty obvious that if you have a micronutrient deficiency causing low levels of testosterone, simply eliminating these deficiencies is the easiest way to increase your testosterone, leading to easier muscle gain, fat loss, sexual health, and general well-being.

Since we've covered a lot of ground here, I'd like to recap one of the really important findings here, since these studies also show us that you can see some insanely good results with micronutrient supplementation by combining a few key vitamins/mineral together:

- Vitamin A + Iron
- Vitamin D + Calcium
- Selenium + Zinc

I like to think of micronutrient health as a car metaphor – it's kind of like when your endocrine system is the car and vitamins and minerals are the gasoline. The car will not run properly without the gasoline in the tank; just like your endocrine system will not properly produce healthy levels of all the hormones that keep you feeling great, lean, and strong without the proper micronutrients to fuel it.

You can definitely get all of these nutrients from your diet though – but if you're like me and you value convenient solutions and don't have the patience to count every micronutrient you put into your body, then a high quality micronutrient support supplement may be the answer.

Also, I highly recommend you read the book Nutrient Power by William Walsh PhD if you're interested in further exploring the impact micronutrient therapy can have on your brain and endocrine health.

Next up, boron.

3. Boron as a Testosterone Supplement

Boron is one of my daily testosterone supplements.

Boron is a natural testosterone supplementI freaking love the effect it gives me.

After finding out how consistently effective it is at raising T and free T significantly in just a matter of 1-3 weeks in studies, I decided to try it for myself. And it feels awesome. I've since begun recommending it to friends and they report similar effects.

My buddies reported the same finding.

They felt more dominant, like they were less susceptible to the outside world, and more in control of their inner world.

Good shit.

Boron is a trace mineral located at the top of the periodic table with symbol B and atomic number 5. As a dietary mineral it is essential for healthy bone development, as well as increasing testosterone levels. In addition, it helps metabolize key vitamins and minerals that also affect testosterone and estrogen.

Summary of Boron as a Testosterone Supplement:

The health benefits of Boron have been widely studied for many years. It is a mineral which is found all around us in fruits, vegetables, leafy greens, and even water. (741) As a mineral, it participates as a Lewis Acid which binds to hydroxyl groups and when it binds to three hydroxyl groups, it is referred to as Boric Acid. (742) As with many minerals it is absorbed in the intestines, however Boron has a very high absorption which means it is easily metabolized. (743) It is essential for normal growth and health of the body and when deficient causes serious and dangerous conditions such as arthritis, osteoporosis, sex hormone imbalance and neural malfunctions.

Why It's Important:

Borons role on human health is vital! When the body is deficient in Boron, a slew of serious conditions arise. Deficiencies affect many areas of the body such as the brain. A boron deficiency has shown to alter brain wave activity which is associated with cognitive impairment. Borons role within the bone and skeletal mass is also critical with deficiencies causing many major health issues such as osteoarthritis, and other bone and joint diseases. (745)(746)

What You Should Know:

- Boron is a chemical element found on the periodic table.
- Boron can be found in fruits, vegetables, drinking water, avocados, ground cinnamon, apples,broccoli and many other foods.
- When Boron binds to three hydroxyl groups, it forms a new structure called Boric Acid.

- Boron is essential for human health and deficiencies of Boron cause serious health problems.
- Boron helps preserve neuronal functions.
- Boron is used as a supplement to increase testosterone levels.
- Boron supplements interact with Vitamin D metabolism.

Why We Need Boron / The Benefits:

Boron is essential for life. It's essential for humans, animals as well as plants. Deficiencies of Boron cause serious health issues such as neurological issues, bone and skeletal mass damage, and decreased testosterone. Our bodies use Boron to keep the brain function well and when deficiencies occur, the brain wave activity is altered. (747) The bones rely on Boron for many functions, such as keeping calcium levels high so that bones don't become weak. (745) (746) It is also beneficial as an anti-inflammatory and helps reduce negative side effects of rheumatoid arthritis. Boron is highly sought after for its important role in enhancing testosterone levels. (748)

Boron, Bones and Skeletal Mass:

Boron has shown to positively affect bones and inflammation. (746) Some studies have shown that regular Boron supplementation may help alleviate joint inflammation and have a positive impact on osteoarthritis. (745)

Boron and Testosterone:

Studies have shown that testosterone levels may increase with Boron supplementation. One study in particular showed that after just 7 days, testosterone levels increased by 28%. Testosterone is a hormone responsible for many important functions within the body. Hence, if a testosterone deficiency exists within the body, it causes many serious health issues.

Boron and Osteoarthritis:

Boron has many positive effects on bones and the skeletal mass. Studies have shown that boron supplementation alleviates joint inflammation and has healing benefits on osteoarthritis. Supplementation with Boron reduces excretions of calcium which suppresses osteoporosis.

Interesting Boron Facts:

- Boron is a chemical element literally from out of space because it formed after the big bang by a process called cosmic ray spallation.
- Boron may have played a key role in the evolution of life on Earth.
- The largest boron deposits are in Turkey.
- Boron plays an important function in testosterone development.
- When Boron binds to three hydroxyl groups, it forms Boric Acid which is used by women to alleviate yeast infections.
- Boron in its crystalline form is the second hardest element on earth after carbon in its diamond form.
- We recommend boron chelate or boron glycinate.

4. Phosphatidylserine as a Testosterone Supplement

Beat cortisol and produce testosterone with this one supplement.

- Are you feeling stressed out?
- Do you feel as though your brain isn't functioning as well as it should be?

Then you may want to consider getting a daily dose of phosphatidylserine in your life.

What is Phosphatidylserine?

Phosphatidylserine (PS) is a naturally occurring phospholipid nutrient found in the cell membrane of all species.

It is mostly found in organs with high metabolic activity, such as the brain, the liver, the lungs, the heart, and skeletal muscle. Around half of the body's supply of PS is in the neural tissue.

PS does a lot of awesome things for your body. According to a study in found in the International Journal of Sports Nutrition, phosphatidylserine modulates the activity of receptors, ion channels, enzymes and signaling molecules and is involved in governing membrane fluidity.

Due to the fact that such a large portion of the body's PS supply is contained in the neural tissue, it is widely believed that PS can also improve brain function.

This would qualify phosphatidylserine as a nootropic.

A large number of research studies support the idea that PS can help brain function.

In this study, (771) 157 elderly participants who had previous complaints of failing memory were given PS or a placebo for 15 weeks. At the end of the period, cognitive memory was found to be much better in the PS group than the control group.

In another study, (772) 36 children who had been previously diagnosed with ADHD and had received no previous drug treatment were given PS for 2 months. Results showed that PS improved symptoms of ADHD and also improved short-term auditory memory.

The studies and positive results go on and on, all showing positive conclusions that PS does indeed improve cognitive function in the forms of memory, speed, accuracy, and attention.

New results involving PS were found in this study, (773) where 14 healthy males were asked to partake in a session of intermittent cycling on different percentages of energy until exhaustion. After controls were tested, a different group of males were given PS before the workout. Breath by breath respiratory data and heart rates were recorded throughout the workout and after the workout was completed.

The results were rather fantastic. The time to exhaustion in the workout went from 7:51 in the placebo group to 9:51 in the group that supplemented PS. This suggests that PS can actually increase exercise capacity.

Aside from all of these amazing effects of taking phosphatidylserine, PS has also been found to reduce stress and fatigue.

This leads perfectly into an investigation as to the effects of PS on testosterone levels, considering reducing stress and fatigue should indeed boost testosterone levels.

Phosphatidylserine and Testosterone:

So far, we have only discussed PS and its effects on cognitive abilities, but there are a few clues that would lead us to believe that PS also has a positive effect on boosting testosterone. (774)

First, PS is a message sender between cells. Communication between cells is a key component in hormone production.

Second, PS is known to protect cells from any oxidative damage. For testosterone, the most important cells to protect are those in the testicles and the brain and guess what, the testes and the brain hold most of the body's PS.

This enough should clue us in on the idea that PS is awesome for testosterone production, but to make sure, let's look at some research.

In this study, (775) 9 healthy men were supplemented 800mg of PS for 10 days. All 9 men took part in physical exercise during the trial and compared to a control, researchers found a significant drop in physical stress induced cortisol levels among the group taking PS.
This would in turn increase the amount of flowing testosterone during the workouts.

If you are looking for a study that directly shows results in the testosterone to cortisol ratio, then look no further.

In this study, (776) 10 healthy males were either given a placebo or PS and were asked to complete a moderate intensity interval exercise. Blood samples were taken before, at various points throughout, and after the workout.

The results were very telling of the power of PS. The PS group not only had lower cortisol levels, but the PS group had an improved testosterone to cortisol ratio by 184%.

So basically PS is a killer way to get the testosterone to cortisol ratio you need to build lean muscle mass.

So how can you get phosphatidylserine in your diet?

Ways to Ingest Phosphastidylserine:

You can either get your daily dose of PS by taking supplements or eating foods that contain enough PS to have an effect.

One is a little more difficult than the other.

Let's start with food. Here is a list of foods/sources you could find that contain phosphatidylserine:

Cow Brains
Interestingly enough, when the first studies on phosphatidylserine's effects on cognitive ability, the PS used was derived from cow brains. When the Mad Cow Disease scare hit though, researchers moved to a PS derived from soy.

For our purposes, you probably want to stay away from soy due to the high levels of estrogen.'

Lucky for us, the Mad Cow Disease scare is virtually over/has severely declined in the last decade, so you can fairly safely get your desired dose of PS from bovine brains again. Yum!

This is good because the highest concentration of PS you can get in a food is from bovine brains.

In a 100g serving of bovine brain, you can get over 700mg of PS, which is about the dose of PS used in the studies above (between 600-800mg).

Just watch out for diseased cows!
Nobody wants Mad Cow Disease.

Organ Meats

If you are still scared of getting that Mad Cow Disease, you can also get a fairly high (but not as high) dose of PS from organ meats.

I'm talking liver, heart and kidney.

In comparison to the cow brains, a 100g serving of chicken heart contains just over 400mg of PS, so you'd have to almost double the amount of chicken heart to get the same amount of PS as the cow brain.

If pig kidney is more your speed, you can get around 218mg PS per 100g.

Lecithin

Lecithin – while soy derived – is currently the only reliably safe way to get high doses of PS in supplement form. And even though it is soy-derived, it actually doesn't contain phytoestrogens, due to the extensive extraction process, so there is no need for worry.

How to take it (recommendations and dosages):

The standard Phosphatidylserine (PS) dose is 100 mg, taken 3 times a day totaling 300 mg. Based on current research, 300 mg a day seems to effectively prevent against cognitive decline and improve cognitive functioning.

You should not exceed 550 mg a day.

If you notice any unwanted energy boosts or experience insomnia in the evenings, lower your dose and eliminate any doses in the afternoon.

Phosphatidylserine may be one of the best supplements out on the market.

Not only does it have some amazing effects on your cognitive health and abilities (not to mention healing effects on dementia and Alzheimer's), it can also optimize your testosterone to cortisol ratio.

Having a great testosterone to cortisol ratio is extremely vital to men who want to gain lean muscle mass, reduce depression, have less stress, and have better general wellbeing.

The Best Natural Testosterone Booster Supplement Available

During these years of running the Anabolic Men website, several supplement manufacturers have asked us to:

- Formulate a supplement for them.
- Promote their supplements on our site.
- And even bash their competitors on our articles.

However, we have never done any of the things above. Simply because we have never found a supplement which we could fully trust and promote as the #1 testosterone booster. And obviously, were not in the business of smearing other companies reputation for our own (or someones else's) gain.

But now as the AM website has stabilized its place as the leading men's hormonal health resource, we are finally able to actually formulate our own supplements.

With complete control of the quality of the ingredients, the use of the ingredients, and the dosaging of the ingredients.

This allowed us to finally produce the #1 natural testosterone booster supplement on the market. And if you look through the ingredients and the research behind them below, I think you'll agree with us.

The Perfect Formulation

Unlike many brands manufacturing supplements for increasing testosterone levels, we don't hide behind proprietary blends. Our ingredients and where they are derived are easily accessible information.

We also refuse to use ingredients that aren't proven in science or inhibit some other crucial hormones or enzymes in the body (like 5-ar or DHT).

Supplement Facts		
Serving Size: 3 Capsules		
Servings Per Container: 30		
Amount Per Serving		%Daily Value
Magnesium (as Magnesium Citrate)	150 mg	38 %
Zinc (as Zinc Gluconate)	15 mg	100 %
KSM-66® Organic Ashwagandha Root Extract	400 mg	*
Forskohlii Root Extract	250 mg	*
Inositol	200 mg	*
Glycine	200 mg	*
L-Theanine	100 mg	*
Boron (as Boron Citrate)	10 mg	*
Bioperine® Black Pepper Fruit Extract	10 mg	*
*Daily Value not established		

This is why we decided **NOT TO** include the following common ingredients:

- Tribulus terrestris (it doesn't work) (777)
- Maca root (it doesn't work either) (778)
- Fenugreek (it only raises T because it inhibits DHT) (779)
- Saw palmetto (same story as with fenugreek) (780)
- D-Aspartic acid (which actually lowers testosterone). (781)

Here's what we **DID** include:

Magnesium Citrate

Magnesium can benefit testosterone levels by reducing the levels of sex hormone binding globulin (SHBG).

When SHBG is inhibited, more free-testosterone remains bioactive in the bloodstream and is able to bind into receptor sites.

This is likely the reason why magnesium supplementation and high magnesium levels in the serum are consistently linked to:

- Higher free-testosterone levels in test-tube studies. (782)
- Higher free-testosterone levels in exercising men. (783)
- Higher testosterone levels in elderly males. (784)
- Positively correlated with anabolic hormones in review studies. (785)
- And deficiency – as to be expected – is linked to lowered testosterone. (786)

Magnesium is highly beneficial for male hormonal health, which is why we decided to include 150mg of well absorbing magnesium citrate into the formula of Testro-X (no higher amount since mega-dosing magnesium is associated with gastric upset, and 150mg on top of average diet is well enough for benefits).

Zinc Gluconate

Zinc is without a doubt the most important mineral for healthy testosterone production.

Aside from being one of the 24 essential micronutrients for human survival and regulating more than 100 bodily enzymes, zinc plays a crucial role in the production of testosterone, in its utilization by the androgen receptor sites, in DHT production, and at keeping estrogen levels low.

Here's some research about the importance of zinc for hormonal optimization:

- Supplementation results in higher total and free testosterone and thyroid hormones in exercising men. (787)
- Supplementation results in higher total T, free T, and thyroid hormones T3 and T4 in sedentary subjects. (788)
- Correcting zinc deficiency has been found to lead to rapid and significant increases in testosterone (789) and DHT levels. (790)
- Animal studies have found zinc supplementation to elevate LH levels, testosterone levels, and thyroid hormones. (791)
- One study noted that zinc deficiency led to 59% reduction in androgen receptors (36% of those being in testicles). (792)
- There are three extremely bio-available forms of zinc to use in supplementation: picolinate, citrate, and gluconate. We decided to go with 15mg dose of zinc gluconate for Testro-X, as it's known to be the form of zinc containing the lowest amounts of cadmium (793) (a testosterone lowering heavy-metal found in high amounts on low quality zinc supplements).

KSM-66 Ashwagandha

Ashwagandha (Withania Somnifera) is primarily used in the Indian herbal medicine.

Therefore one could think that its effects are not proven in science and only folklores told by the neighborhood shaman.

But fear not, there actually is Western medicine clinical research behind this herb. Just take a look at these:

- Several studies have found ashwagandha to reduce feelings of stress, as well as significantly lower the levels of the stress hormone cortisol. (794)
- Ashwagandha has been associated with significant increases in sperm quality and testosterone levels on infertile subjects (up to 40% in 90 days). (794)
- In a non-sponsored peer-reviewed study with 57 young healthy male subjects, ashwagandha supplementation raised the average testosterone levels from 630 ng/dL to 726 ng/dL. (795)
- The highest-quality ashwagandha on the market is a patented water-extract called KSM-66 Ashwagandha, we decided to include a potent 400mg dose of it in Testro-X based on the dosages used in majority of the human studies.

Forskohlii Root Extract

Forskohlii root extract (Forskolin), rose to popularity after the notorious fool Dr. Oz proclaimed that it would be a "magical fat-loss miracle".

This obviously was just hype to sell the product, and even though Forskolin works by stimulating certain enzymes necessary for fat oxidization, it isn't exactly as effective as Oz claims.

Now, although that sneaky salesman of a doctor has done his best to make forskolin look like a scam, there actually is some scientifically found benefits for the root in terms of testosterone optimization.

For instance:

- Forskolin is well known for increasing the levels of intracellular cAMP (cyclic adenosine monophosphate). (796)
- Increased cAMP is known for its stimulatory effect on testosterone production (797) and androgen receptor (AR) activation. (798)
- Forskolin in cell-culture studies has been linked to significant and consistent increases in testosterone. (799)
- 250mg's of Forskolin was able to increase T levels by 33% when compared to placebo in overweight males. (800)
- Based on the human study (801) which showed nice increases in testosterone levels, we decided to include 250mg's of high-quality Forskolin in Testro-X formulation.

Boron Citrate

You may or may not have heard about boron before.

It's a trace-mineral, not considered absolutely essential for survival, and honestly, not that popular as a supplement.

Here at Anabolic Men we absolutely love boron, and we believe it deserves more attention than what it is getting now.

Here's why:

- In rodent studies, boron has been found to dose-dependently increase testosterone levels. (801)
- 6mg's of boron for 2 months in human subjects was associated with a nice 29% increase in testosterone levels. (802)

- 10mg's of boron for 7 days in humans was able to increase free-testosterone by 28%, while reducing estrogen by 39% and boosting DHT by 10%. (803)

Boron deserves more attention as an essential trace-mineral for maintaining male hormonal balance. We are proud to include 10mg's of highest-quality boron citrate in Testro-X.

GnRH Surge Blend

When your body naturally produces testosterone, the whole cascade starts from the brain substrate called hypothalamus, which releases a hormone called GnRH.

GnRH then stimulates the release of luteinizing hormone (LH) from the pituitary gland. Which then travels down to your testicles via the spine and triggers the leydig cells to synthesize testosterone.

Our idea with the specific "LH Surge Blend", was to identify natural compounds that can stimulate the release of GnRH and LH, for higher amount of natural testosterone production.

That's why we included 200mg's of inositol, a precursor needed for the natural synthesis of GnRH. (804)

That's also why we included 100mg's of L-theanine, which excites the GABA-neurons in the brain and stimulates GnRH release. (805)

And finally the blend was completed with 200mg's of glycine, which increases the pulsatile release of GnRH. (806)

Bioperine®

Bioperine is a patented extract of the black pepper fruit.

Although there's animal research suggesting that black pepper fruit extract may be beneficial for androgenic hormones in rodents, (807) we didn't include bioperine in Testro-X because of those studies.

Instead, we formulated bioperine into the supplement as it is known to significantly enhance the absorption of many herbs, minerals, vitamins, and amino-acids. (808)

We wanted to make sure that the ingredients in the supplement, actually absorb into the body to provide real effects.

Hence the bioperine, and if it boosts testosterone as it did in the rat studies, that's obviously just another plus.

Conclusion

When we say that Testro-X is the best testosterone booster on the market, we're not joking around.

Every ingredient in this supplement has been scientifically proven to either increase testosterone levels or improve the absorption of other ingredients.

No shady herbs with baseless claims, no hiding behind proprietary blends and ineffective dosages.

Just 100% research-backed men's health supplements.
Available now at store.anabolicmen.com

Chapter 50

7 Best ED Supplements

Erection problems are one of those "silent health hazards" that are rapidly increasing all around the globe, especially in countries where obesity, poor nutrition quality, and lack of exercise are key "attributes" of the population.

Chances are that if you have problems with erection strength all the time or occasionally, and you go to a doctor for help, you'll likely leave with a prescription erectile dysfunction drug for Cialis or Viagra. While both of them do work extremely well, they are also: Ridiculously expensive.

Synthetic prescription pharmaceuticals with a host of side-effects.
Not going to address the original root of the problem, (low T, poor vascular function, etc).

Like so many of the modern-day pharmaceutical erectile dysfunction supplements, they're just a means to mask the real problem with a "robotic erection". There's nothing natural in needing a drug for getting your battle-sword up. What if you forgot the prescribed magic-pill somewhere for example? And what happens when you have poked with the assist of a blue-pill for years, then develop side-effects and have to discontinue the use? Let me give you a hint: nothing good (at least that is if you haven't focused on fixing the root issues of your problem).

Now while I would recommend that you start from fixing certain health and lifestyle factors (sleep, exercise, weight-loss, etc) before jumping head-first into using erectile dysfunction supplements, tThere are 7 (yes, seven!) natural supplements for erectile dysfunction that are alternatives to synthetic pharmaceuticals, and all of these are proven to work with multiple scientific studies. Use them strategically while also doing the things in this book to optimize your overall hormonal and vascular health and I can guarantee you that you're not going to need any pharmaceutical aids after that.

1. Ginseng

Ginseng is a great erectile dysfunction supplement.Ginseng has been titled as the "natural Viagra" due to its impressive results in multiple scientific trials, and while I can guarantee you that ginseng is nowhere near as potent as synthetic Viagra is, the benefit is that it's all natural, costs just a fraction of the price, and actually works unlike many other natural erectile dysfunction supplements out there.

The roots of ginseng are best known as "adaptogens," a blanket term coined by the scientist in Soviet Russia for identifying compounds that can promote the body to adapt into stressful situations and maintain the bodily homeostasis naturally by balancing stress and steroid hormones. The theorized reasoning for these effects is often claimed to be the high amount of phytonutrients (mainly ginsenosides) and antioxidants found in the roots.

While the evidence on ginseng's ability to increase testosterone levels is mixed (raising the hormone on infertile men, (809) but not on men with no infertility), (810) the research behind its erection promoting effects is stronger than a steel pipe.

In a Korean double-blind placebo study, (811) 900mg's of ginseng taken 3 times per day for 8-weeks was able to significantly improve erectile quality of subjects with clinically diagnosed erectile dysfunction. These effects were noted by a questionnaire, as well as RigiScan measurement (yes, that's an actual device that measures erection quality.)

Another study conducted five years later (812) found similar results with 1000mg of ginseng taken 3 times per day, across the board patients receiving the ginseng had noticeably improved their quality of erection rigidity, maintenance, and penetration efficacy.

In a research-study of ginseng saponin's (813) it was also noted that ginseng has the ability to significantly improve erection quality when compared to a placebo solution. This time the researchers used another erection strength monitoring device called "AVS-penogram". The underlying mechanism of ginseng's actions is not fully understood, but its likely a combination of multiple compounds (saponins, antioxidants, ginsenosides). What has been seen in animal studies is that many of the ginsenosides have the ability to raise nitric oxide levels in the blood, (814) and thus widen the blood vessels and improve circulation.

We have recently added a high-quality liquid ginseng extract to the Anabolic Men Marketplace (store.anabolicmen.com), consisting of American, Korean & Chinese red, and Siberian ginseng's all dissolved into alcohol solution to derive maximum amount of the active ingredients from the roots.

2. Pycnogenol

Pycnogenol is a great supplement for erectile dysfunction.

Pycnogenol is a patented water-extract of the bark of the French maritime pine tree. It's standardized to contain 65-75% procyanidin, which is a compound known to stimulate nitric oxide synthesis (815) and therefore greatly increase vascular health and blood flow.

And that is the mechanism of how pycnogenol works as an erectile dysfunction supplement. It is used to improve erection strength and the promotion of arterial relaxation with a boost in nitric oxide.

40mg's of pycnogenol was used alongside with 1700mg's of arginine and aspartic acid in a Bulgarian trial. (816) The study had 40 subjects suffering from clinically evaluated erectile dysfunction, and they took the combination of these supplements for erectile dysfunction, 3 times per day (so 120mg's of pycnogenol). Three months into the study, 92,5% of the test subjects reported that their ability to regain erections had returned. In 2003, another group of researchers replicated the study with similar results using 120mg's pycnogenol with 21 subjects. (817)

In 2007, 180mg's of pycnogenol was found (818) to increase arterial expansion of young male subjects by a staggering 42%. Another trial noted that in patients with coronary artery disease, pycnogenol is a potent compound for greatly improving vascular health and blood flow. (819)

Since pycnogenol is so well-documented to promote vascular health and blood flow, we formulated 100mg's of it into one Redwood capsule to be taken for every 12-hours, giving you a scientifically solid dosage of 200mg's pycnogenol daily.

3. Garlic Extract + Vitamin C

Garlic extract and vitamin C increase erection quality. Both garlic and vitamin C have been studied for their effects in promoting blood flow, reducing inflammation, and dropping blood-pressure. In fact, garlic is often more potent at relieving high blood-pressure than pharmaceutical solutions. (820)

The thing that many people don't know, is that when you combine vitamin C with garlic extract, you can expect massive improvements in your circulation due to elevated nitric oxide production.

This effect was seen in a study concluded by Mousa et al. (821) when they administered 2 grams of vitamin C in combination with 4 capsules of garlic extract daily for 10-days to their patients with mild hypertension (high blood-pressure).

They saw the following improvements:

- Endolethial nitric oxide output increased by a staggering 200% (that's 3-fold increase!).
- On average systolic blood pressure dropped from 142 to 115.
- On average diastolic blood pressure dropped from 92 to 77.
- For this very reason we decided to add 300mg's of garlic extract, along with 1 gram of vitamin C to one capsule of Redwood, which is taken twice per day, resulting in 2 grams of vitamin C and 600mg's of garlic extract.

4. Citrulline or Arginine

Arginine is an amino acid that acts as a precursor to nitric oxide, citrulline on the other hand is also an amino acid (found in watermelons for example), which naturally converts to arginine in the kidneys.

For these reasons both are generously used in pre-workout supplements to increase "pump" of the muscles and improve blood flow.

The science behind these compounds is pretty solid, they both seem to very reliably increase nitric oxide output (822, 823, 824, 825), however for some reason citrulline seems to be more potent at this. (826) Maybe your body converts it into a more potent form of arginine than that of which can be found in arginine supplements, who knows.

Whatever the case, both of them seem to work, citrulline is just better.

I have for years recommended this powder (827) which contains 5 potent ingredients for increased circulation; arginine, citrulline, Coenzyme Q10, resveratrol, and pomegranate extract.

It's sold as a cardiovascular health formula, but can be used as an erectile dysfunction supplement to improve erection quality as well as a pre-workout booster before workouts.

5. Horse Chestnut Extract

Horse chestnut extract can be used to cure erectile dysfunctionHorse Chestnut Extract (HSE) is often standardized to 10-20% of the active ingredient escin, which has been found to be extremely beneficial for vascular health.

The mechanism at which horse chestnut extract improves erection quality is two-fold. Firstly its able to increase nitric oxide levels, and secondly it improves the function of the "vascular valves" and thus prevents and relieves the formation of varicoceles (half-blocked veins with poor valve function leading to testicles and thus impairing testosterone production).

The latter mechanism of HSE is particularly interesting due to the fact that roughly 20% of men have varicose veins in their testicles, sometimes noticeable, but often so mild that they go unnoticed. These veins can be surgically operated, but so far escin (the active compound in horse chest nuts) has been identified as the only compound that has proven research backing up its use as a natural varicocele treatment.

There are three studies which all found that standardized escin is able to significantly "resolve" varicose veins all around the body (828, 829, 830), and most importantly one which showed that escin derived from HSE was able to reduce the rate of varicoceles and thus improve the sperm counts and testosterone levels of infertile patients. (831) One study (832) has also experimentally varicocele'd rodents just to find out that standardized escin can reverse the negative effects.

We included horse chest nut extract in Redwood simply because we feel that improving the valve function and reducing the rate of varicoceles can bring massive improvements to the erection quality of many men who are not aware of the fact that they might have varicose veins, plus it also increases NO production so it was a no-brainer anyway.

6. Grape Seed Extract

Grape seeds are often extracted to get a standardized amount of the active ingredient; procyanidin. It's the same nitric oxide stimulating compound that can be found in pycnogenol.

Aside from increasing nitric oxide, grape seed extract (GSE) has been found to inhibit the activity of the aromatase enzyme, (833) which is an enzyme that converts testosterone molecules into estrogen.

The mechanism of action in grape seed extract makes it a great erectile dysfunction supplement as it can benefit erectile health by boosting nitric oxide and preserving testosterone.

The research behind GSE is interesting. In rats for example, 100mg/kg has been able to increase nitric oxide levels by 125% at rest and 138% after exercise. (834) Human studies consistently show how GSE increases NO-production and thus reduces blood-pressure, leg swelling, heart rate, and cardiovascular disease risk (835, 836, 837, 838).

Because of its clinically proven use to improve nitric oxide output, we recently added this high-quality high potency grape seed extract product to the marketplace.

7. Icariin

Icariin is the active ingredient found in a herb called horny goat weed (epidemium). There's research showing that it can act similarly to a testosterone mimetic in the body while also increase nitric oxide output and serving as a PDE-inhibitor.

Since icariin is a PDE-inhibitor, one could compare it to Viagra, due to the fact that the mechanism at which sildenafil (the active ingredient in Viagra) works is also PDE-inhibition.

I'm sad to say that when compared to its synthetic relative, icariin is not nearly as potent, but again, it's natural and a significantly cheaper alternative.

The research shows that when male rats are administered 80mg/kg of icariin, their testosterone levels increase 3-fold, (839) and this occurs without significant changes in LH or FSH, suggesting that icariin has a direct testicular effect on testosterone production.

When icariin was tested in cell-cultures, (840) the researchers noted that it was able to inhibit the PDE5 enzymes, thus many supplement manufacturers have started selling it as an aphrodisiac or under the name of "natural Viagra", again though, icariin is not as potent as the blue-pill.

Some other studies have found that icariin can increase the nerve growth and circulation of the pelvic region, (841) significantly increase nitric oxide output, (842) and blunt the rise in stress-hormone cortisol. (843)

Icariin might be an useful addition to your erectile dysfunction supplement arsenal, but I doubt it has even remotely similar effects as Viagra does, unless you also make sure that you optimize your lifestyle, body composition, and diet towards healthier erections. If your problems are due to performance anxiety, the stress-reducing effects of icariin might be particularly useful.

Conclusion on The Best Supplements for Erectile Dysfunction

There you go, 7 compounds with science backing up their use as great supplements for erectile dysfunction. None of the compounds alone might not be as effective as Viagra or Cialis, but heck, at least you're not poking around with a robotic erection.

Just to recap, you can get clinically effective dosages of pycnogenol, garlic extract + vitamin C, and horse chestnut from REDWOOD (see, told you we formulated it science-first, haha). If you're interested in the ginseng, icariin, citrulline, arginine, and grape seed extract, you can find them in the AM marketplace. store.anabolicmen.com

— Chapter 51 —

Stress-Lowering Supplements

Stress is the "silent killer" of our time. So you must know how to lower stress naturally.

Stress, whether physical or psychological, manifests itself physiologically in our body... negatively effecting our hormones, chronically elevating cortisol levels – our main stress hormone – which leeches the body of essential micronutrients over time: fuel it desperately needs for daily metabolic processes.

Most of us, in some way, shape, or form, experience significant physical or psychological stress on a daily basis. This chronic elevation in cortisol levels leaves us with any number of the following symptoms:

- Insomnia
- Crippling Anxiety
- Loss Of Libido/Sex Drive
- Low Testosterone
- Extreme Reactions To Common Stimulants Like Caffeine
- Lack of Focus
- Difficulty Recalling Recent Memories
- Lack Of Motivation and Stamina For Training

If you're experiencing any of these symptoms, don't fret because the 5 little-known all natural ingredients I'm about to show you will put a stop to all of this, and will help cure your problem from it's roots – eliminate stress naturally. Each of them have a lot of research to back their cortisol-balancing effects and I'm excited to show them to you. They're especially potent when taken in the right dosages altogether. Phosphatidylserine (PS) cell membrane building block, molecular model. PS is also important in apoptosis (programmed cell death).

1. Non-GMO Phosphatidylserine

Phosphatidylserine is one of the most widely researched stress reduction agents on the supplement market. It has research that backs up claims that it can reduce stress and increase mental performance. Researchers have gone to great lengths to look at how this supplement can affect both physical and mental performance – so much so, that the FDA has approved health claims for PS, which is incredibly rare for nutritional supplements – a true testimony to its effectiveness (they usually reserve FDA approval for pharmaceuticals).

In this study, (844) researchers looked at phosphatidylserine's effect on cortisol release after an intense bout of exercise. The study utilized a clinically effective dose of 600mg of PS. Using Cortigon you could easily reach the 600mg per day mark. The difference is the synergistic effect the other ingredients in Cortigon cause when combine with phosphatidylserine.

In this study researchers looked at the effect PS supplementation had on cognitive performance. (845) While this is a difficult to measure, scientists looked at calmness as measured by the types of brain waves present in the participants. What they noticed was that the participants who had undergone PS supplementation were able to maintain a calmer state while performing different tasks designed to challenge the participants "cognition".

2. Gingko Biloba Leaf Extract

Ginko Biloba is another heavily researched supplement ingredient that was a no brainer for inclusion in Cortigon, the worlds #1 stress reducing compound. In studies performed on animals (846) Ginko Biloba is shown to attenuate the affects of acute stress. Researchers often perform studies on rats as their response to many drug and supplement compounds mimics that of humans. In multiple studies done on rats, researchers have found that Ginko Biloba not only reduces the level of circulating cortisol, (847) but actually reduces the activity of the glands associated with cortisol and adrenaline production.

Beyond Ginko Biloba's ability to reduce cortisol and other stress hormones, it attenuates the negative affects of oxidative stress as well. In this study researchers looked at the affects of Ginko Biloba on the onset of Alzheimer's disease. (848)

What the research showed was that many of the negative symptoms of Alzheimer's disease, caused by oxidative damage, were slowed when patients underwent supplementation with Ginko Biloba. Alzheimer's disease generally is caused by a degradation in nervous system functioning which can largely be attributed to oxidative damage. Taking measures to slow this type of damage ensures greater mental acuity and performance over time.

3. L-Carnitine

Choline and L-Carnitine have been shown to reduce the negative affects of free radical damage in the body. This should be a huge concern for anyone that enjoys exercise as one of the only consistently negative aspects of exercise is the free radical damage that it forces on the body. Many people look to their diets to provide all the free radical fighting anti-oxidants they can get.

Unfortunately, the amount of anti-oxidants you get from your food is entirely dependent on the state and quality of the food at the time you eat it. Between transportation, storage, refrigeration and cooking, food can loose quite a bit of its free radical fighting potency.

4. Choline

One of the first orders of business in designing Cortigon was to ensure that it would be able to protect against both the physical and psychological causes of stress. In terms of physical stress, few supplements have a larger body of research to support their use in the fight against stress induced damage. In this illuminating study, using human subjects, researchers noticed significantly lower levels of oxidative damage after 21 days of supplemental Choline and L-Carnitine. (849)

In another human study, (850) Choline was shown to reduce oxidative stress in patients with compromised respiratory function due to asthma. These patients were able to reduce their higher then normal levels of oxidative stress over the course of 6 months even in a compromised state of health.

5. Omega-3 (DHA Powder)

Omega 3 fatty acids are essential to your overall health. DHA (the Omega provided from fish oil), or docosahexaenoic acid, not only provides incredible heart protection, but also feeds your brain and accentuates the effects of substances like Phosphatidylserine and L-Carnitine, making even smaller doses of those substances more potent. Healthy doses of DHA can even provide a noticeable nootropic (brain enhancing) effect when taken alone.

The inclusion of DHA in Cortigon was a no-brainer because of its synergistic power with the other ingredients. When stacked together the sum of these ingredients has a stress-crushing effect.

Bonus: Inositol

Inositol has been shown to decrease the severity or occurrence of a number of mental conditions from panic attacks (851) and depression (852) to anxiety and nervousness. (853) This has to do with inositol's ability to balance the functioning of the nervous system and brain. While Inositol has been used as an assistant for the treatment of many health issues, there is evidence to support its stand alone use in treating mentally based conditions such as anxiety.

Inositol has proven to be an effective compound through research and anecdotal experience. When creating the short list of compounds that needed to be in Cortigon, Inositol was another one that quickly made the roster. Though the affects of Inositol are more subtle then those of a substance like say PS, we challenge anyone who has not tried it to take it on its own to feel its effects.

Prior to the creation of Cortigon, Inositol first made its round with the AnabolicMen team as a fantastic addition to our morning coffee routine! This is one of the best ways to notice its affects on calmness as the experience of caffeine vs. caffeine and Inositol is clear.

How To Use Cortigon for Lower Stress

Cortigon uses a host of different ingredients that are powerful enough to form the basis of their own supplement. What do you mean....? The above stress-fighting supplements are often the main ingredient in other companies products. Basically any compound that can be used effectively is more expensive to purchase. Supplement manufacturers know this......so they charge accordingly.

Many supplement companies will build a product around 1 or 2 high cost ingredients and then include a whole host of lower cost ingredients who's effectiveness is questionable at best. This makes for an impressively long ingredient list that provides relatively lackluster results.

The Cortigon formulation is comprised of only ingredients that are effective enough to form their own supplements. We know....most of the AnabolicMen.com team has been taking the majority of the ingredients on their own as individual supplements. Supplements like Ginko Biloba and Phosphatidylserine are all fantastic on their own.

Using our team as Guinea Pigs we figured out which supplements and which doses were effective enough to be purchased and used on their own. We then combined them to form a supplement that could replace them all.

In Cortigon, you will never find an ingredient that is included to justify a higher price.

There is no Shark Cartilage, desiccated bovine liver or space dust extract. Just the supplements that most fitness enthusiasts or nootropic users will recognize.

The difference is that the Cortigon formulation is made with only clinically effective doses of each ingredient.

Unlike many manufacturers that only include clinically effective doses of the few ingredients that consumers will be keeping their eyes on, we have included it for every one.

— Chapter 52 —

Estrogen-Lowering Supplements

In this chapter, I break down the 5 estrogen supplements that are proven to help lower high estrogen levels. Now, there are many reasons why high estrogen levels are no good news for men. Sure you need some for bone & joint health, and brain function, but most men these days have their levels completely overblown due to high exposure to xenoestrogenic chemicals, storing too much fat in their bodies, and consuming a diet that is not hormonally beneficial in any way shape or form.

In men, 95% of the time elevated estrogen levels are due to having too high level of aromatase enzyme activity. That is, an enzyme directly converting testosterone molecules into estrogen. (854)

High estrogen on the other hand has been found to suppress testosterone production by inhibiting the luteinizing hormone release from the pituitary gland. (855) This vicious cycle eventually causes very low levels of testosterone, with overblown estrogen – and thus – the testosterone to estrogen ratio shifts far too much to the right, resulting in:

- Feminization of the physique and face.
- Retaining of subcutaneous water under the skin.
- Weakened libido and dramatically increased emotionality.
- In the worst case scenario; development of man-boobs, prostate issues, and hot flashes.

This list consists of five scientifically proven supplements that work by either inhibiting the aromatase enzyme or by down regulating the activity of estrogen towards its receptors.

> NOTE: Do remember, that outside of using estrogen supplements, the hands-down the best way to lower high estrogen levels is to get lean, eat real food, and avoid exposure to man-made estrogen-mimic chemicals.

The 5 Natural Estrogen Supplements to Lower High Estrogen Levels

1. Zinc

Zinc as an estrogen supplement lowers estrogen levels and aromatase enzymeZinc is one of the 24 essential micronutrients necessary for human survival.

It's known to regulate hundreds of bodily enzymes, as well as being absolutely necessary for the proper functioning of the immune system.

Some of the scientifically proven benefits of zinc supplementation include (seen up to the point where bodily zinc levels are saturated):

- Reduced activity of estrogen receptors and inhibition of aromatase enzyme. (856)
- Increased thyroid hormone production (857) and lower levels of SHBG. (858)
- Increased levels of DHT, (859) total, and -free testosterone. (860)

For best results consume 15-30mg's of high-quality zinc supplement or have large amounts of some good meat in your diet, best if you do both.

2. Boron

Boron is an anti estrogen supplement and estrogen suppressantBoron is a mineral and estrogen supplement that can pack an estrogen-lowering punch.

Although it's a trace mineral, and not considered absolutely essential to human survival, it still has some interesting benefits for us.

Study from Naghii et al. (860) for example showed the following results after men consumed 10mg's of boron for a week:

- Free-testosterone levels increased by 28%.
- Free-estrogen levels had decreased by -39%.
- Dihydrotestosterone (DHT) levels rose by 10%.
- Inflammation biomarkers (hsCRP, TNF-α) dropped significantly.

Another study saw that 6mg's/day of boron for 2-months can increase testosterone levels by 29% as well as improve serum vitamin D by increased absorption of the vitamin.

> NOTE: For best results consume 6-10mg's of high-absorption boron glycinate or eat plenty of raisins.

3. Grape Seed Extract

Grape seeds are high in a valuable compound called procyanidin, this phenol is mostly hailed due to its ability to naturally increase nitric oxide levels (and therefore improve circulation).

One of the lesser-known benefits of grape seed extract is its ability as a natural estrogen supplement to reduce estrogen levels by inhibiting the activity of aromatase enzyme.

Researchers studying ways to prevent and cure breast cancer have identified grape seed extract as a natural compound that blocks estrogen biosynthesis by inactivating the aromatase enzyme (862, 863, 864).

Due to grape seed extract having low bio-availability in the human body, high doses (up to 2000mg/day) of the extract are needed to see these positive effects in studies. This would translate to about a gallon of grape juice or five pills of high-potency grape seed extract supplement.

To counteract the low absorption rate of GSE, take it in fasted-state, one study saw that this improved the bio-availability by up to 5x! (865)

4. Resveratrol

Resveratrol is the antioxidant polyphenol found in red grapes. It's one of the main reasons why red wine is considered healthy. It is also a great estrogen blocker supplement.

Many studies have shown that resveratrol can increase testosterone levels and suppress estrogen by inhibiting the aromatase enzyme in test-tubes (866, 867, 868).

The problem with resveratrol however is that it doesn't seem to work as well in living organisms, ie. when people take it orally. This is due to low bio-availability.

The only two types of resveratrol I've seen to actually work and be properly absorbed in studies are the conjugated form of resveratrol, and this patented resveratrol delivery system called VESIsorb® (absorption rate 100x that of pure resveratrol powder). (869)

5. Tongkat Ali

Tongkat Ali (Eurycoma Longifolia, Pasak Bumi) comes from Malaysia, it has huge popularity as a pro-erectile testosterone booster due to multiple studies supporting its effect at increasing testosterone levels and suppressing the stress hormone cortisol. (870)

There seem to be many claimed mechanisms of action in which Tongkat Ali works, but three of the scientifically proven ones include; stimulation of testicular CYP17-enzymes, suppression of SHBG, and inhibition of aromatase enzyme.

The inhibition of aromatase enzyme has actually been shown in only one rodent study (871) so far, but the results were staggering.

Injected Tongkat Ali blocked estrogen with comparable potency to Tamoxifen, which is a synthetic – and extremely powerful – prescription aromatase inhibitor.

Chapter 53

Androgen Receptor Supplements

Before androgens (testosterone or DHT) can make any changes in your body, they have to enter DNA. In order for them to actually get to the DNA, they have to be bound from blood circulation by androgen receptors in cells.

This happens naturally all day long around your body, but did you know that you can actually increase androgen receptor density, as well as enhance their activity at utilizing male hormones?

That's right, there are a handful of supplements, few specific training methods, meal timing pattern, and one pretty popular drink that have all been scientifically proven to increase androgen receptor density.

1. Intermittent Fasting

intermittent fasting to increase androgen receptor sensitivityIntermittent fasting (IF) is gaining popularity like a rolling snowball. It's an eating pattern where you fast for majority of the day and consume all of your daily calories in a short eating window.

The most common method of this is the Lean Gains style where you fast for 16 hours and feast for 8 hours. This cycle repeats everyday.

There are many benefits to IF, things like improved insulin sensitivity, weight loss due to easier maintenance of the calorie deficit, and sharper cognitive functions.

But did you know that insulin is not the only thing that your body becomes more responsive to after short-term fasting?

Androgen receptors seem to have the same effect towards testosterone and DHT after fasting, when you start eating. There are two studies which showcase this, one from Sweden (872) which showed that fasting for 12-56 hours can increase the responsiveness to testosterone by up to 180%.

How fasting increases androgen receptor activity naturally...And another one where the subjects actually did a 10-day water fast, then resumed eating and they were followed for 5 days as they consumed their normal meals, as you can see from the graph on right, their testosterone levels shot up like crazy (873) and kept climbing for the 5-day post-fasting follow up. The likely explanation here is that their bodies became more sensitive towards androgens during the ruthless 10 days of no calories whatsoever.

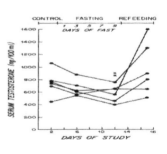

> NOTE: No, I do not recommend anyone to do a 10-day water fast, shorter fasts like the 16:8 method should still do the trick.

2. Resistance Training

Resistance training increases androgen receptor density. Resistance training is a reliable way to increase testosterone levels. Not only does it boost the production of the big-T, it also increases its utilization by up-regulating the activity and density of androgen receptors in muscle tissue.

Research has shown that trained men have significantly higher AR content in their muscles than non-trained individuals, (874) and that different types of weight-lifting methods yield different degrees of AR activation. (875) Since androgen receptors are a factor in muscle protein synthesis, it's only logical that their density and activity increases after the body adapts to resistance training.

There are few "training rules" you should follow in order to maximize the androgen receptor increase, testosterone and DHT release, and of course, muscle & strength gains:

1. Activate large amounts of muscle mass, with proper form, and still remain somewhat "explosive".

2. Do it rather quickly in order to avoid increases in cortisol (which decreases AR content of muscles). (876)

3. Progress with your lifts on a weekly basis, and rest accordingly to actually be able to do that.

Luckily, this all has been explained in a detailed manner with actual exercise routines and periodization schemes in the THOR Program.

3. Carnitine

Carnitine is an androgen receptor activator. Carnitine occurs naturally in meats and fish. In fact it might be one of the most hormonally useful compounds that vegans miss in their diets.

The simplified mechanism of action for how it can increase androgen receptors naturally is as follows:

Carnitine transports lipids (fat) into the cellular mitochondria to be used as energy -> androgen receptor (AR) activity within those same cells is increased.

These effects were shown in a study (877) where 3-weeks of L-Carnitine L-Tartrate supplementation at 2g/day was able to significantly increase the amount of active androgen receptors in human subjects at rest.

The same researchers later replicated the study with exercising subjects to prove – this time with actual muscle biopsies – that in trained males, L-Carnitine L-Tartrate is even better at boosting AR content than what is seen at subjects who are sedentary. (878)

Bottom line is that <u>carnitine increases androgen receptors at rest and even more so after exercise</u>. Using 1-2g/day of a similar tartrate for as used in the studies should do the trick.

4. Levodopa

L-DOPA (levodopa) is a naturally occurring amino acid found in high amounts in mucuna pruriens (velvet bean). It's a direct precursor to dopamine, can bypass the blood-brain barrier, and effectively raise serum dopamine levels.

In my article about mucuna pruriens on AnabolicMen.com, I linked few studies which showed how L-DOPA from mucuna pruriens was able to increase testosterone levels, raise dopamine, boost sperm health, enhance cognitive ability, and reduce prolactin levels.

And as an icing to the cake, there's the fact that levadopa acts as a co-activator protein to the androgen receptors, effectively enhancing their activity in in-vitro studies (879, 880).

Using 250-500mg's per day of quality M.Pruriens extract with standardized amount of L-DOPA should do the trick.

5. Caffeine

Caffeine, the principal alkaloid and active ingredient of coffee beans, is not only good at boosting your creativity and energy levels. The good stuff can also increase workout performance as well as increase androgen receptors and testosterone!

Studies on rodents have shown that chronic low-dose caffeine intake can increase testosterone levels, DHT levels, and androgen receptor (AR) expression. (881)

The mechanism of action is that caffeine stimulates cAMP enzyme inside the cells that host the androgen receptor, (882) and cAMP then stimulates another enzyme called protein kinase A (PKA), which then regulates the glycocen, sugar, and lipid metabolism inside the receptors, enhancing their activity at binding DHT and testosterone.

Caffeine activates AR with the same mechanism as forskolin does, by increasing intracellular cAMP levels. For better results, take your forskolin and caffeine in a fasted-state (insulin inhibits cAMP).

Conclusion on Androgen Receptors

There you go pal, five ways to maximize and increase androgen utilization at the receptor sites. To recap, here's your five-step natural AR optimization stack:

- Drink some coffee in the morning in fasted-state
- Pop few caps of forskolin, also in fasted-state
- Crush a heavy THOR workout in the evening (preferably still at fasted-state if u can).
- Break the fast with a big post-workout meal and 1-2 grams of L-Carnitine L-Tartrate.
- Before you go to sleep, consume 250-500mg's of mucuna pruriens extract.

Bonus: For poor guys who can't get the supplements; double the coffee, get the carnitine from red meat, and L-DOPA from fava-beans.

PART 8:
APPENDICES

The 30 Item Grocery List

A few of the most often asked questions we get are: what do I eat to maintain high testosterone levels, and if I have a specific list of recommended foods that boost testosterone. While there are many food related posts scattered around this blog, I've never really made an all-around post about what I would put into a high T pantry. Until now.

In this appendix, you will basically get a 30 item shopping list of foods that boost testosterone in men with all the nitty-gritty explanations about why the foods are great for the endocrine system. Think of it as a grocery list that your balls would write if they had hands.

1. All Kinds of Potatoes

Potatoes are a great food that boosts testosterone. If you're a frequent reader here at AM, you already know that carbohydrates are hugely important for healthy testosterone production.

You also know that grains are not the preferred source of carbs, mainly due to problems with gluten, which can significantly increase prolactin levels, effectively messing up T production.

Simple sugars are also not the preferred carbohydrate sources on a high T diet, since they have been linked to lowered testosterone levels in multiple studies.

Ruling out grains and simple sugars, may make it look like you can't eat any carbs, except for salad, but that's not the case.

You can – and should eat – potatoes as part of a testosterone boosting diet!

Sweet potatoes, white potatoes, russets, red potatoes, purple potatoes, etc. If it's a potato, you should be eating it. Potatoes are excellent no-gluten source of testosterone boosting carbohydrates, and also very dense in nutrients. Stock pile your pantry full of them, and make potatoes your main carbohydrate source.

2. Macadamia Nuts

Dietary fat, in general, is known for its testosterone increasing effect, and nuts in general, are very high in fats. So one could easily assume that all nuts are pro-testosterone. However, that's not the case.

The kinds of fats that have been linked to increased T production are saturated fatty-acids (SFAs) and monounsaturated fatty-acids (MUFAs). Polyunsaturated fatty-acids (PUFAs) on the other hand tend to lower testosterone levels.

Most nuts are – unfortunately – loaded with PUFAs.

Not macadamia nuts though. 100 grams of these wonderful little fat balls contain ~75 grams of dietary fat, out of which 60 grams are MUFAs, 13 grams are SFAs, and less than 2 grams are PUFAs.

3. Epic Bar

I couldn't believe my eyes when I first saw 100% grass-fed bison bars on the market.

Not only bison, but also lamb, turkey, and beef.

Why are the epic bars so epic then? Well, despite their high price point, they're exactly the kind of protein your endocrine system craves for. Animal-based. Grass-fed. And free of antibiotic, hormone, and pesticide traces.

I know for sure that my pantry is always loaded with bison bars. Or should I say testosterone bars. Either way, they're epic.

4. Beef Gelatin

In traditional societies, the bones and connective tissue of meat-giving animals were generously enjoyed, giving the consumer a great balance of amino acids.

In more recent cultures, we have started eating only the muscle-meat, tossing away the connective tissue, bones, and organ meat.

The problem with that is the fact that we are getting too much of the amino acids tryptophan and cysteine, and too little of the amino acids proline and glycine (both of which act as crucial neurotransmitters for the body).

To correct this, you could eat some bone broth and animal organs, but there's also an easier way.

Gelatin. It's an incredibly dense source of connective-tissue protein, providing you with ~27% glycine and ~15% proline. It's also tasteless, so you can easily scoop it straight on with a spoon.

Why would gelatin be pro-testosterone then? For starters, once you balance out the neurotransmitters in your body, your sleep quality and hormonal signaling will improve, this alone will lead to significant increases in testosterone and life-quality.

5. Coffee

Coffee is a great drink to boost testosterone levels. Who doesn't love a cup – or five – of strong coffee?

Coffee is great. It gives you the caffeine which stimulates the nervous system and jolts you up, while also boosting cAMP levels, leading to increased testosterone production.

Sure coffee can also increase cortisol levels (which is a stress hormone notorious for lowering testosterone), but it's crucial to understand that the cortisol boost from caffeine is very short in duration, not like the T suppressing long-term (usually stress-related) cortisol elevation.

Oh, and coffee is also loaded with antioxidants. So again, there's no need to start avoiding coffee, just don't drink it 15 cups a day for every hour of your time awake.

6. Brazil Nuts

Brazil nuts are an essential part of a testosterone boosting food list. Brazil nuts are shelled in a thick cone, so technically they're seeds, but due to their nut-like taste and structure, people have always called them nuts.

They do not have as good fat ratios for testosterone production as the macadamia's do (100 grams of brazil nuts has 15g SFAs, 25g MUFAs, and 19g PUFAs), but their true testosterone boosting potential is not in the fat ratio.

It's in the ridiculously high selenium content. 100 grams of Brazil nuts contains 1917 mcg's of selenium, which is 2739% of the RDA%! Selenium – mostly due to its glutathione stimulating effects – is directly linked to increased testosterone production, and just a handful of Brazil nuts a day is easily enough to cover your selenium needs, naturally.

NOTE: Most of the selenium is in the skin of the nut, so don't buy your Brazil nuts unshelled.

7. Extra Virgin Olive Oil

Extra virgin olive oil can be straight on labeled as a testosterone booster.

Since there's literally a study where young Moroccan men changed to extra virgin olive oil as their main source of fat, and in 2 weeks their testosterone levels increased by 17%.

This could have been caused by the fact that olive oil has a pretty darn great fat ratios for T production (73% MUFAs, 14% SFAs, 13% PUFAs), or it could also be the fact that olive oil is anti-inflammatory, or that it's ridiculously high in antioxidants. It also contains the possibly testosterone boosting bitter glycoside; oleuropein.

Just make sure your olive oil is the real deal. Organic. Extra Virgin. And from a trusted brand. Many cheaper olive oils have been heated, processed, and adulterated with cheaper oils (usually high PUFA ones too).

8. Raisins

Raisins are a great food that boost testosterone levels for multiple reasons.

Firstly, they're anti-inflammatory and chock-full of antioxidants, such as resveratrol, which has been linked to increased testosterone and lowered estrogen levels in few studies.

Secondly, 100 grams of raisins contain ~3 mg's of boron, which is a not too popular mineral that has increased testosterone levels quite significantly in few scientific studies.

So, it's not a bad idea to make your own testosterone boosting snack trail mix with raisins, macadamia nuts, and brazil nuts.

9. Parsley

Parsley is a great little plant. That's because of a compound in it called apigening.

The researcher at Texas tech found out that apigening increases the amount StAR (steroidogenic acute regulatory protein) inside the testicular leydig cells.

Why is this great you might ask? Well, StaR is the binding protein that transports cholesterol into the mitochondria inside your ballsack, essentially converting it to free testosterone.

So, more parsley -> more StaR -> better conversion from cholesterol to free testosterone -> more free testosterone.

Bottom line: You better be consuming parsley.

10.Ginger

Ginger is a common household spice, but it can be used to many other things than just to add flavor to foods.

Ginger contains the active ingredient, gingerol, which is a potent anti-inflammatory agent in the body.

Not only that, but several animal studies have identified ginger as an androgenic compound, while one Iraqian human study noted a 17% increase in testosterone levels after ginger supplementation.

So not a common household spice alone, but also a powerful androgenic anti-inflammatory agent. And cheap as fuck.

11. Raw Cacao Products

Raw cacao, cocoa, or chocolate products are nutritionally dense testosterone boosting superfoods.

However, I'm not talking about the chocolate or cacao that most people identify as chocolate. Real chocolate is not heated (this destroys the antioxidants and many vitamins), it's not processed, and it's definitely not refined.

It's this unheated, minimally processed, and essentially RAW version of chocolate that maintains the antioxidants, enzymes, and friendly gut bacteria. It's also the RAW chocolate that is linked to increased cardiovascular health, lowered blood pressure, and lowered blood glucose levels. Not the junk on the candy shelves.

But why are raw chocolate and cacao products an awesome food that boosts testosterone production?

First of, they're loaded with antioxidants and jam-packed with minerals, such as magnesium, zinc, manganese, iron, and copper.

And not only that but raw cacao products have pretty much perfect fat ratios for testosterone production too. For example, out of the dietary fat in raw chocolate ~61% is saturated fats, ~37% is monounsaturated fats, and only ~2% is polyunsaturated (depending bit on the manufacturer).

So, chock-full of antioxidants, live bacteria, and enzymes. Full of testosterone boosting minerals. It also has perfect fat ratios, making raw cacao products a powerhouse food that boosts testosterone levels.

12.Eggs

Eggs are a nutrition powerhouse and great for testosterone production. Eggs are considered as "the perfect protein" since they contain a nearly perfect balance of amino acids for human needs.

Eggs are also highly nutritious, containing nearly all of the recognized vitamins (with the exception of vitamin C).

They also have good fatty-acid ratios for testosterone production. 38% saturated fats, 44% monounsaturated fats, and only 18% polyunsaturated fats.

The most important factor that makes eggs a high-T food, is the fact that the yolk contains hefty doses of cholesterol, which like you might already know, is the direct precursor of testosterone.

> NOTE: I know that many people get scared about cholesterol and fats in the yolk, but there's no need to. It has been scientifically proven that regular egg consumption on a daily basis does not negatively influence your cardiovascular health.

13.Real Salt

Real salt is great as part of a testosterone boosting foods listThere's a huge difference between real crystal, sea, or rock salt when compared to the usual "table salt".

That is, real unrefined and unaltered salts are bit clumpy and they have about 60+ trace minerals in them.

The basic table salt on the other hand? It's usually got 2. Sodium and chloride. Rest is stripped away.

What more? Well, the processed table salts can have up to 3% anti-caking agents, which are often unhealthy heavy metals like aluminum silicate or sodium ferrocyanide.

This is all done because of increased profits, aka. longer shelf-life. When salt is stripped from its natural minerals, it's no longer salt. It's processed shit.

So, would you rather consume the shitty purified table salt that has mere 2 minerals and heavy-metal caking agents, or the real deal that contains 100% real salt and 0% caking agents, with a taste that explodes in your mouth? Your call.

14. Argan Oil

Argan oil is a great addition to a testosterone boosting diet. Argan oil is the oil pressed from the argan tree kernel. It's heavily used in the Mediterranean diet.

Previously in this chapter, I mentioned a study where olive oil, a main source of fat for 2 weeks, was able to increase testosterone levels by 17% in healthy young Moroccan men.

Well, in that same study there was another group too. A group that used virgin argan oil as their main source of dietary fat for 2 weeks. Their testosterone levels increased by ~20%.

Much like olive oil, argan oil is anti-inflammatory and has a lot of antioxidants. It also has pretty good fatty-acid ratios for T production (not as good as olive oil does, though).

Anyhow, there's clinical evidence showing how it boosts testosterone by 20%, so you better be eating this.

15.Avocados

Avocados are a food that boost testosterone naturallyThese fatty fruits are often deemed "bad" by the low-fat idiots. And this is because unlike many other fruits, 77% of the calories in an avocado come from fats.

If you're a frequent reader of AnabolicMen.com, you already know that increased dietary fat intake is directly correlated with increased testosterone production. And not only that, but the types of fat that increase T seem to be saturated fats (SFAs) and monounsaturated fats (MUFAs), while polyunsaturated (PUFAs) actually tend to lower testosterone.

In the view of the above, we can see that avocados are a great food that boosts testosterone naturally. Since they contain a lot of dietary fat, from which 16% is SFAs, 71% is MUFAs, and only 13% is PUFAs. Avocados are also loaded with fat-soluble vitamins, many of which are crucially important for healthy testosterone production.

16.White Button Mushrooms

White button mushrooms increase testosterone levelsI used to eat these only as a pizza topping, and since they are mostly water, I was under the notion that white button mushrooms probably won't do Jack-shit health wise.

As usual, I was wrong.

White button mushrooms are loaded with polysaccharides, and in multiple studies, they have been found to exert anti-estrogenic effects, since they seem to naturally block the aromatase enzyme which converts testosterone to estrogen.

Similar anti-estrogenic effects have been noted with other mushroom varieties too, but white button mushrooms seem to be the strongest shroomy aromatase inhibitors identified so far.

17.Baking Soda

I use baking soda (sodium bicarbonate) more as a supplement (pre-workout, and for increased T) than a grocery item, but since it can be bought at any supermarket, it fits perfectly to this list.

Why baking soda you might ask? Well, firstly because it is a great ergogenic aid that can dramatically improve your squat and bench press performance, cellular adaptation to HIIT, and can be used to supercharge your creatine supplements.

And then there's also the fact that sodium bicarbonate tends to act as a molecular switch for the cyclic adenosine monophosphate (cAMP). And increased cAMP levels – as you might already know – correlate with increased T production since cAMP activates protein kinase A and serves as a secondary messenger between cells and hormones.

It's also about $7 per lb.

18. Yogurt

As of late, there has been a lot of evidence suggesting that prebiotics, probiotics, live enzymes, and other kinds of friendly bacteria could have a positive impact on testosterone production.

Few examples: In a 2014 study, a bunch of researchers tested multiple different diets with added Lactobacillus reuteri on male rodents. In every single case, the addition of L.Reuterii to the feed increased testosterone levels, increased luteinizing hormone levels, increased testicular size & weight, prevented age-related testicular shrinkage, improved semen parameters, and even increased markers of social domination.

Another rodent study found out that increased exposure to healthy gut microbiomes led to elevated testosterone levels. And one even saw that the probiotic Clostridium scindens can literally convert the stress hormone cortisol into androgens inside the gut.

So, how do you nourish the gut flora and colonize those healthy probiotics, prebiotics, and friendly enzymes into your intestines more effectively? Simple, by eating fermented foods, which naturally have the friendly bacteria and enzymes.

Yogurt is a great example and an awesome food that boosts testosterone levels. It contains the L. Reuterii and C. Scindensis, and several other – yet unresearched – probiotic strains.

19. Grass-Fed Beef Jerky

There's just no way around the fact that grass-fed beef is the number #1 source of testosterone boosting protein.

It's high quality, not corn-fed, has awesome amino-acid balance, and even the fat in it is saturated, which is the kind of fat linked to biggest increases in testosterone production.

Not to mention that grass-fed and organically grown animals are not exposed to testosterone-lowering pesticides, fungicides, herbicides, or insecticides. They're also not pumped full of estrogen, like conventional cattle often is.

I developed a deep love for beef jerky in the military since it's probably one of the healthiest foods you can carry as a "snack". And there's no way I would leave it out from a testosterone boosting foods list.

20.Minced Meat

Minced meat is great for increasing testosterone levels. Every time I visit my local grocery store, I leave with at least 2 kilos worth of organic minced meat.

There's a good reason for that. Minced meat is fucking awesome.

Whether it's beef or a mix of beef and pork or even lamb, you're getting plenty of high-quality testosterone boosting fats, along with some animal protein that your endocrine system craves for.

Minced meat is almost like a staple in many testosterone boosting recipes. It's so easy to use, tasty, and pro-testosterone. Why not load up with it?

NOTE: I use organic meat since I don't want to eat meat that has been treated with estrogen (to make the meat-giving animal fat). If you can't afford organic/grass-fed minced meat, it's better to buy the kind with the lowest amount of fat, since that's where the trace hormones tend to accumulate.

21.Pomegranates

There have been some very interesting study results about pomegranates as of late.

In one human study, daily pomegranate juice consumption for 2 weeks increased salivary testosterone levels by 24%, while also dropping diastolic and systolic blood pressure.

Another human study associated long-term (1-3 years) pomegranate juice consumption to -35% reduction in arterial plague. Pomegranate juice also protected LDL cholesterol from oxidative damage and dropped blood pressure as seen in the above study.

In test-tubes, few compounds extracted from pomegranates have found to be anti-estrogenic.

On top of that, pomegranates and the juice tastes like heaven.

22.Blue Cheese

Blue cheese is a great testosterone increasing foodAs you can see from the "yogurt" subheading above, fermented foods are excellent for testosterone production, since they contain the probiotics, prebiotics, friendly bacteria, and enzymes associated with increased T production.

Just like in the case of yogurt, blue cheese is also filled with that friendly gut bacteria, live enzymes, and the like.

On top of that, blue cheese contains hefty amounts of testosterone boosting saturated fat, and certain testosterone boosting fat-soluble vitamins, like the K2 for example.

Blue cheese goes perfectly in dressings, dips, between hamburgers, etc. It's a super simple way to add some T boosting goodness to your meals.

23. Dark Berries

Dark berries like blueberries, blackberries, acai berries, and so forth have always been identified as healthy.

And why wouldn't they be? The darker the berry, the higher the antioxidant content, and the more antioxidants you consume, the less inflammation and oxidative damage takes place in your body.

The result of that should be significantly increased testosterone production and testosterone molecule preservation.

Not only the antioxidants but berries are quite low in calories while being chock-full of nutrients.

They also contain the unique fiber called Calcium-D-Glucarate, which can potentially help your body to remove excess estrogen.

24. Grass-Fed Butter

Real grass-fed butter is an amazing food that boosts testosterone and should be the staple in every testosterone boosting diet.

It's a quality source for T boosting SFAs, while also containing the fat-soluble vitamins A, E, K2, and D, all of which are linked to increased testosterone production.

Just remember that it has to be real butter, and preferably from grass-fed cows. Margarine and other kinds of spread mixes are just rubbish PUFA filled inflammatory junk.

Get the real deal, the same stuff your ancestors used, then use it with cooking, in coffee, as is, whatever. Your balls will thank you.

25. Sorghum

Sorghum is used to boost DHT. Ever since I started seeing evidence of gluten being a potential prolactin booster and thyroid suppressant, I have been limiting my intake of grains and focusing more on potatoes as my main carbohydrate source.

I've seen nothing but good results health-wise from limiting grain consumption, but sometimes I just yearn for some floury grains, bread and the like.

I'm not completely anal about not eating grains, but since I discovered sorghum (a gluten-free androgenic grain), I have been substituting some of the more gluten heavy grains with it.

I was pleasantly surprised to even stumble upon this in-vitro study where sorghum extract increased 5-alpha reductase levels by 54% (this should lead to increased DHT conversion).

26. Coconut Oil

Coconut oil is a testosterone booster. Look no further than the alternative medicine community, and you will see NOTHING but praises about coconut oil. And even though I don't always agree with their ideologies, coconut oil really is kind of damn healthy.

It has been shown to improve cognitive abilities, increase testosterone production, increase thyroid hormones, boost metabolic rate, and so forth.

Being mostly saturated fat, it also fits well to the optimal testosterone boosting fatty-acid ratios.

> NOTE: Despite being high in saturated fat, coconut oil doesn't cause any cardiovascular problems. Does anyone even believe anymore that saturated fat would be the culprit anyway?

27. Organic Bacon

Bacon boosts testosterone in men. Bacon is pretty amazing. Not only does it have a heavenly taste, but it's also packed with high-quality animal protein, testosterone boosting saturated fats, and the direct precursor of testosterone: cholesterol.

In my opinion, you should only eat organic bacon, though.

Because of the mass production, conventional pigs are fed with GMO soy and corn, and they're living in such horrid conditions that they're pumped full of antibiotics to ensure that the pigs won't get any inflammatory diseases, and then they're fed & injected with ridiculous amounts of estrogen and growth hormone to make the pigs fatter and bigger in record times.

That last part is crucial. Because of the high fat content of the pig meat, the hormone residues are much more of a concern. You see, the adipose tissue (fat) is exactly where the hormone traces can be found.

So, organic estrogen-trace free bacon is a great food that boosts testosterone naturally, but the conventionally raised stuff should be avoided. You're better of using some lower fat conventional meats if you can't afford organic bacon.

28. Onions

Pretty much all kinds of onions are loaded with anti-inflammatory phytochemicals and antioxidants. Some of which are potentially testosterone boosting, like apigening and quercetin.

It's not a big surprise that in several rodent studies, onions have increased testosterone and produced androgenic effects.

Possibly the sickest result so far comes from one study where onion juice added to male rodents feed, increased testosterone levels by ~300% on average. Hard to say if the results are skewed or if this applies to humans at all, but it's still quite fascinating.

I have never seen any human data on the hormonal effects of onions, but there's potential and onions can add great punch to many foods, so why not?

29. Garlic

Despite the fact that garlic can give you a foul breath, it's also capable of increasing your nitric oxide levels by ~200% when taken in combination with vitamin C. Making it a stupidly cheap pre-workout booster.

There's also a rat study where rodents on a high-protein diet, saw significant increases in testosterone and drops in cortisol after garlic supplementation.

I have no idea what would cause this rise in testosterone after garlic consumption, but it could be caused by quercetin, anti-inflammatory effects, high amount of antioxidants, or its vasodilating effects.

Whatever it is, garlic is a food that boosts testosterone levels and is definitely worth the money.

30. Oysters

Oysters are a staple in many testosterone boosting foods lists out on the internet.

Not for nothing. They are absolutely jam-packed with zinc, magnesium, selenium, copper, and vitamin D. All of which are crucial for testosterone production.

Oysters also contain high quality protein, including some of the more rare amino acids (like the possible testosterone boosting D-aspartic acid).

The legend says that the 18th-century ladies man – Casanova – ate 50 oysters for breakfast. You know, maybe he was on to something.

— Appendix 2 —

5 Sample T-Boosting Recipes

A huge part of boosting testosterone levels naturally comes down to nutrition.

You want to eat a good amount of starchy carbs, good amount of the right type of fats, and low-medium amount of protein mainly from animal sources (both muscle-meat and collagen-proteins).

On top of all, it's ideal to get plenty of micronutrients (vitamins and minerals) with the foods you eat.

To achieve those goals, I have gathered you these 5 mouth-watering recipes. They're simple, delicious, and most importantly: recipes that nourish the bodily testosterone production.

We just put together a brand-new full color cookbook for **AnabolicMen.com** readers over at **TestosteroneChef.com** if you want an incredible book with all the recipes you need to raise your testosterone to new heights.

(It makes a great gift as well.)

Let's get to it shall we?

1. Spicy Lamb Stew

This spicy lamb shank stew is super-easy to make and it'll last for days. One of my ultimate T-boosting favorites. Look closely to the ingredient list and you'll see that almost everything on it has a positive effect on testosterone production:

- 3 lbs of lamb shoulder meat, cubed
- 3 tablespoons of olive oil
- 2 onions, chopped
- 6 cloves of garlic, minced
- 2 red bell peppers, chopped
- 2 tablespoons of ginger, ground
- 1½ tablespoons of cayenne pepper, ground
- 2 cups of beef stock
- 5 tomatoes, puréed
- 1 handful of fresh parsley
- 1 teaspoon of pure sea salt
- 1 teaspoon of pepper

Preparation:

1. Add the 3 tablespoons of olive oil into a pan or high sided pot. Add the lamb meat cubes and cook for 6-8 minutes until the cubes are evenly brown on all sides. Put the meat into a bowl.
2. Heat the same pan or high sided pot that you cooked the lamb cubes in, but this time put it to medium-high heat and add in the onions and bell peppers. Cook, stirring occasionally, for 5 minutes. Add garlic and continue cooking for 1 more minute.

3. Throw in the beef stock, lamb cubes, cayenne pepper, ginger, puréed tomatoes, and fresh parsley leaves. Bring the pan or pot to boil over high heat, then lower the heat to low and cook partially covered for 3 hours, or until the lamb is tender.
4. Season with salt and pepper. Eat.

Why exactly makes the lamb stew testosterone-friendly?

Lamb meat is a good source of carnitine which is an amino-acid that increases androgen receptor density and sensitivity. There's also saturated fat, cholesterol, high quality protein, zinc, several B vitamins, and CLA in lamb meat and all of which are linked to increased testosterone production.

Olive oil consists mostly of monounsaturated fatty accids, which in this study were shown to be pro-testosterone. A study found out that olive oil converted cholesterol more easily into testosterone. And one study saw that healthy male subjects who switched to using olive oil as their main source of fat noted a 17% increase in their testosterone levels.

Onions contain hefty amounts of quercetin and alliins, compounds that both are linked to increased T production. Moreover this study found out that feeding fresh onion juice to male rats more than tripled their serum testosterone levels.

Garlic is also rich in alliins and quercetin, and it comes not as a surprise that few studies have found out its testosterone boosting effects, such as this and this study.

Ginger increased testosterone levels by 17% in a human study, and it more than doubled testosterone levels in this rat study. One animal study also found out that it works similarly in diabetic rats.

Cayenne pepper, at least according to this study, may have a testosterone boosting effect.

Parsley contains a compound called apigening, which stimulates testosterone synthesis inside isolated leydig cells.

2. Guacamole

Who doesn't love to dip everything in Guac? Nobody! This classic guacamole recipe combines all of the T-boosting goodness into the ultimate Mexican dipping experience. The ingredients speak for theirselves:

- 4 ripe Haas avocados
- 3 tbsp lemon juice (1 lemon)
- 1 tsp cayenne pepper
- ½ cup diced red onion
- 1 large garlic clove (minced)
- 1 tsp coarse sea salt
- 1 diced tomato

Preparation:

1. Cut the avocados in half and remove the pits. Scoop the flesh into a bowl. Add lemon juice, cayenne pepper, diced onions, garlic, salt, and tomatoes.
2. Take a sharp knife and start dicing the avocado halves into smaller pieces. Once done, mix well and you're finished.

Why Guac is Pro-T?

Avocados are loaded with testosterone boosting monounsaturated-fats (MUFAs), while also being a source of a bitter glycoside; oleuropein, which increased T levels by a staggering 250% in this rat study. Add in 20 dietary vitamins and minerals present in the flesh of an avocado. Many which your body uses and requires to produce testosterone: A, K2, C, B2, B5, B6, zinc, magnesium, and copper, and you have yourself one of the possibly best testosterone boosting ingredients as a base for this recipe.

Cayenne pepper, Although not significant, there's a study which suggests that the capsaicin in cayenne pepper can protect your testosterone levels from the stress of a calorie deficit.

Garlic and onions both correlate heavily with increased T production in multiple animal studies.

3. Slow Cooker Swiss Steak

This recipe is courtesy of the Midnight Baker blog, it's quite simple to made in a slow-cooker, and its chock-full of testosterone boosting ingredients:

- 6 beef blade steaks
- 8 oz white button mushrooms, sliced
- 1 onion, sliced
- 1 tbs fresh thyme, minced
- 1 ½ tsp cayenne pepper
- 3/4 cup beef stock
- 1/4 cup dry sherry
- 1/4 cup sorghum flour
- 4 tbs olive oil
- ½ cup heavy cream
- 2 tbs fresh parsley, chopped

- salt & pepper to taste

Preparation:

1. Heat a pan over medium heat. Add in 1 tbs olive oil and the mushroom slices. Cook until the mushrooms start to brown. Remove from pan and put into the slow cooker.
2. Return the pan to medium heat and season the blade steaks with salt and pepper. Add 1 tbs of olive oil again and brown the steaks. Once browned, set them aside on a plate.
3. Once again, return the pan to medium heat, this time add: 2 tbs olive oil, sliced onions, and ground cayenne pepper. Cook and stir for a minute, then add the sorghum flour and dry sherry into the mix. Cook again for a minute, then pour the contents of the pan into the crockpot.
4. Add the blade steak slices on top of the mixture in crockpot, cover, and cook for 6-8 hours on low heat.
5. After 6-8 hours, remove the steaks into a serving plate and cover with foil so that they stay warm. Meanwhile add the heavy cream and chopped parsley into the liquid still in the slow cooker. Heat for another 10 minutes to make a sauce. Pour the sauce on top of the blade steaks, and serve with mashed potatoes.

Here's why the swiss steak boosts testosterone:

Beef steak is easily the best source of animal protein you would want to eat on a high testosterone diet.

White button mushrooms are natural aromatase inhibitors, meaning that they inhibit the conversion from testosterone into estrogen.

Onions have been linked to increased testosterone production in multiple animal studies.

Cayenne pepper has a testosterone protecting effect in testicular leydig cells, that is, at least when you're on a diet.
Sorghum has a potent DHT boosting effect, which was noted in one in-vitro study.

Olive oil is a great source of monounsaturated fatty acids, which are crucially important for healthy testosterone production. Also, a study with young Moroccan men saw that 2 weeks of using olive oil as a main source of fat, increased testosterone levels by 20%.

Heavy cream is a great source for saturated fat, a.k.a, the most testosterone friendly type of dietary fat.

Parsley contains high amounts of a compound called apigening, which has been linked to significant increases in testosterone production, due to its stimulatory effect on testicular StAR protein.

4. The Men's Salad

Salad doesn't have to be a boring experience of rabbit foods. In fact you can whip up a hormonally nourishing health-bomb of a salad in few minutes with this recipe that includes:

- 3 cups leafy greens
- 2 eggs, boiled
- ½ cup blue cheese
- 5 slices bacon, crumbled
- 1 avocado
- 3 tomatoes
- 1 tbsp olive oil

Preparation:

1. Cook the bacon, crumble into a cup. Boil the eggs and peel + slice them to your liking.
2. Combine everything in a large bowl and now you have a salad.

Here's why this salad is your high-testosterone fuel:

If you use spinach as a lettuce base, it's filled with natural nitrates that convert into nitric oxide inside of your body. This occurrence will then increase your blood flow. Spinach is also filled with a natural steroid called ecdysterone, which is linked to elevated testosterone production.

Eggs are packed with cholesterol, which is the direct precursor of testosterone and linked to elevated testosterone production in various studies. Eggs are also filled with choline, which helps your body to chelate (get rid of) estrogens.

Blue cheese is filled with live bacteria, enzymes, and probiotics, and those are all linked to supreme health and elevated testosterone production.

Bacon gives you some natural saturated fat which is the kind of fat that stimulates testosterone synthesis. Bacon will also give you hefty doses of testosterone boosting cholesterol.

Avocado is jam-packed with mono-unsaturated fatty acids, which in this study increased testosterone production. Avocados also contain various T boosting vitamins such as: C, E, D, and K2.

Olive oil will help your testicles to convert cholesterol more easily into testosterone. It also increased testosterone levels by 17% in this study. Olive oil also has a compound called Oleuropein which is shown to be anti-estrogenic in few in-vitro studies.

5. Max-Testo Burger

Every man needs a good burger once in a while. Heck, why not every day? If you make your own, using quality ingredients and T-boosting fats, this delicious recipe is far from "fast food":

- 4 hamburger buns
- 1 lb beef, ground
- 4 bacon slices
- 4 tbsp Dijon mustard
- 1 tsp himalayan or sea salt
- 1 tbsp ground pepper
- ½ red onion, sliced
- 4 white button mushrooms, chopped
- ½ cup blue cheese
- 4 slices cheddar cheese
- 1 cup mayo (olive oil base)
- 1 cup of lettuce

Preparation:

1. Preheat a grill over high heat.
2. In a bowl, mix the ground beef, mustard, salt, and pepper. Then shape the mixture into 4 evenly sized patties and grill for 5 minutes a side or until they're roughly medium doneness. Then add the cheddar cheese slices on top of the patties and grill for 1 more minute.

3. Throw the bacon slices, onion slices, and white button mushrooms into the grill or into a pan, grill/cook until they're all evenly brown.
4. Cut the buns in half and grill for 10 seconds the cut side facing down.
5. Start assimilating the hamburger in the order you prefer.
6. Eat.

Here's the T-boosting magic behind these burgers:

Ground beef is a good source for carnitine which is linked to increased androgen receptor density and sensitivity. Also meat eaters tend to have higher testosterone levels than the fellows who refuse to eat it.

Bacon is an excellent source for testosterone boosting cholesterol and saturated fat.

All kinds of onions are filled with quercetin and alliins, which both are linked to increased testosterone production. Few studies have also examined the effects that onions have on testosterone levels and found only positive correlations.

Blue cheese is filled with probiotics, healthy bacteria, and live enzymes, all of which are linked to elevated testosterone levels.

White button mushrooms have the ability to inhibit the aromatase enzyme. It's an enzyme that converts testosterone molecules into estrogen molecules. Thus, blocking its activity will naturally increase your testosterone levels.

— Appendix 3 —

References

1. http://www.publish.csiro.au/paper/RD01077
2. http://www.ncbi.nlm.nih.gov/pubmed/8855804
3. http://www.ncbi.nlm.nih.gov/pubmed/15466673
4. http://www.centromedicoathenas.com.br/Content/Uploads/Info/127.pdf
5. http://www.ncbi.nlm.nih.gov/pubmed/19625884
6. http://www.ncbi.nlm.nih.gov/pubmed/8855804
7. http://www.ncbi.nlm.nih.gov/pubmed/16210377
8. http://www.ncbi.nlm.nih.gov/pubmed/1730811
9. http://press.endocrine.org/doi/abs/10.1210/jcem.81.10.8855787
10. http://www.ncbi.nlm.nih.gov/pubmed/25105998
11. http://healthland.time.com/2012/02/27/the-secret-to-guys-sex-appeal-low-stress-high-testosterone-strong-immunity/
12. http://www.livescience.com/28812-women-prefer-smell-of-manly-guys.html
13. http://www.telegraph.co.uk/news/uknews/2964139/Men-with-high-testosterone-attracted-to-women-with-feminine-faces.html
14. http://www.ncbi.nlm.nih.gov/pubmed/20194727
15. https://www.researchgate.net/publication/221741578_Testosterone_Deficiency_Accelerates_Neuronal_and_Vascular_Aging_of_SAMP8_Mice_Protective_Role_of_eNOS_and_SIRT1
16. http://www.ncbi.nlm.nih.gov/pubmed/19367574
17. http://psychcentral.com/news/2012/06/25/testosterone-decline-linked-to-depression-smoking-obesity-but-not-aging/40620.html
18. http://www.ncbi.nlm.nih.gov/pubmed/21129941
19. http://www.bioimmersion.com/media/docs/fructoborate_monograph.pdf
20. http://www.ncbi.nlm.nih.gov/pmc/articles/PMC534397/pdf/pnas00650-0279.pdf
21. http://www.sciencedirect.com/science/article/pii/0024320587900865
22. http://www.ncbi.nlm.nih.gov/pubmed/16320174
23. http://www.ncbi.nlm.nih.gov/pubmed/20050857
24. http://www.ncbi.nlm.nih.gov/pubmed/21154195

25. http://www.ncbi.nlm.nih.gov/pubmed/18351428

26. http://www.ncbi.nlm.nih.gov/pubmed/21154195

27. http://www.ncbi.nlm.nih.gov/pubmed/8942407

28. http://www.ingentaconnect.com/content/routledg/nc/ 2011/00000063/00000004/art00004

29. http://www.ncbi.nlm.nih.gov/pubmed/23448151

30. http://www.ncbi.nlm.nih.gov/pubmed/2900627

31. http://www.ncbi.nlm.nih.gov/pubmed/3937735

32. http://www.priory.com/psych/sexdys.htm

33. https://www.anabolicmen.com/how-to-increase-testosterone-levels-naturally/

34. http://www.ncbi.nlm.nih.gov/pubmed/2352035

35. http://www.ncbi.nlm.nih.gov/pubmed/19369047

36. http://www.ncbi.nlm.nih.gov/pubmed/11525593

37. http://www.sciencedirect.com/science/article/pii/S0731708508005955

38. http://www.ncbi.nlm.nih.gov/pubmed/20352370

39. http://www.ncbi.nlm.nih.gov/pubmed/21675994

40. https://www.anabolicmen.com/zinc-testosterone/

41. http://www.sciencedirect.com/science/article/pii/S096007600300195X

42. http://www.sciencedirect.com/science/article/pii/S096007600300195X

43. https://www.anabolicmen.com/alcohol-testosterone/

44. https://www.anabolicmen.com/alcohol-testosterone/

45. https://www.anabolicmen.com/alcohol-testosterone/

46. "What Does Insulin Do?" What Is Insulin? What Does Insulin Do? Learn from Experts! Web. 02 May 2016.

47. Cox, D. J., B. P. Kovatchev, L. A. Gonder-Frederick, K. H. Summers, A. Mccall, K. J. Grimm, and W. L. Clarke. "Relationships Between Hyperglycemia and Cognitive Performance Among Adults With Type 1 and Type 2 Diabetes."Diabetes Care 28.1 (2004): 71-77. Print.

48. "Insulin Resistance Syndrome Symptoms, Signs & Diet."MedicineNet. Web. 02 May 2016.

49. "Increasing Insulin Sensitivity Is the Key to Fat Loss." COACH CALORIE. Web. 02 May 2016.

50. "Carbohydrates and Testosterone: Carbs Are Essential for T." Anabolic Men. 28 Sept. 2015. Web. 02 May 2016.

51. Zhang, Yifei, Xiaoying Li, Dajin Zou, Wei Liu, Jialin Yang, Na Zhu, Li Huo, Miao Wang, Jie Hong, Peihong Wu, Guoguang Ren, and Guang Ning. "Treatment of Type 2 Diabetes and Dyslipidemia with the Natural Plant Alkaloid Berberine."The Journal of Clinical Endocrinology & Metabolism 93.7 (2008): 2559-565. Print.

52. Dong, Hui, Nan Wang, Li Zhao, and Fuer Lu. "Berberine in the Treatment of Type 2 Diabetes Mellitus: A Systemic Review and Meta-Analysis." Evidence-Based Complementary and Alternative Medicine 2012 (2012): 1-12. Print.

53. Yan, Hong-Mei, Ming-Feng Xia, Yan Wang, Xin-Xia Chang, Xiu-Zhong Yao, Sheng-Xiang Rao, Meng-Su Zeng, Yin-Fang Tu, Ru Feng, Wei-Ping Jia, Jun Liu, Wei Deng, Jian-Dong Jiang, and Xin Gao. "Efficacy of Berberine in Patients with Non-Alcoholic Fatty Liver Disease."PLOS ONE PLoS ONE 10.8 (2015). Print.

54. Pérez-Rubio, Karina G., Manuel González-Ortiz, Esperanza Martínez-Abundis, José A. Robles-Cervantes, and María C. Espinel-Bermúdez. "Effect of Berberine Administration on Metabolic Syndrome, Insulin Sensitivity, and Insulin Secretion." Metabolic Syndrome and Related Disorders11.5 (2013): 366-69. Print.

55. "Cinnamon – Scientific Review on Usage, Dosage, Side Effects."Independent Analysis on Supplements & Nutrition. Web. 02 May 2016.

56. "Chromium – Scientific Review on Usage, Dosage, Side Effects."Independent Analysis on Supplements & Nutrition. Web. 02 May 2016.

57. "Office of Dietary Supplements – Chromium." Chromium — Health Professional Fact Sheet. Web. 02 May 2016.

58. https://www.ncbi.nlm.nih.gov/pubmed/2298157

59. http://www.ncbi.nlm.nih.gov/pubmed/14757277

60. http://www.ncbi.nlm.nih.gov/pubmed/9349747

61. http://annals.org/article.aspx?articleid=746453

62. http://www.jci.org/articles/view/119074/version/1/pdf/render

63. http://www.ncbi.nlm.nih.gov/pubmed/11549629

64. https://www.ncbi.nlm.nih.gov/pmc/articles/PMC1472916/

65. http://www.ncbi.nlm.nih.gov/pubmed/7126460

66. https://www.ncbi.nlm.nih.gov/pubmed/10332569

67. http://www.ncbi.nlm.nih.gov/pubmed/11549629

68. http://www.ncbi.nlm.nih.gov/pubmed/11906709

69. http://onlinelibrary.wiley.com/doi/10.1113/jphysiol.2009.182162/abstract

70. https://en.wikipedia.org/wiki/Secondary_sex_characteristic

71. http://www.ncbi.nlm.nih.gov/pubmed/11500254

72. Http://www.ncbi.nlm.nih.gov/pubmed/11932266
73. Principles Of Orthomolecularism https://www.amazon.com/Principles-Orthomolecularism-R-S-Hemat/dp/1903737060?tag=testshock0e-20
74. http://www.ncbi.nlm.nih.gov/pubmed/3622795
75. http://www.ncbi.nlm.nih.gov/pubmed/22970699
76. http://www.ncbi.nlm.nih.gov/pubmed/23425925
77. http://www.ncbi.nlm.nih.gov/pubmed/23507475
78. http://www.ncbi.nlm.nih.gov/pubmed/23121123
79. http://www.ncbi.nlm.nih.gov/pubmed/11399122
80. http://joe.endocrinology-journals.org/content/191/3/637.full
81. http://www.ncbi.nlm.nih.gov/pubmed/3350906
82. http://www.ncbi.nlm.nih.gov/pmc/articles/PMC2701485/
83. http://www.ncbi.nlm.nih.gov/pubmed/8855804
84. http://www.eje-online.org/content/153/2/317.full.pdf
85. http://www.sciencedirect.com/science/article/pii/S0039128X09002670
86. http://www.fasebj.org/content/28/4/1891.short
87. https://www.anabolicmen.com/how-to-increase-testosterone-levels-naturally/
88. http://www.ncbi.nlm.nih.gov/pubmed/23471952
89. http://www.ncbi.nlm.nih.gov/pubmed/26518151
90. http://www.ncbi.nlm.nih.gov/pubmed/19690072
91. http://www.ncbi.nlm.nih.gov/pubmed/21056661
92. http://www.ncbi.nlm.nih.gov/pubmed/16707435
93. http://www.ncbi.nlm.nih.gov/pubmed/1809093
94. http://academy.anabolicmen.com/courses/thor
95. http://www.ncbi.nlm.nih.gov/pubmed/23412685
96. http://www.ncbi.nlm.nih.gov/pmc/articles/PMC3569090/
97. http://www.sciencedirect.com/science/article/pii/0531556581900255
98. https://www.anabolicmen.com/how-to-lose-weight/
99. http://www.ncbi.nlm.nih.gov/pubmed/3573976
100. http://jap.physiology.org/content/82/1/49
101. http://www.ncbi.nlm.nih.gov/pubmed/8495690
102. http://www.ncbi.nlm.nih.gov/pubmed/20091182
103. http://www.ncbi.nlm.nih.gov/pmc/articles/PMC534397/
104. http://www.ncbi.nlm.nih.gov/pubmed/10355847
105. http://www.ncbi.nlm.nih.gov/pubmed/12416261
106. http://www.ncbi.nlm.nih.gov/pubmed/15735098?dopt=Abstract
107. http://jap.physiology.org/content/82/1/49
108. http://www.cancerletters.info/article/S0304-3835(79)80054-3/abstract

109. Http://onlinelibrary.wiley.com/doi/10.1002/pros.20397/abstract
110. Http://www.sciencedirect.com/science/article/pii/0022473189904597
111. Http://www.sciencedirect.com/science/article/pii/0022473184902541
112. Http://jap.physiology.org/content/82/1/49
113. https://www.anabolicmen.com/more-dht-from-diet/
114. https://www.anabolicmen.com/fats-and-testosterone/
115. Http://www.ncbi.nlm.nih.gov/pmc/articles/PMC1132824/
116. Http://raypeat.com/articles/articles/unsaturatedfats.shtml
117. https://www.anabolicmen.com/caffeine-testosterone/
118. https://www.jstage.jst.go.jp/article/endocrj1954/26/3/26_3_345/_pdf
119. Http://www.ncbi.nlm.nih.gov/pmc/articles/PMC3521899/
120. Http://www.ncbi.nlm.nih.gov/pmc/articles/PMC3358932/
121. Http://www.ncbi.nlm.nih.gov/pmc/articles/PMC3358932/
122. Http://www.ajol.info/index.php/wsa/article/viewFile/112127/101887
123. Http://www.ncbi.nlm.nih.gov/pubmed/25324206
124. Http://www.sciencedirect.com/science/article/pii/S0896844611002762
125. https://www.anabolicmen.com/painkillers-testosterone/
126. Http://www.ncbi.nlm.nih.gov/pubmed/16143488
127. Http://www.ncbi.nlm.nih.gov/pubmed/20977699
128. Http://joe.endocrinology-journals.org/content/191/3/637.full
129. Http://www.ncbi.nlm.nih.gov/pubmed/3200111
130. Http://www.ncbi.nlm.nih.gov/pubmed/7962322
131. https://www.anabolicmen.com/creatine-testosterone/
132. Http://www.ncbi.nlm.nih.gov/pubmed/19741313
133. Http://www.ncbi.nlm.nih.gov/pubmed/19741313
134. Http://www.ncbi.nlm.nih.gov/pubmed/19010408
135. Http://www.ijem.in/article.asp?
    issn=2230-8210;year=2012;volume=16;issue=3;spage=485;epage=486;aulast=
    Chaiyasit
136. Http://www.ncbi.nlm.nih.gov/pubmed/22017963
137. Http://www.ncbi.nlm.nih.gov/pubmed/21103034
138. Http://www.ncbi.nlm.nih.gov/pubmed/20523044
139. https://www.ncbi.nlm.nih.gov/pubmed/16394955
140. https://www.ncbi.nlm.nih.gov/pubmed/16118575
141. Http://jissn.biomedcentral.com/articles/10.1186/1550-2783-4-23
142. https://www.ncbi.nlm.nih.gov/pubmed/1325348
143. https://www.ncbi.nlm.nih.gov/pmc/articles/PMC2503954/
144. Http://www.ncbi.nlm.nih.gov/pubmed/3426586

145. http://www.ncbi.nlm.nih.gov/pubmed/3124852

146. http://www.ncbi.nlm.nih.gov/pubmed/11500963

147. http://onlinelibrary.wiley.com/doi/10.1038/oby.2005.162/abstract

148. http://www.ncbi.nlm.nih.gov/pubmed/22393824

149. https://repositories.tdl.org/utswmed-ir/handle/2152.5/755

150. http://www.ncbi.nlm.nih.gov/pubmed/21129941

151. http://www.bioimmersion.com/media/docs/fructoborate_monograph.pdf

152. https://www.anabolicmen.com/probiotics-and-endocrine-health/

153. http://www.wisegeek.com/what-is-aromatization.htm

154. http://drplechner.com/learn/miscellaneous-articles/what-is-aromatase/

155. http://www.ncbi.nlm.nih.gov/pmc/articles/PMC3074486/

156. https://www.anabolicmen.com/foods-that-block-aromatase-enzyme/

157. http://www.ergo-log.com/luteolin-anti-oestrogen-in-celery.html

158. http://www.ncbi.nlm.nih.gov/pubmed/11519862/

159. http://www.ncbi.nlm.nih.gov/pubmed/11739882

160. http://www.ncbi.nlm.nih.gov/pubmed/9690769

161. http://search.proquest.com/openview/
    75ade726227e28f41cf19e02b938b455/1?pq-origsite=gscholar

162. http://www.ncbi.nlm.nih.gov/pubmed/16648789

163. http://www.ncbi.nlm.nih.gov/pubmed/12943704

164. http://www.ncbi.nlm.nih.gov/pubmed/7271365

165. http://www.ncbi.nlm.nih.gov/pubmed/17984944

166. http://www.ncbi.nlm.nih.gov/pubmed/21129941

167. http://www.ncbi.nlm.nih.gov/pubmed/16740737

168. http://www.ncbi.nlm.nih.gov/pubmed/14679019

169. http://www.ncbi.nlm.nih.gov/pubmed/16740737

170. http://www.ncbi.nlm.nih.gov/pubmed/20003617

171. http://www.ncbi.nlm.nih.gov/pubmed/16611627

172. http://www.ncbi.nlm.nih.gov/pubmed/17766065

173. http://www.ncbi.nlm.nih.gov/pubmed/18277612

174. http://www.ncbi.nlm.nih.gov/pubmed/24089405

175. http://www.ncbi.nlm.nih.gov/pubmed/21261651

176. https://www.anabolicmen.com/how-to-increase-testosterone-levels-naturally/

177. http://www.ncbi.nlm.nih.gov/pubmed/20665368

178. http://www.ncbi.nlm.nih.gov/pmc/articles/PMC1476085/

179. http://www.ncbi.nlm.nih.gov/pmc/articles/PMC2770912/

180. http://www.ncbi.nlm.nih.gov/pubmed/19789214

181. http://www.ncbi.nlm.nih.gov/pubmed/1490755

182. http://press.endocrine.org/doi/abs/10.1210/jcem-34-4-756

183. http://www.ncbi.nlm.nih.gov/pubmed/3080462

184. http://press.endocrine.org/doi/abs/10.1210/endo-94-4-1077

185. https://www.anabolicmen.com/mucuna-pruriens-testosterone/

186. http://press.endocrine.org/doi/abs/10.1210/jcem-42-3-603

187. https://www.anabolicmen.com/mucuna-pruriens-testosterone/

188. http://www.ergo-log.com/mucunatest.html

189. http://www.ncbi.nlm.nih.gov/pubmed/20563862

190. http://www.ncbi.nlm.nih.gov/pubmed/2753470

191. https://store.anabolicmen.com/collections/single-ingredient-supplements/
products/zinc-picolinate-15mg?
utm_source=anabolic.link&utm_medium=urlshortener

192. http://suppversity.blogspot.fi/2014/04/common-nutrient-deficiencies-
their.html

193. http://www.reproduction-online.org/content/124/2/173.long

194. http://www.ncbi.nlm.nih.gov/pubmed/3360302

195. http://onlinelibrary.wiley.com/doi/10.1111/j.1365-2265.2004.02034.x/abstract

196. http://press.endocrine.org/doi/abs/10.1210/endo-32-1-97

197. http://press.endocrine.org/doi/abs/10.1210/endo-31-1-109

198. http://press.endocrine.org/doi/abs/10.1210/jcem-45-5-1019

199. http://www.sciencedirect.com/science/article/pii/S0015028201032290

200. http://www.ncbi.nlm.nih.gov/pmc/articles/PMC3134113/

201. http://europepmc.org/abstract/med/8792655

202. http://www.ncbi.nlm.nih.gov/pubmed/22731648

203. http://online.liebertpub.com/doi/abs/10.1089/jmf.2006.9.440

204. http://www.ncbi.nlm.nih.gov/pubmed/16327030

205. http://www.ncbi.nlm.nih.gov/pubmed/21154195

206. http://www.ncbi.nlm.nih.gov/pubmed/18351428

207. http://www.ncbi.nlm.nih.gov/pubmed/20050857

208. http://onlinelibrary.wiley.com/doi/10.1111/j.1365-2265.2012.04332.x/
abstract;jsessionid=39A4EF02A366FD626A4A8A00CD537D8C.f02t04?
deniedAccessCustomisedMessage=&userIsAuthenticated=false

209. https://www.jstage.jst.go.jp/article/endocrj1954/29/3/29_3_287/_article

210. http://www.ncbi.nlm.nih.gov/pubmed/20352370

211. http://www.ncbi.nlm.nih.gov/pubmed/21675994

212. https://www.hindawi.com/journals/ije/2014/525249/

213. http://www.ncbi.nlm.nih.gov/pmc/articles/PMC1164258/pdf/
biochemj00520-0038.pdf

214. http://link.springer.com/article/10.1007%2Fs12011-008-8294-5
215. http://www.ncbi.nlm.nih.gov/pubmed/23678636
216. http://www.sciencedirect.com/science/article/pii/S0022534708027018
217. http://www.ncbi.nlm.nih.gov/pubmed/16648789
218. http://www.ncbi.nlm.nih.gov/pubmed/17984944
219. http://www.ncbi.nlm.nih.gov/pubmed/20446777
220. http://www.ncbi.nlm.nih.gov/pubmed/7271365
221. http://www.ncbi.nlm.nih.gov/pubmed/16648790
222. http://www.ncbi.nlm.nih.gov/pubmed/8613886
223. http://www.bioimmersion.com/media/docs/fructoborate_monograph.pdf
224. http://www.ncbi.nlm.nih.gov/pubmed/21129941
225. http://www.sciencedirect.com/science/article/pii/S0890623806000827
226. http://europepmc.org/abstract/cba/326536
227. https://ods.od.nih.gov/factsheets/VitaminA-HealthProfessional/
228. http://www.ncbi.nlm.nih.gov/pmc/articles/PMC2906676/
229. http://www.ncbi.nlm.nih.gov/pubmed/20364093/
230. https://en.wikipedia.org/wiki/Vitamin_A
231. https://www.anabolicmen.com/fats-and-testosterone/
232. http://www.ncbi.nlm.nih.gov/pubmed/20364093/
233. http://www.ncbi.nlm.nih.gov/pubmed/20650878/
234. http://www.biolreprod.org/content/21/4/891.long
235. http://www.ncbi.nlm.nih.gov/pubmed/3360302
236. http://www.ncbi.nlm.nih.gov/pubmed/11055546
237. http://onlinelibrary.wiley.com/doi/10.1111/j.1365-2265.2004.02034.x/abstract
238. http://www.reproduction-online.org/content/124/2/173.long
239. https://www.anabolicmen.com/vitamin-d-testosterone/
240. Why Is Thiamin So Important? (n.d.). Retrieved June 16, 2015, from http://www.boxingscene.com/supplements/4329.php
241. 5 Foods To Skyrocket Testosterone Levels. (2013, December 29). Retrieved June 16, 2015, from http://www.health-host.co.uk/5-foods-skyrocket-testosterone-levels/
242. Nakayama, O., Yagi, M., Kiyoto, S., Okuhara, M., & Kohsaka, M. (1990).Riboflavin, a testosterone 5.ALPHA.-reductase inhibitor. J. Antibiot. The Journal of Antibiotics, 43(12), 1615-1616. Retrieved June 16, 2015, from National Institute of Health.
243. Nordqvist C (2012-02-23). "What Is DHT (Dihydrotestosterone)? What Is DHT's Role In Baldness?". Medical News Today.

244. Kock, N. (2010, June 7). Niacin turbocharges the growth hormone response to anaerobic exercise: A delayed effect. Retrieved June 16, 2015, from http://healthcorrelator.blogspot.com/2010/06/niacin-turbocharges-growth-hormone.html

245. Sly, B. (n.d.). The ABCs of Vitamins: Vitamin B5 (Pantothenic Acid). Retrieved June 16, 2015, from http://breakingmuscle.com/nutrition/the-abcs-of-vitamins-vitamin-b5-pantothenic-acid

246. Moore, J. (2014, December 8). The Role of Vitamin B6 and B12 in Boosting Testosterone Levels. Retrieved June 17, 2015, from http://www.testosteroneboostersreview.com/research/vitamin-b6-b12/

247. Paulose, C., Thliveris, J., Viswanathan, M., & Dakshinamurti, K. (1989). Testicular Function in Biotin-Deficient Adult Rats. Hormone and Metabolic Research Horm Metab Res, 21(12), 661-665.

248. Jackson, D., & Stoppani, J. (n.d.). 10 Supps You Never Thought of. Retrieved June 17, 2015, from http://www.muscleandfitness.com/supplements/build-muscle/10-supps-you-never-thought/slide/3

249. McAdams, M. (2015, January 27). Foods That Are High in B Vitamins. Retrieved June 17, 2015, from http://www.livestrong.com/article/22253-foods-high-b-vitamins/

250. https://www.anabolicmen.com/combination-of-garlic-and-vitamin-c-for-blood-pressure-and-nitric-oxide/

251. http://www.ncbi.nlm.nih.gov/pmc/articles/PMC3134113/

252. http://europepmc.org/abstract/med/8792655

253. http://www.ncbi.nlm.nih.gov/pubmed/23336340

254. http://www.ncbi.nlm.nih.gov/pubmed/23689303

255. http://www.ncbi.nlm.nih.gov/pubmed/23241495

256. http://www.ncbi.nlm.nih.gov/pubmed/22079541

257. http://europepmc.org/abstract/med/15055539

258. http://www.sciencedirect.com/science/article/pii/S0940299308000365

259. http://www.sciencedirect.com/science/article/pii/S0041008X06004236

260. http://www.tandfonline.com/doi/abs/10.1080/10715760500308154

261. http://www.sciencedirect.com/science/article/pii/S0300483X05002994

262. http://www.sciencedirect.com/science/article/pii/S0300483X01003663

263. http://www.ncbi.nlm.nih.gov/pubmed/23115449

264. http://www.ncbi.nlm.nih.gov/pubmed/22731648

265. http://www.sciencedirect.com/science/article/pii/S0093691X04003528

266. http://online.liebertpub.com/doi/abs/10.1089/jmf.2006.9.440

267. http://journals.lww.com/nsca-jscr/abstract/1998/08000/
effects_of_ascorbic_acid_on_serum_cortisol_and_the.10.aspx

268. http://www.sciencedirect.com/science/article/pii/S0302283804006256

269. http://www.ncbi.nlm.nih.gov/pubmed/16327030

270. http://www.ncbi.nlm.nih.gov/pubmed/12627313

271. http://www.ncbi.nlm.nih.gov/pubmed/19223675

272. http://www.ncbi.nlm.nih.gov/pubmed/18427418

273. http://www.ncbi.nlm.nih.gov/pubmed/14498993

274. https://www.amazon.com/Sari-Foods-Acerola-Cherries-Organic/dp/
B00PJ3WBPA?tag=testshock0e-20

275. http://ajpgi.physiology.org/content/253/3/G390.abstract

276. http://press.endocrine.org/doi/abs/10.1210/jc.2004-1513

277. http://press.endocrine.org/doi/abs/10.1210/jc.2004-1513

278. http://www.ncbi.nlm.nih.gov/pubmed/19786070

279. http://suppversity.blogspot.fi/2014/10/fructose-as-dieting-tool-100g-
fructose.html

280. https://www.anabolicmen.com/bromelain-testosterone/

281. http://www.ncbi.nlm.nih.gov/pubmed/21669584

282. http://www.ncbi.nlm.nih.gov/pubmed/21154195

283. http://www.ncbi.nlm.nih.gov/pubmed/21154195

284. http://www.ncbi.nlm.nih.gov/pubmed/18351428

285. http://europepmc.org/abstract/med/9734509

286. http://onlinelibrary.wiley.com/doi/10.1111/j.1365-2265.2012.04332.x/
abstract?deniedAccessCustomisedMessage=&userIsAuthenticated=false

287. http://press.endocrine.org/doi/pdf/10.1210/endo-25-1-7

288. http://www.ncbi.nlm.nih.gov/pmc/articles/PMC2885316/

289. http://www.ncbi.nlm.nih.gov/pubmed/21427118

290. http://www.ncbi.nlm.nih.gov/pubmed/2723823

291. http://www.ncbi.nlm.nih.gov/pubmed/7625775

292. http://ajcn.nutrition.org/content/84/4/694.full

293. http://www.jabfm.org/content/22/6/698.full

294. http://www.telegraph.co.uk/news/uknews/1486054/Raw-oysters-really-are-
aphrodisiacs-say-scientists-and-now-is-the-time-to-eat-them.html

295. https://www.sciencedaily.com/releases/2015/03/150317122458.htm

296. http://www.ncbi.nlm.nih.gov/pubmed/10804454

297. http://jap.physiology.org/content/82/1/49

298. https://www.anabolicmen.com/erection-boosting-foods-to-cure-erectile-
dysfunction/

299. http://www.ncbi.nlm.nih.gov/pubmed/10804454
300. http://www.ncbi.nlm.nih.gov/pubmed/10804454
301. http://www.ncbi.nlm.nih.gov/pubmed/19085527
302. http://www.sciencedirect.com/science/article/pii/S0731708508005955
303. http://www.ncbi.nlm.nih.gov/pubmed/20352370
304. http://www.ncbi.nlm.nih.gov/pubmed/21675994
305. http://www.ncbi.nlm.nih.gov/pubmed/24723948
306. http://www.ncbi.nlm.nih.gov/pubmed/23031616
307. http://www.ncbi.nlm.nih.gov/pubmed/20537519
308. https://www.anabolicmen.com/magnesium-boosts-free-testosterone/
309. http://www.ncbi.nlm.nih.gov/pubmed/16648789
310. http://www.ncbi.nlm.nih.gov/pubmed/17984944
311. http://www.ncbi.nlm.nih.gov/pubmed/20446777
312. http://www.ncbi.nlm.nih.gov/pubmed/7271365
313. http://www.ncbi.nlm.nih.gov/pubmed/16648790
314. http://www.ncbi.nlm.nih.gov/pubmed/23406764
315. http://www.ncbi.nlm.nih.gov/pubmed/8613886
316. http://www.ncbi.nlm.nih.gov/pubmed/3207614
317. https://www.anabolicmen.com/zinc-testosterone/
318. https://chriskresser.com/natures-most-potent-superfood/
319. http://www.ncbi.nlm.nih.gov/pubmed/21129941
320. http://www.ncbi.nlm.nih.gov/pubmed/9197924
321. http://www.bioimmersion.com/media/docs/fructoborate_monograph.pdf
322. http://www.sciencedirect.com/science/article/pii/0955286396001027
323. http://www.sciencedirect.com/science/article/pii/0041008X78901199
324. http://www.bioimmersion.com/media/docs/fructoborate_monograph.pdf
325. https://www.anabolicmen.com/resveratrol-testosterone/
326. https://www.anabolicmen.com/brazil-nuts-testosterone/
327. http://www.biochemj.org/content/160/3/433
328. http://link.springer.com/article/10.1007%2Fs12011-008-8294-5
329. https://www.anabolicmen.com/milk-testosterone/
330. https://www.youtube.com/watch?v=Icxwwy7a7Sk
331. http://www.ncbi.nlm.nih.gov/pubmed/23678636
332. http://anabolicmen.com/antioxidants-ultimate-guide/
333. https://www.anabolicmen.com/boost-nitric-oxide-naturally/
334. http://www.sciencedirect.com/science/article/pii/S0022534708027018
335. http://www.ncbi.nlm.nih.gov/pubmed/9587151
336. http://www.ncbi.nlm.nih.gov/pubmed/6378607

337. http://www.ncbi.nlm.nih.gov/pubmed/16449843

338. http://ajcn.nutrition.org/content/67/5/965S.abstract

339. http://www.tandfonline.com/doi/abs/10.3109/19396360903582216

340. http://www.scielo.br/scielo.php?
pid=S0102-311X2006000300003&script=sci_arttext&tlng=es

341. http://www.ncbi.nlm.nih.gov/pubmed/6358411

342. http://jn.nutrition.org/content/134/11/3100.short

343. http://link.springer.com/article/10.1023%2FA%3A1017930931736?LI=true

344. http://ajcn.nutrition.org/content/87/4/985.abstract

345. http://www.ncbi.nlm.nih.gov/pubmed/15514282

346. http://ajcn.nutrition.org/content/87/4/985.abstract

347. http://www.ncbi.nlm.nih.gov/pubmed/15514282

348. http://lipidworld.biomedcentral.com/articles/10.1186/1476-511X-10-158

349. http://www.sciencedirect.com/science/article/pii/S0304416506001590

350. http://jn.nutrition.org/content/104/6/660.full.pdf

351. Department of Urology, Johns Hopkins Medical Institutions. "The Role of Nitric Oxide in Erectile Dysfunction: Implications for Medical Therapy." National Center for Biotechnology Information. U.S. National Library of Medicine, 8 Dec. 2006. Web. 27 July 2015. <http://www.ncbi.nlm.nih.gov/pubmed/17170606>.

352. Grossmann, Kayla. "5 Ways to Get More Choline in Your Diet: Secret of Radiant Living." 5 Ways to Get More Choline in Your Diet: Secret of Radiant Living. The Radiant Life Blog, n.d. Web. 27 July 2015. <http://blog.radiantlifecatalog.com/bid/63690/5-Ways-to-Get-More-Choline-in-Your-Diet-Secret-of-Radiant-Living>.

353. Kuoppala, Ali. "Testosterone Boosting Super Nutrient Called Choline." Anabolic Men. Anabolicman.com, 01 June 2014. Web. 27 July 2015. <http://www.anabolicmen.com/choline-testosterone-super-nutrient/>.

354. Nast, Conde. "Foods Highest in Choline." Foods Highest in Choline. SELFNutritionData, 2014. Web. 27 July 2015. <http://nutritiondata.self.com/foods-000144000000000000000-1w.html>.

355. Nootriment, Admin. "The Dangerous Effects of a Choline Deficiency." Nootriment. Nootriment, n.d. Web. 26 July 2015. <http://nootriment.com/choline-deficiency/>.

356. Sahelian, Ray, M.D. "Phosphatidylcholine Supplement Health Benefit, Side Effects." Phosphatidylcholine Supplement Health Benefit, Side Effects. N.p., 28 June 2014. Web. 27 July 2015. <http://www.raysahelian.com/phospha.html>.

357. The World's Healthiest Foods. "Choline." Choline. The George Mateljan Foundation, July 2015. Web. 27 July 2015. <http//www.whfoods.com/genpage.php/genpage.php?tname=nutrient&dbid=50>.

358. Weil, Andrew, M.D., and Brain Beckler, M.D. "Vitamin Library." Choline. Weil Lifesyle, 27 Sept. 2012. Web. 27 July 2015. <http://www.drweil.com/drw/u/ART03240/Choline.html>.

359. Wilson, Mark. "Choline Benefits! Choline Supplements! Choline Diet!" Choline Benefits! Choline Supplements! Choline Diet! Boost-Your-Low-Testosterone.com, 2015. Web. 27 July 2015. <http://www.boost-your-low-testosterone.com/choline-benefits.html>.

360. https://www.anabolicmen.com/caloric-intake-testosterone/

361. http://edition.cnn.com/2010/HEALTH/11/08/twinkie.diet.professor/

362. http://www.ncbi.nlm.nih.gov/pubmed/3573976

363. http://www.nature.com/icb/journal/v78/n5/full/icb200076a.html

364. https://www.anabolicmen.com/how-to-lower-cortisol/

365. http://www.ncbi.nlm.nih.gov/pubmed/21855365

366. http://www.ncbi.nlm.nih.gov/pubmed/20091182

367. http://www.ncbi.nlm.nih.gov/pubmed/8495690

368. http://www.ncbi.nlm.nih.gov/pubmed/24603159

369. http://www.ncbi.nlm.nih.gov/pubmed/15085559

370. http://www.ncbi.nlm.nih.gov/pmc/articles/PMC1476085/

371. http://www.ncbi.nlm.nih.gov/pmc/articles/PMC2821887/

372. https://www.anabolicmen.com/how-to-lower-cortisol/

373. http://www.ncbi.nlm.nih.gov/pubmed/3573976

374. http://www.ncbi.nlm.nih.gov/pubmed/10634401

375. http://jap.physiology.org/content/82/1/49

376. http://www.ncbi.nlm.nih.gov/pubmed/16286871

377. https://www.cambridge.org/core/journals/british-journal-of-nutrition

378. http://jap.physiology.org/content/82/1/49

379. http://www.ncbi.nlm.nih.gov/pubmed/1435181? access_num=1435181&link_type=MED&dopt=Abstract

380. http://www.sciencedirect.com/science/article/pii/0022473189904597

381. http://www.cancerletters.info/article/S0304-3835(79)80054-3/abstract

382. http://ajcn.nutrition.org/content/42/1/127? ijkey=fb34fb0e1260844fb8f4c686bcbc17803aff95f1&keytype2=tf_ipsecsha

383. https://www.cambridge.org/core/journals/british-journal-of-nutrition/article/
testosterone-sex-hormone-binding-globulin-calculated-free-testosterone-and-
oestradiol-in-male-vegans-and-omnivores/
27DDFF5DF01A55EA4E1ECDBA443B7896

384. http://www.sciencedirect.com/science/article/pii/0022473184902541

385. http://www.ncbi.nlm.nih.gov/pubmed/8039147?
access_num=8039147&link_type=MED&dopt=Abstract

386. http://press.endocrine.org/doi/abs/10.1210/jcem-64-5-1083

387. http://www.ncbi.nlm.nih.gov/pubmed/1387870?
access_num=1387870&link_type=MED&dopt=Abstract

388. http://www.ncbi.nlm.nih.gov/pubmed/20071648

389. http://www.artofmanliness.com/2013/01/18/how-to-increase-testosterone-
naturally/

390. http://www.ers.usda.gov/data-products/adoption-of-genetically-engineered-
crops-in-the-us/recent-trends-in-ge-adoption.aspx

391. http://www.ncbi.nlm.nih.gov/pubmed/14728586?dopt=Abstract

392. http://www.ncbi.nlm.nih.gov/pubmed/14681200?dopt=Abstract

393. http://www.ncbi.nlm.nih.gov/pubmed/21353476

394. http://humrep.oxfordjournals.org/content/23/11/2584.short

395. http://cebp.aacrjournals.org/content/5/10/785.short

396. http://www.ncbi.nlm.nih.gov/pubmed/11431339

397. http://www.ncbi.nlm.nih.gov/pubmed/11577007

398. http://www.ncbi.nlm.nih.gov/pubmed/11694625

399. http://www.ncbi.nlm.nih.gov/pubmed/7892297

400. http://www.ncbi.nlm.nih.gov/pubmed/10828262

401. http://www.ncbi.nlm.nih.gov/pubmed/15735098

402. http://www.ncbi.nlm.nih.gov/pubmed/1656395?dopt=Abstract

403. http://www.ncbi.nlm.nih.gov/pubmed/10325492?dopt=Abstract?
access_num=10325492

404. http://www.ncbi.nlm.nih.gov/pubmed/7490559/

405. http://www.ncbi.nlm.nih.gov/pubmed/?term=PMC2752973

406. http://www.ncbi.nlm.nih.gov/pubmed/19064574

407. http://www.ncbi.nlm.nih.gov/pubmed/11445478/

408. http://www.ncbi.nlm.nih.gov/pubmed/8594308/

409. http://www.ncbi.nlm.nih.gov/pubmed/2826899/

410. http://www.ncbi.nlm.nih.gov/pubmed/2850159

411. http://www.nejm.org/doi/full/10.1056/NEJM199910073411515

412. http://jap.physiology.org/content/82/1/49

413. http://www.ncbi.nlm.nih.gov/pubmed/12442909
414. http://www.ncbi.nlm.nih.gov/pubmed/19666200
415. http://www.goldjournal.net/article/S0090-4295(04)00418-2/abstract
416. http://www.sciencedirect.com/science/article/pii/S0278691508004523
417. http://www.ncbi.nlm.nih.gov/pmc/articles/PMC4224956/
418. http://www.ncbi.nlm.nih.gov/pubmed/17310494
419. http://onlinelibrary.wiley.com/doi/10.1002/ptr.2900/abstract
420. http://www.ncbi.nlm.nih.gov/pubmed/3593480
421. http://www.ncbi.nlm.nih.gov/pubmed/219455
422. http://onlinelibrary.wiley.com/doi/10.1111/j.1530-0277.1978.tb05808.x/
     abstract
423. http://www.ncbi.nlm.nih.gov/pubmed/2155675
424. http://www.ncbi.nlm.nih.gov/pubmed/6443186
425. http://www.ncbi.nlm.nih.gov/pubmed/11912073
426. http://jpet.aspetjournals.org/content/202/3/676.short
427. http://www.alcoholjournal.org/article/0741-8329(84)90043-0/abstract
428. http://press.endocrine.org/doi/abs/10.1210/endo-105-4-888?
     url_ver=Z39.88-2003&rfr_id=ori%3Arid%3Acrossref.org&rfr_dat=cr_pub%3
     Dpubmed&
429. http://www.ncbi.nlm.nih.gov/pubmed/19450718
430. http://www.ncbi.nlm.nih.gov/pubmed/9046385
431. http://www.ncbi.nlm.nih.gov/pubmed/17349749
432. http://www.ijpp.com/IJPP%20archives/2006_50_3/291-296.pdf
433. http://onlinelibrary.wiley.com/doi/10.1111/j.1530-0277.2003.tb04405.x/
     abstract;jsessionid=B0E13DCD049737AC03BBE4DE9206648A.f01t01
434. http://onlinelibrary.wiley.com/doi/10.1097/01.ALC.0000125356.70824.81/
     abstract
435. http://www.ncbi.nlm.nih.gov/pubmed/23470309
436. https://www.anabolicmen.com/alcohol-testosterone/
437. http://www.ncbi.nlm.nih.gov/pubmed/10868587
438. http://www.ncbi.nlm.nih.gov/pubmed/16965913
439. http://www.ncbi.nlm.nih.gov/pubmed/18852123
440. https://www.ncbi.nlm.nih.gov/pubmed/16704348
441. http://www.ncbi.nlm.nih.gov/pubmed/15142373
442. https://www.ncbi.nlm.nih.gov/pubmed/14681200
443. https://www.ncbi.nlm.nih.gov/pubmed/16351761
444. http://cebp.aacrjournals.org/content/16/4/829.short
445. http://www.ncbi.nlm.nih.gov/pubmed/15735098

446. https://www.cambridge.org/core/journals/british-journal-of-nutrition

447. http://joe.endocrinology-journals.org/content/170/3/591.short

448. http://www.ncbi.nlm.nih.gov/pubmed/7892297

449. http://www.nature.com/ejcn/journal/v57/n1/abs/1601495a.html

450. http://www.ncbi.nlm.nih.gov/pubmed/21353476

451. http://jn.nutrition.org/content/132/3/570S.short

452. http://www.tandfonline.com/doi/abs/10.1080/01635581.2001.9680610

453. http://www.tandfonline.com/doi/abs/10.1207/s15327914nc4702_1

454. http://www.sciencedirect.com/science/article/pii/S0015028209009662

455. http://journals.cambridge.org/action/displayFulltext?
type=6&fid=906928&jid=BJN&volumeId=84&issueId=04&aid=906924&fullte
xt

456. http://time.com/3922583/trans-fats-hydrogenated-oils/

457. http://www.ncbi.nlm.nih.gov/pubmed/15051604

458. http://www.ncbi.nlm.nih.gov/pubmed/20338284

459. http://www.annualreviews.org/doi/abs/10.1146/annurev.nu.15.070195.002353

460. https://www.cambridge.org/core/journals/british-journal-of-nutrition/article/
effects-of-dietary-trans-fatty-acids-on-reproductive-performance-of-wistar-
rats/CB59DB23E97FD565BC5F1C08FB855D54

461. http://www.andjrnl.org/article/S0002-8223(09)02094-X/abstract

462. http://humrep.oxfordjournals.org/content/29/3/429.short

463. http://www.fertstert.org/article/S0015-0282(10)02735-4/abstract

464. MNT. "What Is Erectile Dysfunction? What Causes Erection Problems?"
Medical News Today. MediLexicon International, 22 May 2015. Web. 05 July
2015.

465. 2. TED Case Studies. "TED Case Studies." Viagra and Species Protection. N.p.,
n.d. Web. 05 July 2015.

466. 3. Theobald, Mike. "8 Lifestyle Changes and Natural Treatments for ED."
EverydayHealth.com. N.p., 17 Sept. 2014. Web. 05 July 2015.

467. 4. Borreli, Lizzete. "6 Ways To Treat Erectile Dysfunction Without
Medication." Medical Daily. N.p., 08 May 2014. Web. 05 July 2015.

468. 5. Mayo Clinic Staff. "Erectile Dysfunction." Herbs: A Natural Treatment for
ED? N.p., 19 Jan. 2013. Web. 05 July 2015.

469. 6. Shiel, William, MD. "Natural Remedies for Erectile Dysfunction (ED,
Impotence)." MedicineNet. N.p., 28 Aug. 2014. Web. 05 July 2015.

470. http://www.dailymail.co.uk/news/article-2239621/Researchers-test-mens-
testosterone-levels-rise-arousal--visiting-sex-club.html

471. http://www.ncbi.nlm.nih.gov/pubmed/1529008

472. http://www.ncbi.nlm.nih.gov/pubmed/7069152

473. http://www.ncbi.nlm.nih.gov/pubmed/7434016

474. http://www.ncbi.nlm.nih.gov/pubmed/15355456

475. http://www.ncbi.nlm.nih.gov/pubmed/11247105

476. http://www.ncbi.nlm.nih.gov/pubmed/16287455

477. http://www.ncbi.nlm.nih.gov/pubmed/11760788

478. http://www.ncbi.nlm.nih.gov/pubmed/12659241

479. http://onlinelibrary.wiley.com/doi/10.1046/j.1365-2605.1999.00196.x/full

480. http://joe.endocrinology-journals.org/content/52/1/51.short

481. http://www.ncbi.nlm.nih.gov/pubmed/11760788

482. http://www.sciencedirect.com/science/article/pii/0003347278900532

483. http://psycnet.apa.org/journals/com/91/1/120/

484. https://www.researchgate.net/profile/Alonso_Fernandez-Guasti/publication/
6536830_Relationship_between_sexual_satiety_and_brain_androgen_recepto
rs/links/54b6c2970cf2e68eb27f0321.pdf

485. http://www.ncbi.nlm.nih.gov/pubmed/17239879

486. http://download.springer.com/static/pdf/473/
art%253A10.1186%252F1477-7827-5-11.pdf?
originUrl=http%3A%2F%2Frbej.biomedcentral.com%2Farticle%2F10.1186%2
F1477-7827-5-11&token2=exp=1473256538~acl=%2Fstatic%2Fpdf%2F473%
2Fart%25253A10.1186%25252F1477-7827-5-11.pdf*~hmac=31ef5d752e0a37
2166092881105c34538f0af5ab709ddbe678f813f0a15ed394

487. http://www.dailymail.co.uk/news/article-2239621/Researchers-test-mens-
testosterone-levels-rise-arousal--visiting-sex-club.html

488. http://www.ncbi.nlm.nih.gov/pubmed/1529008

489. http://www.ncbi.nlm.nih.gov/pubmed/7069152

490. http://www.karger.com/Article/Abstract/122746

491. http://www.sciencedirect.com/science/article/pii/0044848693903656

492. http://www.sciencedirect.com/science/article/pii/S0018506X03001624

493. http://onlinelibrary.wiley.com/doi/10.1002/jez.1402390211/abstract

494. http://press.endocrine.org/doi/abs/10.1210/endo-109-1-185

495. http://onlinelibrary.wiley.com/doi/10.1002/j.1939-4640.2004.tb03170.x/full

496. http://ebm.sagepub.com/content/204/2/231.short

497. http://www.sciencedirect.com/science/article/pii/0018506X9090013N

498. http://www.sciencedirect.com/science/article/pii/0306453094000476

499. http://www.sciencedirect.com/science/article/pii/S0016648097969690

500. http://onlinelibrary.wiley.com/doi/10.1111/j.1439-0272.2000.tb02858.x/full

501. http://www.sciencedirect.com/science/article/pii/0300962989900601

502. http://journals.lww.com/psychosomaticmedicine/Abstract/1969/09000/Androgen_Responses_to_Stress__II__Excretion_of.8.aspx

503. http://www.sciencedirect.com/science/article/pii/S0006322399003078

504. http://www.sciencedirect.com/science/article/pii/S0006322399003078

505. http://archpsyc.jamanetwork.com/article.aspx?articleid=490664

506. http://onlinelibrary.wiley.com/doi/10.1111/j.1365-2605.1978.tb00573.x/abstract

507. http://europepmc.org/abstract/med/15905625

508. http://www.ingentaconnect.com/content/asma/asem/2008/00000079/00000002/art00009

509. http://press.endocrine.org/doi/abs/10.1210/jcem.74.5.1314847

510. http://www.sciencedirect.com/science/article/pii/0165178194900485

511. https://www.researchgate.net/publication/12930648_Testosterone_Gonadotropin_and_Cortisol_Secretion_in_Male_Patients_With_Major_Depression

512. http://onlinelibrary.wiley.com/doi/10.1046/j.0007-1331.2001.00727.x/full

513. http://link.springer.com/article/10.1207/S15324796ABM2603_04

514. http://psycnet.apa.org/journals/bul/133/1/25/

515. http://www.tandfonline.com/doi/abs/10.3109/10253890902874913

516. http://www.eje-online.org/content/78/2/258.short

517. http://press.endocrine.org/doi/abs/10.1210/jcem-35-4-535

518. http://www.eje-online.org/content/65/1/11.short

519. http://bja.oxfordjournals.org/content/85/1/109.short

520. http://www.ncbi.nlm.nih.gov/pmc/articles/PMC1470424/

521. http://www.ncbi.nlm.nih.gov/pubmed/9226731

522. http://www.ncbi.nlm.nih.gov/pubmed/12100842

523. http://link.springer.com/article/10.1007%2FBF02884454

524. http://www.ncbi.nlm.nih.gov/pubmed/19568835

525. http://www.ncbi.nlm.nih.gov/pubmed/9415946

526. http://link.springer.com/article/10.1207%2Fs15327558ijbm0201_2

527. https://www.anabolicmen.com/more-testosterone-in-minutes/

528. http://www.ncbi.nlm.nih.gov/pubmed/3573976

529. http://www.ncbi.nlm.nih.gov/pubmed/8495690

530. http://www.ncbi.nlm.nih.gov/pubmed/16320174

531. http://www.ncbi.nlm.nih.gov/pubmed/17520786

532. http://www.ncbi.nlm.nih.gov/pubmed/19684340

533. http://www.ncbi.nlm.nih.gov/pubmed/15195201

534. http://jama.jamanetwork.com/article.aspx?articleid=412611

535. http://www.ncbi.nlm.nih.gov/pubmed/19085527
536. http://www.ars.usda.gov/SP2UserFiles/Place/80400530/pdf/0506/
     usual_nutrient_intake_vitD_ca_phos_mg_2005-06.pdf
537. http://www.ncbi.nlm.nih.gov/pmc/articles/PMC3703169/
538. http://www.ncbi.nlm.nih.gov/pubmed/12163983
539. http://www.ncbi.nlm.nih.gov/pubmed/21199787
540. http://www.lifeforce.net/pdfs/withania_review.pdf
541. http://www.ncbi.nlm.nih.gov/pubmed/21369449
542. http://www.ncbi.nlm.nih.gov/pubmed/17585686
543. http://www.ncbi.nlm.nih.gov/pubmed/22546655
544. http://www.ncbi.nlm.nih.gov/pubmed/12508132
545. http://www.ncbi.nlm.nih.gov/pubmed/23125505
546. http://www.ncbi.nlm.nih.gov/pubmed/15937373
547. http://www.ncbi.nlm.nih.gov/pubmed/23142798
548. http://onlinelibrary.wiley.com/doi/10.1111/j.1479-8425.2006.00193.x/full
549. http://onlinelibrary.wiley.com/doi/10.1111/j.1479-8425.2007.00262.x/abstract
550. http://www.ncbi.nlm.nih.gov/pubmed/22529837
551. http://www.ncbi.nlm.nih.gov/pubmed/22804755
552. http://www.ncbi.nlm.nih.gov/pubmed/18036082
553. http://www.ncbi.nlm.nih.gov/pubmed/20975054
554. http://www.ncbi.nlm.nih.gov/pubmed/21340475
555. http://www.ncbi.nlm.nih.gov/pubmed/16455366
556. http://www.ncbi.nlm.nih.gov/pubmed/21859051
557. http://ehp.niehs.nih.gov/1408163/
558. http://www.huffingtonpost.com/2013/05/09/bpa-testosterone-bisphenol-a-
     _n_3246042.html
559. http://www.ncbi.nlm.nih.gov/pubmed/20467048
560. http://www.ncbi.nlm.nih.gov/pubmed/24265451
561. http://www.ncbi.nlm.nih.gov/pubmed/24271643
562. http://www.ncbi.nlm.nih.gov/pubmed/24305612
563. http://www.ncbi.nlm.nih.gov/pubmed/24496641
564. http://www.ncbi.nlm.nih.gov/pubmed/24508763
565. http://www.ncbi.nlm.nih.gov/pubmed/23405234
566. http://www.ncbi.nlm.nih.gov/pubmed/11137303
567. http://www.sciencedirect.com/science/article/pii/S0960076010003572

568. http://scholar.google.fi/scholar_url?hl=fi&q=http://www.researchgate.net/
publication/
5441935_A_mixture_of_five_phthalate_esters_inhibits_fetal_testicular_testos
terone_production_in_the_sprague-dawley_rat_in_a_cumulative_dose-
additive_manner/file/
504635294d0f7d7f3e.pdf&sa=X&scisig=AAGBfm234UhBIuae3_AQKz7ssoV
Tw9LMCw&oi=scholarr&ei=WZtaVIa9LoHjO7X4gJAJ&ved=0CCMQgAMo
AjAA

569. http://www.reproduction-online.org/content/127/3/305.short

570. http://content.usatoday.com/communities/greenhouse/post/2011/03/bpa-
free-plastic-products-estrogen/1#.VFqiPvmsXw8

571. http://www.sciencedirect.com/science/article/pii/S0960076010003572

572. http://www.ncbi.nlm.nih.gov/pmc/articles/PMC1240840/

573. http://www.imm.ki.se/Datavard/PDF/
Final%20Phth%20SweEPA%20051111.pdf

574. http://www.ourstolenfuture.org/newscience/oncompounds/phthalates/
2002-0401brocketal.htm

575. http://www.sciencedirect.com/science/article/pii/S1438463913000527

576. https://www.amazon.com/dp/B0040MH642/?tag=testshock0e-20

577. http://www.huffingtonpost.com/2013/05/09/bpa-testosterone-bisphenol-a-
_n_3246042.html

578. http://www.ncbi.nlm.nih.gov/pubmed/24945889

579. http://www.ncbi.nlm.nih.gov/pubmed/24496641

580. http://www.ncbi.nlm.nih.gov/pubmed/24305612

581. http://www.ncbi.nlm.nih.gov/pubmed/24271643

582. http://www.ncbi.nlm.nih.gov/pubmed/24265451

583. http://www.ncbi.nlm.nih.gov/pubmed/24508763

584. http://www.ncbi.nlm.nih.gov/pubmed/20467048

585. http://www.ncbi.nlm.nih.gov/pubmed/23405234

586. http://jama.jamanetwork.com/article.aspx?articleid=1832525

587. http://www.newsweek.com/youre-absorbing-bpa-your-receipts-study-
shows-230178

588. http://www.ncbi.nlm.nih.gov/pubmed/21939283

589. http://www.ncbi.nlm.nih.gov/pubmed/21939283

590. http://www.motherjones.com/environment/2014/03/tritan-certichem-
eastman-bpa-free-plastic-safe?page=1

591. https://www.amazon.com/dp/B003ZF9QES/?tag=testshock0e-20

592. https://www.ncbi.nlm.nih.gov/pubmed/11867263

593. http://www.ncbi.nlm.nih.gov/pubmed/25121464

594. http://www.ncbi.nlm.nih.gov/pubmed/20005209

595. http://www.sciencedirect.com/science/article/pii/S0300483X11002393

596. http://search.informit.com.au/
documentSummary;dn=319040401687055;res=IELHEA

597. https://www.anabolicmen.com/triclosan-testosterone/

598. https://en.wikipedia.org/wiki/Remineralisation_of_teeth

599. http://www.ncbi.nlm.nih.gov/pmc/articles/PMC3890436/

600. http://www.ncbi.nlm.nih.gov/pmc/articles/PMC3890436/

601. http://www.ncbi.nlm.nih.gov/pubmed/?term=19619626

602. http://www.karger.com/Article/Abstract/47443

603. http://link.springer.com/article/10.1007%2FBF02008213#page-1

604. http://www.fluorideresearch.org/424/424/files/FJ2009_v42_n4_p260-276.pdf

605. http://www.tandfonline.com/doi/abs/10.1080/15376520590968824

606. http://en.cnki.com.cn/Article_en/CJFDTOTAL-ZDFB200303001.htm

607. http://www.fluorideresearch.org/411/files/FJ2008_v41_n1_p010-017.pdf

608. http://www.sciencedirect.com/science/article/pii/S0890623802000382

609. http://link.springer.com/article/10.1007/s10534-005-0336-2#page-1

610. http://link.springer.com/article/10.1007/s00114-007-0224-4#page-1

611. http://en.cnki.com.cn/Article_en/CJFDTOTAL-ZDFB406.007.htm

612. http://www.fluoridealert.org/wp-content/uploads/chen-1997.pdf

613. http://europepmc.org/abstract/med/20364589

614. http://www.tandfonline.com/doi/abs/
10.3109/15563659609013768#.VZfHefntlBc

615. http://www.sciencedirect.com/science/article/pii/S0013935103000598

616. https://www.sciencedaily.com/releases/2010/07/100714104059.htm

617. http://www.sciencedirect.com/science/article/pii/S0531556504001275

618. http://www.eje-online.org/content/early/2012/11/15/EJE-12-0288

619. http://www.ncbi.nlm.nih.gov/pmc/articles/PMC3114813/

620. http://pubs.acs.org/doi/abs/10.1021/es403661a

621. http://www.ncbi.nlm.nih.gov/pubmed/16357596

622. http://onlinelibrary.wiley.com/doi/10.1002/tox.21831/abstract

623. https://journals.uplb.edu.ph/index.php/index/index

624. http://tih.sagepub.com/content/23/7/439.abstract

625. http://www.ncbi.nlm.nih.gov/pubmed/22200534

626. http://www.ncbi.nlm.nih.gov/pubmed/17218080

627. http://www.sciencedirect.com/science/article/pii/S0048357598923665

628. http://www.ncbi.nlm.nih.gov/pubmed/15168945

629. http://www.ncbi.nlm.nih.gov/pmc/articles/PMC1469881/

630. http://www.ncbi.nlm.nih.gov/pubmed/2761262

631. http://toxsci.oxfordjournals.org/content/58/1/50.abstract

632. http://www.ncbi.nlm.nih.gov/pubmed/11191080

633. http://www.sciencedirect.com/science/article/pii/S0890623802000199

634. http://www.pnas.org/content/107/10/4612.full

635. https://archive.epa.gov/pesticides/reregistration/web/html/status.html

636. http://www.tandfonline.com/doi/abs/10.1179/oeh.2006.12.4.355

637. http://americannutritionassociation.org/newsletter/high-sperm-density-among-members-organic-farmers-association

638. http://www.sjweh.fi/show_abstract.php?abstract_id=573

639. https://www.scienceopen.com/document_file/0710d58f-d6a3-4b6d-a49a-23d7198704c3/PubMedCentral/0710d58f-d6a3-4b6d-a49a-23d7198704c3.pdf

640. http://www.ncbi.nlm.nih.gov/pubmed/15617990/

641. http://www.ncbi.nlm.nih.gov/pubmed/20005209

642. http://www.sciencedirect.com/science/article/pii/S0300483X11002393

643. http://search.informit.com.au/documentSummary;dn=319040401687055;res=IELHEA

644. http://www.ncbi.nlm.nih.gov/pubmed/11823001

645. http://www.ncbi.nlm.nih.gov/pubmed/15799449

646. http://www.ncbi.nlm.nih.gov/pubmed/16183391

647. http://www.ncbi.nlm.nih.gov/pubmed/12730620

648. http://www.ncbi.nlm.nih.gov/pubmed/15458796

649. http://www.ncbi.nlm.nih.gov/pubmed/11333184

650. http://www.ncbi.nlm.nih.gov/pmc/articles/PMC2453157/

651. http://www.ncbi.nlm.nih.gov/pubmed/16097788

652. http://www.ncbi.nlm.nih.gov/pubmed/15063329

653. http://www.ncbi.nlm.nih.gov/pubmed/11333184

654. http://www.sciencedirect.com/science/article/pii/S037842740300016X

655. http://www.endocrine-abstracts.org/ea/0011/ea0011oc60.htm

656. http://www.ncbi.nlm.nih.gov/pubmed/15142373

657. http://search.informit.com.au/documentSummary;dn=319040401687055;res=IELHEA

658. http://www.sciencedirect.com/science/article/pii/S0960076001001741

659. http://www.ncbi.nlm.nih.gov/pubmed/15799449

660. http://www.dr-baumann.ca/science/Concentrations%20of%20Parabens%20in%20Human%20Breast.pdf

661. http://www.ncbi.nlm.nih.gov/pubmed/12419695

662. http://www.ncbi.nlm.nih.gov/pubmed/15799449

663. http://onlinelibrary.wiley.com/doi/10.1111/j.1365-2605.2012.01280.x/abstract

664. https://en.wikipedia.org/wiki/Octyl_methoxycinnamate

665. http://www.ncbi.nlm.nih.gov/pubmed/15908756

666. http://www.ncbi.nlm.nih.gov/pubmed/15799449

667. http://www.ncbi.nlm.nih.gov/pubmed/16112788

668. http://search.informit.com.au/
documentSummary;dn=319040401687055;res=IELHEA

669. http://www.ncbi.nlm.nih.gov/pubmed/15799449

670. http://www.ncbi.nlm.nih.gov/pubmed/22513303

671. http://www.ncbi.nlm.nih.gov/pmc/articles/PMC1661631/

672. http://www.ncbi.nlm.nih.gov/pubmed/19663879

673. http://www.ncbi.nlm.nih.gov/pubmed/21631527

674. https://www.ncbi.nlm.nih.gov/pubmed/2568579?dopt=Abstract

675. https://www.ncbi.nlm.nih.gov/pubmed/11953750

676. http://www-staro.vef.unizg.hr/vetarhiv/papers/2011-81-4-9.pdf

677. http://www.karger.com/Article/Abstract/123243

678. http://www.sciencedirect.com/science/article/pii/003193849190408G

679. http://spp.sagepub.com/content/1/1/57.short

680. http://www.sciencedirect.com/science/article/pii/S1090513808000676

681. http://www.sciencedirect.com/science/article/pii/S0018506X10002989

682. http://onlinelibrary.wiley.com/doi/10.1002/bdm.671/
abstract;jsessionid=9BA9A99C17A2CED8978F9F87BCCCFB71.f01t03?
deniedAccessCustomisedMessage=&userIsAuthenticated=false

683. http://www.sciencedirect.com/science/article/pii/S0306453010000958

684. http://www.sauder.ubc.ca/Faculty/Divisions/Finance_Division~kaili/
llz_MS.pdf

685. https://www.theguardian.com/science/2008/apr/15/medicalresearch.gender

686. http://www.ncbi.nlm.nih.gov/pubmed/3593480

687. http://www.ncbi.nlm.nih.gov/pubmed/11912073

688. http://www.ijpp.com/IJPP%20archives/2006_50_3/291-296.pdf

689. http://www.ncbi.nlm.nih.gov/pubmed/17349749

690. http://www.ncbi.nlm.nih.gov/pubmed/11163119

691. http://www.ncbi.nlm.nih.gov/pubmed/3593480

692. http://www.ncbi.nlm.nih.gov/pubmed/219455

693. http://onlinelibrary.wiley.com/doi/10.1111/j.1530-0277.1978.tb05808.x/
abstract

694. http://www.ncbi.nlm.nih.gov/pubmed/2155675

695. http://press.endocrine.org/doi/abs/10.1210/endo-105-4-888?
url_ver=Z39.88-2003&rfr_id=ori%3Arid%3Acrossref.org&rfr_dat=cr_pub%3
Dpubmed&

696. http://www.ncbi.nlm.nih.gov/pubmed/6443186

697. http://www.ncbi.nlm.nih.gov/pubmed/11912073

698. http://jpet.aspetjournals.org/content/202/3/676.short

699. http://www.alcoholjournal.org/article/0741-8329(84)90043-0/abstract

700. http://www.ncbi.nlm.nih.gov/pubmed/19450718

701. http://www.ncbi.nlm.nih.gov/pubmed/9046385

702. http://www.ncbi.nlm.nih.gov/pubmed/17349749

703. http://www.ijpp.com/IJPP%20archives/2006_50_3/291-296.pdf

704. http://onlinelibrary.wiley.com/doi/10.1111/j.1530-0277.2003.tb04405.x/
abstract;jsessionid=B0E13DCD049737AC03BBE4DE9206648A.f01t01

705. http://onlinelibrary.wiley.com/doi/10.1097/01.ALC.0000125356.70824.81/
abstract

706. http://www.ncbi.nlm.nih.gov/pubmed/23470309

707. http://onlinelibrary.wiley.com/doi/10.1111/j.1530-0277.1996.tb01676.x/
abstract

708. http://www.ncbi.nlm.nih.gov/pubmed/11134162

709. http://www.newswise.com/articles/hops-compound-may-prevent-prostate-
cancer

710. https://en.wikipedia.org/wiki/Reinheitsgebot

711. http://www.newswise.com/articles/hops-compound-may-prevent-prostate-
cancer

712. http://www.ncbi.nlm.nih.gov/pubmed/11134162

713. http://www.ncbi.nlm.nih.gov/pubmed/9211568

714. http://www.hormones.gr/8449/article/cigarette-smoking-has-a-positive-
and%E2%80%A6.html

715. http://www.ncbi.nlm.nih.gov/pubmed/19473474

716. http://www.biomed.cas.cz/physiolres/pdf/62/62_67.pdf

717. http://www.sciencedirect.com/science/article/pii/S0024320588800018

718. http://www.sciencedirect.com/science/article/pii/002432059090032M

719. http://www.ncbi.nlm.nih.gov/pubmed/9043499?dopt=Abstract

720. http://humrep.oxfordjournals.org/content/17/12/3275.full#ref-9

721. http://www.eurekalert.org/pub_releases/2012-06/tes-dtl062212.php

722. http://www.clinsci.org/content/100/6/661

723. http://www.bioline.org.br/request?bk08005

724. http://www.iasj.net/iasj?func=fulltext&aId=5261

725. http://www.ncbi.nlm.nih.gov/pubmed/20188349

726. http://www.ncbi.nlm.nih.gov/pubmed/3711333

727. http://www.ncbi.nlm.nih.gov/pubmed/8313352

728. http://www.ncbi.nlm.nih.gov/pubmed/6296360

729. http://www.sciencedirect.com/science/article/pii/S0041008X06000093

730. http://www.ncbi.nlm.nih.gov/pubmed/6090909

731. http://www.nejm.org/doi/pdf/10.1056/NEJM197404182901602

732. http://www.sciencedirect.com/science/article/pii/0091305786905150

733. http://www.sciencedirect.com/science/article/pii/0022519383902552

734. http://www.tandfonline.com/doi/abs/10.1080/02791072.1982.10471911?
journalCode=ujpd20

735. http://europepmc.org/abstract/med/1158438

736. http://www.nejm.org/doi/full/10.1056/NEJM197411142912003

737. http://www.sciencedirect.com/science/article/pii/037687169190068A

738. http://www.ncbi.nlm.nih.gov/pubmed/19501822

739. http://www.ncbi.nlm.nih.gov/pubmed/24371462

740. http://www.lifeextension.com/Magazine/2006/6/report_ashwa/Page-01

741. Starks, Michael A., Stacy L. Starks, Michael Kingsley, Martin Purpura, and Ralf Jäger. "The Effects of Phosphatidylserine on Endocrine Response to Moderate Intensity Exercise." Journal of the International Society of Sports Nutrition. BioMed Central, 28 July 2008. Web. 24 July 2015.

742. Kuoppala, Ali. "Phosphatidylserine and Testosterone: Anabolic Nootropic?" Anabolic Men. N.p., 19 Apr. 2015. Web. 24 July 2015.

743. Elsass, Paul. "Foods That Contain Phosphatidylserine." LIVESTRONG.COM. LIVESTRONG.COM, 10 Feb. 2014. Web. 24 July 2015.

744. Ahmad, MK, AA Mahdi, KK Shukla, N. Islam, S. Rajender, D. Madjukar, SN Shankhwar, and S. Ahmad. "Withania Somnifera Improves Semen Quality by Regulating Reproductive Hormone Levels and Oxidative Stress in Seminal Plasma of Infertile Males." National Center for Biotechnology Information. U.S. National Library of Medicine, Aug. 2010. Web. 05 Aug. 2015. <http://www.ncbi.nlm.nih.gov/pubmed/19501822>.

745. Ambiye, VR, D. Langade, S. Dongre, P. Aptikar, M. Kulkarni, and A. Dongre. "Clinical Evaluation of the Spermatogenic Activity of the Root Extract of Ashwagandha (Withania Somnifera) in Oligospermic Males: A Pilot Study." National Center for Biotechnology Information. U.S. National Library of Medicine, n.d. Web. 05 Aug. 2015. <http://www.ncbi.nlm.nih.gov/pubmed/24371462>.

746. Axe, Josh, Dr. "Ashwagandha Benefits Thyroid and Adrenals – DrAxe.com."
DrAxecom. DrAxe.com, 10 Oct. 2013. Web. 04 Aug. 2015. <http://draxe.com/
ashwagandha-proven-to-heal-thyroid-and-adrenals/>.

747. Biswajit, Auddy, PhD. "A Standardized Withania Extract Significantly Reduced
Stress-Related Parameters in Chronically Stressed Humans." Lifeforce.net.
JANA, 2008. Web. 5 Aug. 2015. <http://www.lifeforce.net/pdfs/
withania_review.pdf>.

748. Keifer, Dale. "Ashwagandha Stress Reduction, Neural Protection, and a Lot
More from an Ancient Herb." LifeExtension.com. Life Extension Magezine,
June 2006. Web. 04 Aug. 2015. <http://www.lifeextension.com/Magazine/
2006/6/report_ashwa/Page-01>.

749. Kuoppla, Ali. "Ashwagandha Testosterone Booster Proven by Human Studies."
Anabolic Men. Anabolic Men, 26 Dec. 2014. Web. 05 Aug. 2015. <http://
www.anabolicmen.com/ashwagandha-testosterone/>.

750. Saunders, Jenna. "What Is Ashwagandha?" Chopra.com. Chopra Centered
Lifestyle, n.d. Web. 04 Aug. 2015. <http://www.chopra.com/ccl/
ashwagandhahttp://www.chopra.com/ccl/ashwagandha>.

751. Singh, Narendra, Mohit Bahalla, Prashanti De Jagar, and Marilena Gilca.
"Ashwagandha Stress Reduction, Neural Protection, and a Lot More from an
Ancient Herb." LifeExtension.com. African Journal of Traditional
Complementary and Alternative Medicines, 3 July 2011. Web. 04 Aug. 2015.
<http://www.lifeextension.com/Magazine/2006/6/report_ashwa/Page-01>.

752. Livera, et al., "Regulation and Perturbation of Testicular Functions by Vitamin
A" (Review), Reproduction (2002) 124, 173-180

753. Zadik, et. al., "Vitamin A and iron supplementation is as efficient as hormonal
therapy in constitutionally delayed children," Clin Endocrinol (Oxf). 2004 Jun;
60(6):682-7

754. http://www.ncbi.nlm.nih.gov/pubmed/15477012

755. http://www.ncbi.nlm.nih.gov/pubmed/7942581

756. http://www.ncbi.nlm.nih.gov/pubmed/21154195

757. http://www.ncbi.nlm.nih.gov/pubmed/18351428

758. http://www.ncbi.nlm.nih.gov/pubmed/20050857

759. https://www.jstage.jst.go.jp/article/endocrj1954/29/3/29_3_287/_pdf

760. http://press.endocrine.org/doi/abs/10.1210/endo-32-1-97

761. http://press.endocrine.org/doi/abs/10.1210/endo-31-1-109

762. http://press.endocrine.org/doi/abs/10.1210/jcem-45-5-1019

763. http://www.fertstert.org/article/S0015-0282(01)03229-0/abstract?cc=y=

764. http://www.ncbi.nlm.nih.gov/pubmed/8613886

765. http://www.ncbi.nlm.nih.gov/pubmed/20352370

766. http://www.hindawi.com/journals/ije/2014/525249/

767. http://www.ncbi.nlm.nih.gov/pubmed/21675994

768. http://www.ncbi.nlm.nih.gov/pubmed/23678636

769. http://www.jurology.com/article/S0022-5347(08)02701-8/abstract

770. http://www.jurology.com/article/S0022-5347(08)02701-8/abstract

771. http://www.ncbi.nlm.nih.gov/pubmed/20523044

772. http://www.ncbi.nlm.nih.gov/pubmed/23495677

773. http://www.ncbi.nlm.nih.gov/pubmed/16394955

774. https://store.anabolicmen.com/products/cortigon

775. http://www.ncbi.nlm.nih.gov/pubmed/1325348

776. http://www.ncbi.nlm.nih.gov/pmc/articles/PMC2503954/

777. https://www.anabolicmen.com/tribulus-terrestris/

778. https://www.anabolicmen.com/maca-testosterone-libido/

779. https://www.anabolicmen.com/fenugreek-testosterone/

780. https://www.anabolicmen.com/saw-palmetto-testosterone/

781. https://www.anabolicmen.com/do-testosterone-boosters-work/

782. http://www.sciencedirect.com/science/article/pii/S0731708508005955

783. http://www.ncbi.nlm.nih.gov/pubmed/20352370

784. http://www.ncbi.nlm.nih.gov/pubmed/21675994

785. http://www.ncbi.nlm.nih.gov/pubmed/24723948

786. http://www.ncbi.nlm.nih.gov/pubmed/23031616

787. http://www.ncbi.nlm.nih.gov/pubmed/16648789

788. http://www.ncbi.nlm.nih.gov/pubmed/17984944

789. http://www.ncbi.nlm.nih.gov/pubmed/20446777

790. http://www.ncbi.nlm.nih.gov/pubmed/7271365

791. http://www.ncbi.nlm.nih.gov/pubmed/16648790

792. http://www.ncbi.nlm.nih.gov/pubmed/8613886

793. https://medlineplus.gov/druginfo/natural/982.html

794. https://www.anabolicmen.com/ashwagandha-testosterone/

795. http://www.ncbi.nlm.nih.gov/pubmed/26609282

796. http://www.ncbi.nlm.nih.gov/pubmed/22393824

797. http://www.ncbi.nlm.nih.gov/pubmed/2160383

798. http://www.jbc.org/content/271/33/19900.short

799. http://www.ncbi.nlm.nih.gov/pubmed/11500963

800. http://onlinelibrary.wiley.com/doi/10.1038/oby.2005.162/abstract

801. http://www.sciencedirect.com/science/article/pii/0955286396001027

802. http://www.bioimmersion.com/media/docs/fructoborate_monograph.pdf

803. http://www.ncbi.nlm.nih.gov/pubmed/21129941

804. http://www.ncbi.nlm.nih.gov/pubmed/18436713

805. http://www.ncbi.nlm.nih.gov/pubmed/20071623

806. http://press.endocrine.org/doi/full/10.1210/jcem.82.6.4018

807. http://pubs.sciepub.com/ajmbr/4/1/1/

808. http://www.bioperine.com/index.php/researchhighlight

809. http://www.ncbi.nlm.nih.gov/pubmed/9063034

810. http://www.ncbi.nlm.nih.gov/pubmed/16855773

811. http://www.ncbi.nlm.nih.gov/pubmed/12394711

812. http://www.ncbi.nlm.nih.gov/pubmed/16855773

813. http://www.ncbi.nlm.nih.gov/pubmed/8750052

814. http://www.ncbi.nlm.nih.gov/pmc/articles/PMC1573065/

815. http://www.ncbi.nlm.nih.gov/pubmed/23057780

816. http://aminoacidstudies.org/pine-bark-extract-and-arginine-highly-effective-
    erectile-dysfunction-treatment/

817. http://www.nrjournal.com/article/S0271-5317(03)00126-X/abstract

818. http://www.ncbi.nlm.nih.gov/pubmed/18037769

819. http://www.ncbi.nlm.nih.gov/pubmed/22240497

820. http://www.ncbi.nlm.nih.gov/pmc/articles/PMC2442048/

821. http://www.sciencedirect.com/science/article/pii/S027153170700022X

822. http://www.ncbi.nlm.nih.gov/pubmed/21067832

823. http://www.ncbi.nlm.nih.gov/pubmed/20499249

824. http://www.ncbi.nlm.nih.gov/pubmed/9809945

825. http://jap.physiology.org/content/early/2010/08/19/japplphysiol.00503.2010

826. http://www.ncbi.nlm.nih.gov/pubmed/17953788

827. https://www.amazon.com/dp/B00972QT66/?tag=testshock0e-20

828. http://www.ncbi.nlm.nih.gov/pubmed/11292962

829. http://www.ncbi.nlm.nih.gov/pubmed/23152216

830. http://www.ncbi.nlm.nih.gov/pubmed/9828868

831. https://www.researchgate.net/publication/
    26744088_Escin_improves_sperm_quality_in_male_patients_with_varicocele
    -associated_infertility

832. http://www.ncbi.nlm.nih.gov/pubmed/23682825

833. http://www.ncbi.nlm.nih.gov/pubmed/16740737

834. http://www.ncbi.nlm.nih.gov/pubmed/22745005

835. http://www.ncbi.nlm.nih.gov/pubmed/19608210

836. http://www.ncbi.nlm.nih.gov/pubmed/21802563

837. http://www.ncbi.nlm.nih.gov/pubmed/21802563

838. http://www.ncbi.nlm.nih.gov/pubmed/15577189
839. http://www.ncbi.nlm.nih.gov/pubmed/16751992
840. http://www.ncbi.nlm.nih.gov/pubmed/17169663
841. http://www.ncbi.nlm.nih.gov/pubmed/20141584
842. http://www.ncbi.nlm.nih.gov/pubmed/16281085
843. http://www.ncbi.nlm.nih.gov/pubmed/17142971
844. http://www.ncbi.nlm.nih.gov/pmc/articles/PMC2503954/
845. http://www.ncbi.nlm.nih.gov/pubmed/18616866
846. http://www.ncbi.nlm.nih.gov/pubmed/14643848
847. http://www.ncbi.nlm.nih.gov/pubmed/15886416
848. http://www.ncbi.nlm.nih.gov/pubmed/22784423
849. http://www.ncbi.nlm.nih.gov/pubmed/15930482
850. http://www.ncbi.nlm.nih.gov/pubmed/19897276
851. http://www.ncbi.nlm.nih.gov/pubmed/7793450
852. http://www.ncbi.nlm.nih.gov/pubmed/7726322
853. http://www.ncbi.nlm.nih.gov/pubmed/11386498
854. http://www.ncbi.nlm.nih.gov/pubmed/11399122
855. http://www.ncbi.nlm.nih.gov/pubmed/9690769
856. http://search.proquest.com/openview/
    75ade726227e28f41cf19e02b938b455/1?pq-origsite=gscholar
857. http://www.ncbi.nlm.nih.gov/pubmed/16648789
858. http://www.ncbi.nlm.nih.gov/pubmed/12943704
859. http://www.ncbi.nlm.nih.gov/pubmed/7271365
860. http://www.ncbi.nlm.nih.gov/pubmed/17984944
861. http://www.ncbi.nlm.nih.gov/pubmed/21129941
862. http://www.ncbi.nlm.nih.gov/pubmed/16740737
863. http://www.ncbi.nlm.nih.gov/pubmed/14679019
864. http://www.ncbi.nlm.nih.gov/pubmed/16740737
865. http://www.ncbi.nlm.nih.gov/pubmed/20003617
866. http://www.ncbi.nlm.nih.gov/pubmed/16611627
867. http://www.ncbi.nlm.nih.gov/pubmed/17766065
868. http://www.ncbi.nlm.nih.gov/pubmed/18277612
869. http://www.ncbi.nlm.nih.gov/pubmed/21261651
870. https://www.anabolicmen.com/how-to-increase-testosterone-levels-naturally/
871. http://www.ncbi.nlm.nih.gov/pubmed/20665368
872. http://www.ncbi.nlm.nih.gov/pubmed/2686332
873. http://press.endocrine.org/doi/abs/10.1210/jcem-53-2-258?
    journalCode=jcem&

874. http://link.springer.com/article/10.2165/00007256-200535040-00004
875. https://www.researchgate.net/publication/
8359974_Effects_of_Sequential_Bouts_of_Resistance_Exercise_on_Androgen
_Receptor_Expression
876. http://www.ncbi.nlm.nih.gov/pubmed/15219414
877. http://www.ncbi.nlm.nih.gov/pubmed/16826026
878. http://www.ncbi.nlm.nih.gov/pubmed/12930169
879. http://www.ncbi.nlm.nih.gov/pubmed/16997353?
dopt=Abstract&holding=npg
880. http://www.ncbi.nlm.nih.gov/pubmed/17553164?
dopt=Abstract&holding=npg
881. http://www.ncbi.nlm.nih.gov/pubmed/23136995
882. http://www.sciencedirect.com/science/article/pii/S1567576904001924

Thank You For Reading!

In conclusion, we want to thank you for picking up a copy of this testosterone bible. Hopefully you now know everything you will ever need to know to increase your testosterone naturally, and greatly enhance your health.

Feel free to send your friends and family copies of this book as gifts, or refer them to **MasterYourTestosterone.com** where they can get their own copy.

If you have any testimonials or stories to share about your experiences with information from this book, or something you may have learned on the Anabolic Men Youtube channel or **AnabolicMen.com**, please let us know!

Send us an email to **support@anabolicmen.com**

Probiotics Food List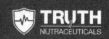

1. Sauerkraut
2. Pickles
3. Yogurt (No added sugar)
4. Kefir
5. Fermented Cheeses
6. Kombucha
7. Fermented Fish
8. Lassi

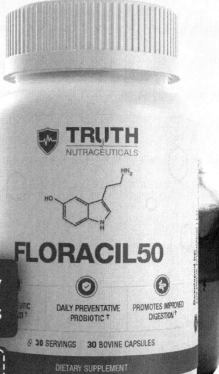

Testosterone Food List

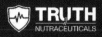

1. Potatoes
2. Macadamia Nuts
3. Epic Bars
4. Beef Gelatin
5. Coffee
6. Brazil Nuts
7. Extra Virgin Olive Oil
8. Raisins
9. Parsley
10. Ginger
11. Raw Cacao
12. Eggs
13. Real Salt
14. Arian Oil
15. Avocados
16. White Button Mushrooms
17. Baking Soda
18. Minced Meat
19. Pomegranates
20. Raw Blue Cheese
21. Dark Berries
22. Grass Fed Butter
23. Sorghum Flour
24. Coconut Oil
25. Garlic
26. Oysters

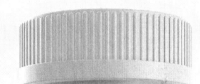

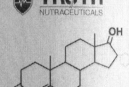

Get 10% off
TESTRO-X BOTTLES

TESTRO10

AIDS MASSIVE ENERGY BOOSTS †

HELPS INCREASE TESTOSTERONE RELIABILITY †

30 SERVINGS   90 BOVINE CAPSULES

DIETARY SUPPLEMENT

N.O. Food List

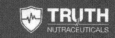

1. Watermelon
2. Spinach
3. Beets
4. Celery
5. Arugala
6. Carrots
7. Parsley
8. Cabbage
9. Radishes
10. Purple Grapes
11. Garlic
12. Oranges
13. Mixed Berries
14. Cayenne Pepper
15. Light Roast Coffee
16. Raw Cacao Nibs
17. Wild Caught Salmon
18. Black Pepper

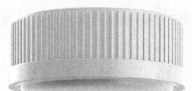
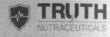

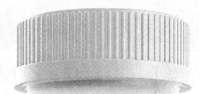

Brain Food List

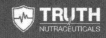

1. Beef Liver
2. Wild Cod
3. Shiitake Mushrooms
4. Egg Yolks
5. Beef Steak
6. Coconut Oil

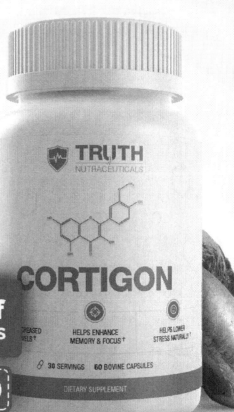

Made in the USA
San Bernardino, CA
02 February 2018